# REPERTORY

## OF THE

# BIOCHEMIC REMEDIES

*by*

## Dr. S. R. Phatak
*M.B.B.S.*

Arranged Alphabetically
with
Many Additions

*by*

## Dr. D. S. Phatak
*M.B.B.S*

# B. Jain Publishers (P) Ltd.
## New Delhi

Part 2 includes Materia Medica of Twelve Tissue
Remedies by Dr. D.S. Phatak

First Edition - 1937
Second Edition - 1986
Third revised edition - 1997
Reprint Edition: 2003

© Dr. D.S. Phatak
177 B Station Avenue Road
Chembur, Bombay - 400 071

*Published by :*
**Kuldeep Jain**
*For*
**B. Jain Publishers (P.) Ltd.**
1921, Street No. 10, Chuna Mandi,
Paharganj, New Delhi 110 055 (INDIA)
*Phones:* 2358 0800, 2358 1100, 2358 1300, 2358 3100
*Fax:* 011-2358 0471
Email: bjain@vsnl.com

*Printed in India by:*
**J.J. Offset Printers**
522, FIE, Patpar Ganj, Delhi - 110 092

**Price: Rs. 110.00**

**ISBN : 81-7021-723-7**
**BOOK CODE: BP-2418**

# PREFACE

Alphabetical arrangement of the entire Repertory has now come to stay. The ease and convenience it offers to the reader, overshadows the minor drawbacks.

Biochemic Repertory of Dr. S. R. Phatak is now arranged alphabetically. Certain additions are made. His Concise Homoeopathic Repertory is taken as a model to copy.

Certain rubrics are kept blank. The author thought them to be worthy of inclusion, but could not find suitable biochemic remedy. If any reader can suggest that (with proper evidence in support) it is most welcome.

Some repetition is obvious. Chicken-pox, small-pox are given as separate headings as well as under Fever. Callosities and Corns, Hurry and impatience are overlapping each other. Similar instances are too many to mention.

Dr. S. R. Phatak, long before his death (in April 1981) had revised his Biochemic Repertory. The idea of arranging it alphabetically was approved by him. For reasons of health, he was reluctant to do it himself.

This Biochemic Repertory, in its present from, is offered to the practitioners, with all humility at my command. Reactions, adverse or favourable are welcome. These suggestions will go a long way in improving the book, if and when need to second edition arises.

B. Jain Publishers deserve congratulations for undertaking the publicaton of this book.

*Bombay: June 1986*

**D. S. Phatak**

In prescribing these remedies the prescriber should take into consideration what are known as "Essentials of Symptoms". These are three in number:

1. Sensation of symptom and its character. (Mental symptoms and sensations are to be given the highest value in prescribing).

2. Location i.e. the part or the organ of the body to which the symptom is referred.

3. Modalities i.e. the conditions and circumstances under which the given symptom becomes worse or better.

# PREFACE

## (Excerpts from the first edition)

The want of a compact and complete Repertory of the twelve tissue remedies useful for ready reference has long been felt by the users of these medicines. When the Bombay Homoeopathic Medical Association started a one year's course for training students in the use of these remedies, and the teaching of their Materia Medica was entrusted to the author, this want was more keenly felt by him.

In compiling the present volume the author is extremely indebted to the following :

1.  Dr. Shanon's Complete Repertory of Twelve Tissue Remedies (Old Edition).

2.  Dr. Kent's Repertory of Homoeopathic Materia Medica.

3.  Twelve Tissue Remedies by Drs. Boericke and Dewey.

4.  Twelve Tissue Remedies by Drs. Carey and Perry.

5.  Dr. Boericke's Pocket Book of Homoeopathic Materia Medica.

6.  Dr. Boger's Synoptic Key.

7.  Dr. Boger's Timing of Remedies.

8.  Original manuscript of Dr. Boenninghausen's Characteristics and Repertory edited by Dr. Boger, and

9.  Other materia medicas in which provings of these biochemic remedies were given.

It is not claimed for this book that it is in any way intended to supercede any of the other useful books on the subject, and the question of how far the author has been successful in compiling a handy book for ready reference is left to the users of the book to judge.

*Bombay*
*October 1937*

**S. R. Phatak**

# ABBREVIATIONS

| | | | | |
|------|-----|-----|----------|------------------|
| Cf | CF | **CF** | stand for | CALCAREA FLUOR |
| Cp | CP | **CP** | stand for | CALCAREA PHOS |
| Cs | CS | **CS** | stand for | CALCAREA SULPH |
| Fp | FP | **FP** | stand for | FERRUM PHOS |
| Km | KM | **KM** | stand for | KALI MUR |
| Kp | KP | **KP** | stand for | KALI PHOS |
| Ks | KS | **KS** | stand for | KALI SULPH |
| Mp | MP | **MP** | stand for | MAGNESIA PHOS |
| Nm | NM | **NM** | stand for | NATRUM MUR |
| Np | NP | **NP** | stand for | NATRUM PHOS |
| Ns | NS | **NS** | stand for | NATRUM SULPH |
| Sil | SIL | **SIL** | stand for | SILICA |

# INTRODUCTION

## (Excerpts from Dr. S.R. Phatak's Introduction to Biochemic Repertory)

It is now an established fact that Dr. Schuessler's twelve tissue or biochemic remedies are capable, not only of alleviating, but in many cases curing many of the sufferings, which human flesh is heir to. One of the main factors in the construction or destruction of body cells is the proportion of the inorganic salts in them. Whenever a deficiency of one or more of these salts occurs in the body, it gives rise to various diseased conditions, and when this deficiency is supplied by giving these salts in an easily assimilable form, the diseased conditions are removed. This was in short the original theory of Dr. Schuessler. Later, these salts were proved on homoeopathic lines and they have now taken their due place in the Homoeopathic Materia Medica, so that in addition to the tested values of these medicines, the force of a systematic and scientific observation has been added to our knowledge of these salts and they can now be administered according to the principles of the law of "Similia Similibus Curentur" with greater advantage and precision.

The prescriber of these twelve remedies is sometimes at a disadvantage as the field of selection of these remedies is limited, but this disadvantage can be removed by giving two or more salts in alteration (or sometimes in combination also) provided they are given in potencies below 12x. Sometimes they are better in high potencies, but when such high potencies are selected it is desirable to given them singly after carefully matching their symptoms to the totality of the symptoms of the patient. In almost all these cases most of the work can usually be done with potencies upto 12x. Dr. Schuessler preferred the use of low potency.

# ABDOMEN

**Affections** In General: Cp; Kp; NP; Ns; MP; SIL.

**Upper**, Drawn in: NM.

**Lower:** See Hypogastrium

**Sides: CP; KP; MP; SIL.**

Left: Cf; Fp; Ns; SIL.

Right: **CP;** Fp; **Ns;** SIL.

Rigidity: Nm.

Distension: NM.

**Backward:** Kp; Mp; Sil.

**Downward:** Cp; Nm.

Anus, to: Nm.

Rectum: Nm.

Testicles: Nm; Ns; Sil.

Thigh: MP; Nm.

Urethra: Nm.

**Upward:** Ns.

Axilla, to: Ns.

Chest, to: Cp; Np; Ns.

Shoulder, to: Ns.

Throat, to: Cp.

**Afternoon** Agg: NM.
Amel: Ns.

**Alive** In, as if something: Cp; Nm; Sil.

**Alternating,** Head, with: Cp.

**Arm** Pain in, With: Nm.

**Back: NM;** Ns.

Small of: Sil.

**Ball**: See Lump.

**Bandaging** Amel: Nm.

**Bending Double**, Amel: Cf; Kp; MP.

**Bending** To one side Agg: NM.

**Bending** Body to side Amel: Nm.

**Bending** Forward, Amel: Cf; MP; Nm.

**Body** Soft, were lying in: Ns.

**Breathing**, As if: Kp.

**Breathing** Deep Agg: CP; Nm; Ns; Sil.

**Bubbling**: Nm.

**Clothes** Amel: Nm.

**Clothes,** Pressed him: Sil.

**Clothing** Sensitive, to: Fp; NS.

**Coldness,** In: Cs; Kp; KS.

Colic, with: Ks.

Painful: Sil.

**Cold** to touch: Ks.

**Cold** Things, Drinking Agg: Cp; Mp.

**Colitis,** Mucous: Kp.

**Constipation**, With: Sil

**Constriction, Bend, Hoop:** NM; Ns; Sil.

Bladder to, before stool: NS

Flatus, Passing Amel: Sil.

Stool During, desire for: Nm; Ns.

Walking: Nm.

**Contraction:** Mp: Nm; Ns; Sil.

Flatus passing, amel: Sil.

Menses after: Nm.

before: NM.

Muscles of: Nn.

Stool, desire for, during: Nm Ns.

Urination, After: Nm.

Walking Agg: Nm.

**Coughing** Agg: Fp; Kp; NM; NS; Sil.

**Cracks** On surface: SIL.

**Damp** Weather Agg: NS; Sil.

**Diarrhea,** As if, would come: NS.

During: Cp; Kp; Ks; Ns.

Followed by: Cp.

**Diarrhea**: As of: NS.

Stool, after abnormal: KS.

**Dinner** Amel: Nm.

**Disagreeable** Feeling: Nm.

**Discolouration,** Inflamed spots: Nm.

**Distended,** Tympanitic, etc: Cp; Cs; Fp; KP; KS; Mp; **NM; NP;** SIL.

Beer, after: NM.

Breakfast after: Nm.

Children, in: Sil.

Clothes, loosen must: Mp.

Flatus passing, Amel: Nm; Sil.

Heat, during: Sil.

Hemicrania, during: Nm.

Menses, during: Kp.

Night: NS.

Painful: Nm.

Stool after: Nm.

amel: Cp; Nm.

Tympanitic: Cp; KP; Ks; Ns; Sil.

Whooping cough, in: Ks.

**Distension,** As of: Nm.

**Dragging,** Down: Nm; Ns.

**Drinks,** Hot Amel: Mp.

Ice-cold Agg: Cp.

**Dropsy** (Ascites): Kp; Ks; Sil.

Diarrhea, frequent, with: Sil.

**Eating,** While, Agg: Cp.

**On every attempt to: Cp.**

**Eating,** Amel: Kp.

**Empty:** Cp; KM; Kp; NP.

Flatus passing Amel: KS.

Lower part: Ks.

Stool, after: KS; NP.

**Enlarged,** Children, in: **SIL.**

**Eructations,** Amel: Cp; Km; Mp; Sil.

With: MP.

**Eruptions,** Pimples, etc.: Nm.

**Eye symptoms,** With: Km; NM.

**Falling,** Out, of: Nm.

**Fasting,** Amel: Sil.

**Fermentation,** In: NM; NS

**Flabby** (Pot-bellied): **CP;** SIL.

**Flatus,** Passing, Amel: Cp; Km; NM; NS; Sil.

**Foetus,** Movements of: **SIL.**

Painful: Mp.

Violent: Sil.

**Frozen** Food Agg: CP.

**Fullness:** Cs; Fp; KM; KS; Nm; Np; NS; **SIL.**

Diarrhea, during: NS.

Eating, after: KM.

Urinating, after: Nm.

**Gurgling** (Meteorism): Fp; NM; NP; SIL.

Gushing stools, then: NS.

Motion, Amel: Nm.

**Hands,** Yellow, blue nails with: **Sil.**

**Hard:** Fp; Kp; Ks; Mp; Nm; Np; **SIL.**

Children, in: Sil.

with thin legs: SIL.

**Hardness,** In spots: Fp.

**Heat** (Burning): Kp; KS; Nm; **SIL**

Extending to head: Ns.

**Heat** of Body, with: Nm.

**Heaviness,** As from load: Cs; Fp; Kp; Ks; NM; SIL.

Menśes, during: Ks; Nm.

**Hernia,** Appear, as if would: Sil.

**Hollow:** See Empty.

**Inflammation** (Peritonitis, enteritis): Fp; Km; Kp; Ks; SIL.

**Intestines,** Ulceration of: Cp; NP.

Typhoid fever, in: Cs.

**Jarring** Agg: Ks; NS; **SIL.**

**Jerks:** Nm.

**Kneading** Amel: NS.

**Knots,** Felt In: Mp.

**Laughing** Agg: Nm.

**Layer** of Hard substance: Fp.

**Leucorrhea,** With: Nm; **SIL.**

Burning, followed by: Cp.

**Lifting,** From: Sil.

**Loose,** Intestines were, as if: Nm.

**Lump,** As if: Nm.

**Lying** On Agg: Ns.

Abdomen, Amel: Cp; Kp.

Back, Agg: Mp.

legs extended, with: Nm

Left side, Agg: NM; NS.

Painful side, Agg: NM; **SIL.**

" Right side, Agg: Cf; Nm; Sil.

**Malaria** after. Nm.

**Marble,** Dropped down in descending colon, as if, while at stool: Np.

**Menses,** After Agg: Nm.

Before Agg: KP; Ks; Mp.

During Agg: **CP;** Fp; Kp; Ks; NM; NS; Sil.

**Menses,** Appear would, as if: Km; Nm.

**Menses,** Flow becomes free, when, Amel: Kp.

**Morning** Agg: Ns.

Rising on: Ns.

**Motion,** Agg: Ks; Mp; Nm; Sil.

**Movements,** In: CP; Nm; Ns;

Flatus from, something alive, as if: Cp.

Morning after: Nm,

Stool, before: Ns; Sil,

**Movements** of Foetus, painful: **SIL.**

Violent: SIL.

**Nails,** Blue with. Sil.

**Nausea,** With: Nm.

**Night,** Agg: Mp; Nm; NP; NS; Sil.

**Numbness:** CP.

Sacrum and lower limbs with: **CP.**

**Pain:** CP; CS; Fp; Kp; Ks; NM; Np; **NS;** SIL.

Left to Right: Kp.

Burning: Cp; Cs; Kp; Ks; NM; Np; **NS;** SIL.

Children, in: Cp; Mp; Np;

Coffee, after: Nm.

Cold drinks, from: CP; Cs.

Constipation, from: NM; **SIL.**

Cramping, griping: CP; Cs; Fp; Km; Ks; **MP;** NM; NP; NS.

 wandering: Ns.

Cutting: Cp; Cs; Kp; **KS;** MP; **NM;** Np; **NS; SIL.**

 tenesmus with, extorting cries: Km.

Damp weather, from: NS.

Diarrhea, like that of: NM; Ns.

Digging: NM; NS.

Dragging, bearing down: Cs; Fp; NM; NS.

Drawing: NM.

Drinking, Agg: Nm.

Exertion from: Nm.

Flatulent colic: Ks; MP; Np; NS.

Fruits from: CP; Ns.

Ice-cream, after: CP.

Lead colic: NS.

Malaria, after: Nm.

Menstrual: CP; KP; Ks; MP; Nm; Sil.

Paroxysmal: Kp; MP; Np.

Periodical, Every day: Nm.

Pinching: NM; Ns; SIL.

Pressing: Cp; Cs; Fp; KS; NM; SIL.

Radiating: MP.

Riding in carriage: Cf; Nm.

Sore, bruised, tenderness: Cs; Fp; KP; Ks; Nm; Np; Ns.

Stitching, shooting: CS; KP; KS; Nm; Np; Ns; SIL.

Tearing: Nm; Sil.

Tossing about, anxiety, no relief, from flatus: Mp.

Twinging: SIL.

Twisting: Sil.

Violent: Sil.

Wandering: Cs; NS.

Worms: Np; Sil.

**Pendulous:** Cf.

**Pressure** Amel: MP; Nm; NS.

Of clothes Agg: Ns.

 Amel: Nm.

**Pulsations:** Cs; Ks; Ns.

Eructations, Amel: Cp.

Walking, while: Ns.

**Relaxed** Feeling, while walking: NM.

**Restlessness,** Uneasiness: NM; NS.

**Retraction:** NM; Sil.

**Rising** From seat, Agg: Nm.

**Rough** Substance, As if a: Nm.

**Rubbing** Amel: Nm; NS.

And warmth amel: Mp.

**Rumbling:** Cp; Cs; Fp; Kp; Ks; NM; Np; **NS; SIL.**

Breakfast, during: Nm.

Drinking, after: Kp.

Eating, after: Nm; Ns.

Flatus passing, amel: **NS.**

Menses, before: Cp.

during: Kp.

Stool, after: Nm.

before: Km; Ks; NM; NS.

diarrheic, before: Nm.

**Screwing:** Nm.

**Sensitive,** Tender: Fp; Kp; Ns.

**Shaking,** Quivering: Sil.

Cough, from: Sil.

**Shattering,** As if a: Sil.

**Shocks:** Nm.

**Sitting** While, Agg: Cf; NM.

**Spasms** In: Mp; Sil.

**Squeezing:** NM.

**Stool,** Before, Agg: Cp; Fp; Km; Kp; Np; NS.

During, Agg: KM; Nm; Sil.

Diarrheic, after: NM; Sil.

**Stool,** After, Amel: **NS.**

Diarrheic, after: CP; NS; Sil.

**Stone,** As of a: Nm.

**Stooping** Agg: NM.

**Storm,** During, Agg: Ns.

**Straining** At stool, Agg: Nm; **SIL.**

**Stretching** On Agg: Nm.

**Swashing:** NM.

**Swelling:** Km.

**Tension:** Cs; FP; Km; Kp; NM; Np; Ns; **SIL.**

Thigh to: Mp.

**Touch,** Agg: Fp; NS.

**Trembling:** KS.

**Twitching,** Jerking: Nm.

**Ulcers:** SIL.

**Urging** To stool, urine: Nm.

**Urination,** During Agg: Cp; Nm.

**Volvulus:** Sil.

**Walking,** Agg: Fp; KS; NM; Np; **NS; SIL.**

Open air, in: Ns; Sil.

**Walking,** Amel: Cf; Mp.

**Warm** Drinks, food, Amel: MP.

**Warmth,** Amel: Mp; Sil.

**Water-Brash,** With: **SIL.**

**Weakness,** Sense of: CP; Fp; NM.

Eructations, Amel: KM.

Stool, after: NP.

**Yawning** Amel: Nm.

**ABORTION:** Cs; Fp; Kp; KS; SIL.

**Grief,** Suppression, from: Nm.

**Habitual:** Sil.

**Haemorrhage,** After: Sil.

**Threatened:** Kp; Mp.

**Weakness,** From, sheer: Sil.

**ABRUPT:** Nm.

**ABSCESS** (Suppuration): Cf; **CS;** Fp; Km; Kp; Nm; **SIL.**

Bones, About: Cf; Cp; Nm; Sil.

Chronic: Cf; Cp; SIL

Fistulous: Ns; SIL.

Glands, of: CS; SIL.

Impending: Sil.

Multiple, Fever, during: Sil

Periosteum: Cf; SIL.

Recurrent: CS.

Retro-Pharyngeal: SIL

Running: CS.

Slow: Sil.

To hasten: Sil.

ABSENT-MINDED,

Absorbed: CP; Cs; KP; KS; NM; Np; SIL.

As to what would become of him: Nm.

ABSENT, Parts of the body were: Sil.

ABSORBENT Action: Km.

ABSTRACTION of mind: NM; Sil.

ABUSIVE: Sil.

ACHING: See under PAIN.

ACIDITY: See Sour.

ACIDOSIS: Np.

ACNE: See Eruptions.

ACRIDITY, Excoriations: Cs; Km; NM; NS; SIL.

ACTIVE, Agile: Cp; Fp; NM.

When, Amel: Fp; NS.

ACTS As if Born Tired: KP.

ACUMINATE: SIL.

ADDISONS Disease: Cp; NM; Ns; SIL.

ADENOIDS: CF; CP; Ks.

Removal, After: Ks.

ADHERENT Internal Sensation: Mp; SIL.

ADYNAMIA: See Weakness.

AFFECTIONATE: NM..

AFTER-PAINS: Cf; Fp; Kp; Mp; NM.

Child, Nurses when: Sil.

Woman, Who has borne many children: KP.

AGILITY (Active): Cp; Fp; NM

AGITATION: See Excitement.

AGONY: Nm; Ns.

AGUE: See Fever intermittent.

AIR BLOWING, On part: Nm.

Cold: CP; Fp; Km; Kp; MP; Nm; NP; SIL.

Draft Agg. (See Wind): Cp.

Hunger: See Open Air Amel.

Hot, As if: Ks.

Night: Ns.

Open, Cool Agg: Cp; Np; SIL.

Open, Amel, Room Agg: CS; KS; NM; NS.

AIR CASTLES: SIL.

AIR SICKNESS: Fp; Sil.

ALBUMINOUS, Glairy: Cp; Np; NM; NS.

ALBUMINURIA: CP; Fp; Km; Kp; NM; NP; NS.

Heart Disease, Consecutive to: Kp.

Pregnancy, During: Cp; Km; NM.

Scarlet Fever, after: KS; NS.

**ALCOHOLISM:** Km; NM; SIL.
**Delirium** Tremens: Kp; NM.
**ALIVE SENSATION:** Nm; SIL.
**ALL GONE:** See Empty.
**ALONE** When AGG: Fp; Kp; NM; Sil.
**When Amel:** Nm.
**Likes to be:** Cp; Nm.
**ALTERNATING** Effects,
States: Cp; Fp; Nm.
**Contradictory:** Nm.
**AMAUROSIS:** See Under Vision.
**AMBITION** Loss of: CP; Fp; Ks; NM; Np.
**AMENORRHEA:** See Under Menses.
**AMOROUS, Lewd, Lascivious:** Cp; Nm; SIL.
**ANAEMIA:** CP; FP; KP; NM; NP; NS; Sil.
**Children,** Infants: Sil.
**Grief,** From: Nm.
**Haemorrhage,** After: NM.
**Menstrual** Derangements: Cp; Nm.
**Nutritional** Disturbances: CP.
**Skin** Affections, With: Km.
**ANALGESIA:** See Numbness.
**ANASARCA:** See Dropsy.
**ANEURISM:** CF; Cp; Fp.
**Capillary:** CF.
**ANGER, Vexation, Irritability:** CP; CS; Fp; KM; KP; KS; NM; Np; NS; Sil.

**Answer,** When obliged to: Nm.
**Coffee,** Agg: Cp.
**Consolation,** Agg: NM; Sil.
**Contradiction,** From: SIL.
**Evening:** Km.
**Flies** Into Passion, can hardly articulate: Kp.
**Grief,** Silent with: NM.
**Indignation,** With: NM.
**Morning,** Does not wish to be spoken to nor to speak: Ns.
**Trembling,** With: Fp.
**Trifles,** At: Km; Np.
**ANGLES** (skin, folds): Nm; Sil.
**ANGUISH,** Empty feeling in head with: Nm.
**Night:** Ns.
**ANIMATION:** See Cheerful.
**ANKLES:** Nm; Np.
**Abscess:** Sil.
**Band,** Around as if: Nm.
**Caries:** Sil.
**Cold:** CF.
**Cramps:** Cp.
**Dislocation,** Easy: **NM.**
**Eruptions:** Cp; Nm; Np.
Eczema: NP.
Herpes: NM.
Pimples: Cp.
Urticaria: NM.
**Fistulous** Opening: Cp; Sil.
**Itching:** NP.
**Lameness,** Sitting while: NM.
Walking, while: NM.

**Numbness:** Nm.
**Pain:** Fp; Nm; Np; NS.
Aching: Np.
Anterior part: Cp.
Boring: Ns.
Dislocated, as if: CP.
Drawing: Nm; Ns; Sil.
Extending upward: FP; Ns.
Gnawing: Nm.
Lying, while Agg: Ns.
       Amel: Sil.
Menses after: Ns.
Motion, Agg and amel: Ns.
Paralytic: NP.
Pressing: Nm; Ns.
Shooting: CP; FP.
Sitting, agg: Ns.
Sore, bruised: **NM.**
Sprained, as if: Nm; NS;
    SIL.
prevents walking: Ns.
Stepping, when, Agg: Nm;
    Np; Sil.
Stitching: Cp; Fp; Nm; Sil.
internal malleolus: Nm.
Tearing: CP; NS; Sil.
malleoli: Nm; Sil.
Touch, Agg: Nm.
Ulcerative: Nm.
Walking, while Agg: Cp;
    Nm.
**Paralysis:** Nm.
Sensation: Nm.
Sitting, walking, while: Nm.
**Stiffness:** Nm; **SIL.**

**Swelling:** Sil.
**Tension:** Sil.
Sitting, while: Sil.
**Turned,** Easily: Nm.
**Turning,** of: Sil.
**Ulcers:** CP; Nm; Sil.
Foetid: CP.
Fistulous: CP; Sil.
Malleoli: CP.
**Weak:** Cs; Nm; NP; NS; Sil.
Children, learning to walk:
    Np.
**ANOREXIA:** See Appetite,
    Wanting.
**ANSWERS,** Aversion, To: Cs;
    KP; NM.
**ANTHRAX:** Kp; Sil.
**ANTHROPHOBIA** (Bashful): CS;
    Kp; NM; Sil.
**ANTICIPATIONS,** Complaints
    from: Nm; SIL.
**ANUS:** See Rectum & Anus.
**ANXIETY** (Cares): **CP; CS;** Fp;
    **KP; KS;** NM; NP; SIL.
**Alternating,** With Indifference:
    Nm.
**Children,** in: Cp.
Lifted from cradle, when:
    CP.
**Conscience** Of (As if guilty of
    crime): Fp; NM; SIL.
**Dreams,** On Waking from
    frightful: NM.
**Fever,** With: Cs; Fp; KP; Ks;
    NM; Np.

**Fever,** During: Cs; Fp; Kp; Nm; Np.

**Fright,** After: Nm; Sil.

**Future,** About: Cs; **Fp;** Kp; Np.

**Health,** About: Cs; Kp; Np; Sil.

Climacteric, about: Sil.

**Lying,** While: Sil.

**Menses,** Before: Nm.

During: NM; **SIL.**

**Money Matters,** About: CF; Kp.

**Motion,** Amel: Sil.

**Salvation,** About: Kp.

**Shut Up,** In Dark Cellar, as if: NP.

**Sleep,** On going to: Nm.

During: Nm.

**Trifles,** About: Sil.

**Uneasiness,** And must uncover: Nm.

**APATHY:** See Indifference.

**APHONIA:** See Voice, Lost

**APHTHAE** See Mouth.

**APOPLEXY:** KM; SIL.

**Pre-Disposition,** To: Cf.

**APPARITION:** See Vision, Fantastic.

**APPENDICITIS** (Ileo-caecal region): CS; Km; **SIL.**

**Flatulence** In: Ns.

**Inflammation** (Typhlitis): FP; Km; NS; SIL.

**Pain,** Cutting: Np.

Stitching: Sil.

**APPETITE** Affected, In General: Nm; Sil.

**Better,** After, beginning to eat: Nm; Sil.

**Capricious,** Variable: Nm.

**Changeable:** Nm.

**Constant:** Kp; NM.

**Easy** Satiety: Ks; NM; SIL.

**Increased,** Ravenous, Canine: CP; CS; Fp; Km; Kp; Ks; Mp; NM; NP; NS; SIL.

Afternoon, 4 P.M.: Cp.

Alternating, with loss of: Nm; NP.

Attacks, of: Km; Sil.

drinking water, amel: Km.

Between regular periods of eating: Km.

Chill, during: SIL.

Constant desire to nurse: Cp.

Eating after, soon: Kp; Nm; Sil.

Emaciation, with: **NM.**

Empty feeling in stomach with: Np.

Evening: NM; Sil.

Forenoon, 10 A.M.: Nm; **SIL.**

eructations, after: Km.

nausea, with: Sil.

Marasmus, with: CP; **NM; SIL.**

Menses, during: Kp.

Night: Sil.

Pain in stomach, with: SIL.

Ravenous: Nm; SIL.

Relish, without: **NM.**

Satiety and fulness, easy: Nm; Sil.

Stool, after: Kp.

Sweets, only, for: Kp.

Vanishing, on attempting to eat: Sil.

at sight of food: Kp.

on drinking water: Km.

Wants to eat every hour: Km.

Wine, after: Nm.

**Wanting,** Diminished: Cp; Cs; Fp; Ks; NM; Np; Ns; **Sil.**

Drinking water, after: Km.

Food, at sight of: Kp.

Habitual: Km.

Hunger, with: **NM; SIL.**

Menses, before and during: Cp.

Returns, after thinking of food: Cp.

Thirst, with: Sil.

Vexations, after: Nm.

**ARMS** (Upper Limbs): SIL.

Right: Sil.

Left shakes, before epilepsy: Sil.

**Alternate,** With Lower: Km; **SIL.**

**Upper Arm**

Blood rushes, to: Sil.

Cold, Sensitive to: Nm.

Coldness: Nm.

internal, right: Km.

Deltoid: Fp; Nm.

Eruptions, Boils: SIL.

herpes: Nm.

Heat: Cp; Nm.

Jerking: Nm.

Pain: Kp; MP; Nm; Sil.

aching: Kp.

bone, external condyle: Sil

burning: Nm; NS.

clothes wearing, Agg: Fp.

drawing: Fp; Nm; Ns; Sil.

cramps, like: Nm.

evening, Amel: Ns.

′ jerking: Sil.

inner side: Ns; Sil.

lower part: Sil.

lying on it Agg: Nm; SIL.

motion Agg: Fm; SIL.

backward and forward: NM.

motion Amel: Kp.

slow: Fp.

posterior part: Sil.

pressing: Ns.

agg: Sil.

pulsating: Nm.

raising arm, agg: CP.

rheumatic: Cp; Fp; Nm.

sore, bruised: NM.

bone, in: Sil.

stitching: Cp; Ns; Sil.

burning: Cp.

tearing: Fp; Kp; Nm; Np; Ns; SIL.

bone in: NS.

Paralysis: Cp.
Sinking down: Nm.
Swelling: Cp.
nodular: Nm.
vaccination, due to: SIL.
Twitching: Nm; Sil.
Weakness: Nm; Sil.
Bones: CF; SIL.
Chilliness: NM.
Coldness: CP; Cs; FP; KP;
Ks; NM; Np; SIL.
Fever, after: Sil.
Joints, of: NM.
Menses, during: Sil.
Painful parts: Sil.
Compression: Ns.
Constriction, Joints of: NM;
Sil.
Contraction of Muscles and
Tendons: NM; Np; SIL.
Extensor muscles, when writ-
ing: NP.
Flexor tendons: Sil.
Joints, of: NM.
Writing, when: Np.
Convulsions: Nm; Sil.
Cracked Skin: Sil.
Cracking, Joints in: KS; NM;
Np; NS.
Tendons, in: Fp; Km.
Cramps: KM; KP; KS; NM;
SIL.
Chill during: SIL.
Exertion after: Mp.
Curving, Bowing of Bones:
CP; SIL.

Discolouration, Mottled: Nm.
Dislocation Joints of, easy:
Nm.
Emaciation: Nm; Sil.
Paralysed parts: KP.
Eruptions: NM; SIL.
Areola, red: Nm.
Blotches: Nm.
Boils: SIL.
Eczema: SIL.
Elevation: Nm.
Gritty: Nm.
Groups, in: Nm.
Hard: Sil.
Herpes: NM; SIL.
Hot water, amel: Ks.
Joints, on: Cp; NM; Np.
bends of: NM.
pimples: CP.
vesicles: Np.
Lumps, hard, bluish, oozing:
CP.
Moist: Nm.
Pimples: CP; Cs; Ns.
burning: Ns.
depressed, head black: Cs.
inflamed: Cs.
sensitive: Cs.
Psoriasis: KS; Sil.
Pustules: NM; SIL.
Rash: Mp; Nm; Sil.
Scabs: KS; SIL.
Urticaria: Nm; Ns.
Vesicles: Cp; NM; SIL.

red, small: NM.

White: Nm.

**Exostoses,** of Bones: **CP;** Sil.

**Fistulous,** Opening in joints: **SIL.**

**Formication:** Nm; Np.

**Hair,** On as if: Nm.

**Heat:** NM.

Flashes of: Sil.

**Hanging** Down, Amel: Sil.

**Heaviness,** (Tired Limbs): Cp; Fp; **KP; NM;** Np; Ns; SIL.

Menses, during: Nm.

Must let them drop: Np.

Numbness, with: Sil.

Pregnancy, during: CP.

**Incoordination:** Kp; Sil.

**Jerking:** Fp; Ks; NM; Sil.

Falling asleep, on: Sil

Lying, back on: Cp.

**Lameness:** Cp; Ns; **SIL.**

Flexor muscles of: Cp.

Joints, of: SIL.

Rheumatic: Cp.

**Light,** As if: Nm.

**Motions,** Of Agg: Nm.

Convulsive: Cp; Nm.

Involuntary: Nm.

Loss of power, on waking: Sil.

Lying, back on: Cp.

side, on amel: Cp.

**Mouse,** Running up limb, sensation of: SIL.

**Nodes:** Nm; Sil.

**Numbness:** Cp; **KM;** Kp; KS; Nm; Np; NS; Sil.

Left: NM.

Leaning on it: Sil.

Lying on it: NM; SIL.

Right: Kp; Sil.

Rubbing amel: Nm.

**Pain:** CP; Cs; Km; MP; Nm; Sil.

Aching: Cp.

bones, in: CP.

extending to fingers: Cp.

Air, open amel: KS.

Bed, warmth of agg: Km.

Chill, during agg: Cs; Ks; Nm; Sil.

Coition, after agg: **SIL.**

Drawing: Cp; Kp; Nm; Ns; Sil.

downwards and to fingers: Sil.

extending to bones: Nm.

Exertion, after Agg: NM; Sil.

Extending to bones: Cp; Nm.

flexors, to grasping, when: NS.

joints, to on motion: Nm.

Festering: Cp; SIL.

Fever, during: Nm.

Grasping, anything, Agg: Ns.

Hanging down, letting arm: Nm.

Amel: Sil.

Heat Agg: Ks.

joints, in: **CP;** Cs; FP; KP; Nm; Np; NS; SIL.

gouty: **CP; CS;** Fp; KP; NM; Np; Ns; SIL.

night, amel: MP.

rheumatic: **CP;** CS; **FP;** Km; Ks; NM; NP; Ns.

Leaning upon, when agg: Nm; **SIL.**

Lying bed in agg: NM; **SIL.**

customary side, on: **SIL.**

Motion, on Agg: Cp; Fp; NM; SIL.

Amel: Kp; **KS;** Nm; NS.

Move, on beginning to: KP; SIL.

Playing piano and violin: Mp.

Pressing: Ns; Sil.

together: Ns.

Pressure, Amel: MP.

Rest, Amel: Nm; Sil.

Rheumatic: CP; Cs; Kp; KS; Fp; MP; SIL.

acute: Cs.

diarrhea, chronic, in: Sil.

Shooting: Cp.

Sore, bruised: Cp; Cs; Nm; Ns; Sil.

Sprained, as if: CP; NM; Sil.

Stitching: Cp; Fp; Nm; Sil.

as if asleep: Sil.

joints, in: Kp; KS; NM; Sil.

Stooping, Agg: Sil.

Stretching, Amel: NM.

Taking hold of something Agg: Sil.

Tearing: CP; KP; Ks; Nm; NP; **NS; SIL.**

jerking: Sil.

joints, in: Ks; Nm; Np; NS; SIL.

Tendons, in: CP.

Touch, agg: Sil.

Uncovering, agg: NM; Sil.

Up and down: Sil.

Walking, amel: KS.

Wandering, shifting: CP; **KS;** MP; NS.

Warmth, amel: **KP; MP; SIL.**

Weather, change of, agg: CP; SIL.

wet, agg: Ns; SIL.

Writing, while: MP; Sil.

**Paralysis:** Cp; Cs; KP; Sil.

Fever, suppressed, from: Nm.

Flexural muscles: Nm.

Mental, emotion from: Nm.

Pain, from: Nm.

Painless: Nm; Sil.

Post-diphtheric: Kp; NM.

Right: Sil.

Sensation, of: Nm; Ns; Sil.

Sexual excess, from: NM.

Stiffness, with: Nm; Sil.

**Pulsation:** Nm; Sil.

Eating, after: Sil.

**Raise,** Impossible to: Nm.

**Restlessness:** Km; KP; NM; **SIL.**
Evening: Km.
**Sensitive:** FP.
Cold, to: Cp.
**Shaking,** Left, Epilepsy before: Sil.
**Shocks:** Nm.
**Sinking,** Down: Nm.
**Smuttiness:** Sil.
**Spotted:** Nm.
**Sprains,** Tendency, to: Nm; SIL.
**Stiffness:** Cp; Cs; NM; NS; **SIL.**
Chill, during: **NS.**
Convulsive: Sil.
Joints, of: Ks; NM; Np; **SIL.**
Menses, during: Cp.
Move, on beginning to: Kp
Paralytic: Nm.
**Suppleness,** lack of: Nm; **SIL.**
**Swelling:** Fp; Kp; NS; Sil.
Bones of: SIL.
Dropsical: Fp; Kp; Sil.
Joints, of: Cf; FP; NM; Sil.
around: Km.
dropsical: NM.
white: Ks; SIL.
Nodular: Nm; Sil.
**Tension:** Mp; Nm; Ns; Sil.
Joints, in: NM.
Tendons, in, as if short: Nm.
Writing, when: **MP.**

**Tingling,** Prickling: NM; Ns; **SIL.**
Right: Sil.
Side, laid on: Sil.
**Trembling:** Kp; Ks; MP; SIL.
Cold, taking, from: Cp.
Emissions, after: **NP.**
Epilepsy, before: SIL.
Exertion, after: Nm; Sil.
Motion, on slight: MP.
Writing, while: Nm; NS.
**Twitching:** Fp; Kp; Ks; NM; NP; Ns; SIL.
Electric shocks, as from: Nm.
Joint, of: Nm; Sil.
Sleep during: Nm; Sil.
falling to, on: NM.
Wandering: Ns.
**Ulcers:** Sil.
Joints. on: Sil.
**Warts:** Nm; NS; SIL.
**Water cold,** Poured over, as if: Cp.
**Weakness:** Cp; CS; Ks; NM; NP; Ns; SIL.
Anger, after a fit of: Nm.
Joints of: Fp; KS; NM; SIL.
Menses, during: CP.
Morning: Km.
Pregnancy, during: Cp.
Rising from bed, amel: Nm.
Stiffness, with: Nm; Sil.
Sudden: Np.
Taking hold of something: Nm; Sil.

**ARROGANCE** (pride): Sil.
**ARTHRALGIA:** See Joints, Rheumatic etc.
**ARTHRITIS DEFORMANCE:** CF; CP; Ks; SIL.
**ARTHRITIC NODOSITIES:** CF; CP; CS; Ks; Nm; SIL.
**ASCENDING** AGG: CP; Kp; **NM;** NP; Sil.
**ASCITES:** See Abdomen, Dropsy.
**ASTHMA:** Fp; KM; KP; KS; NM; Np; NS; **SIL.**
Air, Draught of Agg: Sil.
Ascending, Steps Agg: Kp.
Bronchial catarrh, with: Ns.
Soreness, in, with: Fp.
Children, in: **NS.**
Humid: **NS.**
Cold, From taking Agg: Sil.
Damp weather, Agg: Ns.
Heated, when: Sil.
Coryza, with: NS.
Cough, with: Nm.
Eating, after: KP.
Food, least, Agg: Kp.
Eructations, with: Mp.
Evening Agg: Nm.
Exertion, Agg: NS; Sil.
Expectoration, Difficult, with: Cf; Ks.
Flatulence, From: MP.
Gastric derangement, with: Km.
Hay, Asthma: **KP; NS; SIL.**
Hectic Fever, with: Cs.

Humid: NS.
Lying Down Agg: Ns; Sil.
Midnight After, 4 to 5 a.m.: Ns.
Nervous: Kp; Sil.
Night: Fp; Km; **KP; NS.**
3 a.m.: Km.
4 to 5 a.m.: NS.
morning towards Agg: SIL.
Over Heated, Being after: Sil.
Room, Warm: Ks.
Spasmodic: Fp; MP; Ns.
Sycotic: NS; Sil.
Thunderstorm, During: Sil.
Wet Weather: NS; Sil.
Winter, Agg: Nm.
**ASTIGMATISM:** See under Vision.
**ATHEROMA** (Arteriosclerosis): Cf; Np; Ns; Sil.
**ATROPHY:** See Emaciation.
Glands of: Kp; Sil.
**ATTACKS** recurrent: See Relapses
**ATTENTION** AGG: Cp; Nm; Sil.
**ATTITUDE** Bizarre: NS.
**AURA** Coldness: Sil.
Arms in: Sil.
Extremities, In: Sil.
General, Nervous: NM.
Premonitions, Mental: Nm.
**AUTOMATIC** Acts: Sil.
Hand, Right, towards mouth: Sil.
**AVARICIOUS,** Greedy: Cf.

**AVERSIONS** Acids, To: Fp; Np.
**Alcoholic** Beverages: Sil.
**Answer,** To: Kp; NM; Sil.
**Bathing:** Cs; Mp.
**Beer:** Nm; Ns.
**Boiled Food:** Sil.
**Bread:** Kp; Ks; **NM;** NP; NS.
Black (sour): Nm.
Butter, and: Np.
**Butter:** NM.
**Coffee:** NM.
**Colours,** Bright: SIL.
**Company:** CP; Cs; Fp; Kp;
Ks; **NM;** Np.
**Drinks,** Hot: KS.
**Eggs:** Ks; Np.
**Fats:** Ks; Np.
Rich food, and: Km; NM.
**Females:** Nm.
**Fish:** Nm.
**Food:** Fp; Km; Kp; Ks; Nm;
**NP; NS; SIL.**
Cooked: SIL.
Eat, attempting to: SIL.
Hunger, with: Nm; SIL.
Seen, if: Sil.
Warm: Sil.
**Fuss,** To: Nm.
**Meat: CS;** Fp; Km; NM; Np;
Ns; **SIL.**
**Members,** Family of: Kp.
Wife: Ns.
**Men:** Nm.
**Milk:** CS; Fp; Np; NS; SIL.
Mother's: **SIL.**

**Motion:** FP; Kp; Nm.
**Persons,** Who do not agree
with him: Cs.
**Reading:** Sil.
**Salty,** Food: NM; Sil.
**School,** To: Cp; Nm.
**Spoken,** To be: Kp; Nm; Ns;
SIL.
Morning: Ns.
**Sweets:** Kp.
**Tobacco:** Nm.
Smoking accustomed cigar:
Cp; Nm; Ns.
**Touched,** Being: **SIL.**
**Washing:** MP; NS; Sil.
**Water:** NM.
Cold: Nm.
**Wine:** Nm.
**Women:** NM.
**Work,** For: NM.
Mental: Cp; Cs; Fp Ks; Mp;
NM; SIL.
**AWAKES:** See Waking under
'Sleep.'
**AWKWARDNESS:** Cs; **NM;** Sil.
**Drops,** Things: Nm.
**Knocks** Against things: Nm.
**Stumbles,** When walking: MP;
NM; Sil.
**AXILLAE:** NM; **SIL.**
**Left:** NS; SIL.
**Right:** SIL.
**Abscess: Nm;** NS; SIL.
**Eruptions:** Nm.
Boils: NS; SIL.

Crusts: **NM.**
Eczema: NM.
Herpes: Nm.
Moist: Nm.
Scabs: NM.
**Glands,** Affections of: **NM;**
Sil.
Indurated: **SIL.**
Swelling: Kp; NM; NS; **SIL.**
**Itching:** NM.
**Lump,** Hard in: CP.
**Pain,** Burning: Cp; Nm.
Drawing: Sil.
Stitching: NS; Sil.
Tearing: NM.
**Perspiration:** Kp; KS; NM;
Ns; **SIL.**
Offensive: Ns; **SIL.**
garlic like: Kp.
onions, like: Kp.
**Swelling,** of Glands: Kp; NM;
NS; SIL.
**BACK:** Nm; Ns; **SIL.**
**Left: SIL.**
**Right** to left: Cp; KP.
**Alternating** Sides: Cp.
**Changing,** Here and here:
Ks; MP.
**Chest,** Into, right: Cp.
**Head,** To: Nm; Sil.
**Heart,** To: Nm.
**Hips,** To: Km.
**Leg,** To: Km.
**Ache:** Cf; Cp; Cs; Fp; KS;
NM; NP; SIL.
**Air,** Draught of Agg: **CP;** Sil.

**Bed,** Early in, Agg: Nm.
Warm, when getting: Sil.
**Bending,** Backwards Agg: CP.
Amel: Nm; Sil.
**Blowing** Nose Agg: CP.
**Boring:** Mp.
**Breaking,** Broken Pain: NM.
**Burning:** Kp; Ks; SIL.
Downward: Cp.
Walking in open air: Sil.
**Carried** When, Amel: Cp.
**Chill** During, Agg: **Nm;** Sil.
**Coition** Agg: CP; Nm; **SIL.**
**Coldness** (Chill included): Cs;
Fp; Km; Kp; Ks; **NM; NS;
Sil.**
Eating, after: Sil.
Extending down: SIL.
Up: CP; Kp; NS.
Lying down, amel: Sil.
Up and down, shivering with:
Mp.
**Cold** Weather, Change to:
**CP.**
**Coughing** When Agg: CS;
Ns; Sil.
**Cramp** Like, Pain: Cp; MP.
**Crick** In: Fp.
**Cutting** Pain: Cp; MP; **NM;**
NS; Sil.
Upward like a fan: NS.
**Drawing** Pain: Cp; Cs; Kp;
Ks; NM; Np.
**Driving** Agg: Sil.
**Eating** After Agg: NM.
**Eruptions:** Kp; Nm; SIL.

Carbuncles: SIL.
Crusts: Nm.
Eczema: Sil.
Impetigo: NM.
Pimples: NM; Sil.
Pustules: Nm; SIL.
painful: SIL.
small-pox: Sil.
Evening Agg: CP; Ks; Ns.
Exertion From, Agg: CP; Kp.
Fever, During: NM; Ns.
Fistulae: Cp; SIL.
Flatulence From, Agg: Sil.
Heat: Cs; Nm; SIL.
Heaviness (Weight): Kp; NM; Np.
Injury, Fall etc. Agg: NS; Sil.
Itching: Kp; Nm; Np; NS; Sil.
Night: KP.
Undressing, while: NS.
Jarring Agg: SIL.
Jerking: CP; Nm;
Lameness: Kp; NM.
Leaning, Back Agg: Kp.
Leaning, On something Amel: Kp; Nm.
Lifting Agg: CP.
Lying, while Agg: Nm; Ns.
Back on Agg: Kp; NM.
Side on Agg: NS.
Lying, When Amel: Cp; Km; NM; Sil.
Back on: NM; Sil.
flat, with firm pressure: NM.
right side on: Ns.
something hard on: NM.

Menses, After Agg: Cp.
Beginning of: KS.
Before: CP; Nm.
During: CP; Cs; Fp; KP; KS; Np; Sil.
Mental Exertion Agg: SIL.
Motion on Agg: Cp; Cs; Fp; Np; NS; Sil.
Motion on Amel: Cf; Cp; Kp; KS; Ns.
Gentle: Cp; Kp.
Moving Arms, Agg: Sil.
Head, Agg: Ns.
Neck, Stretching on Agg: Ns.
Night Agg: Fp; Nm; Np; SIL.
2 a.m.: Ns.
3 a.m.: Km.
Numbness: CP; Sil.
Nursing while, Agg: SIL.
Opisthotonos: Cp: Mp; Ns.
Overlifting, From Agg: Cp.
Pain, In General: CP; Cs; Fp; Km; Kp; KS; Mp; NM; Np; NS; SIL.
Paralytic: Kp; Nm; Sil.
Periodical: Ks.
Pressing: Cs; Kp; Nm; Ns; Sil.
stone, as of a: Sil.
Rheumatic: CP; SIL.
Perspiration: Np; Sil.
Emission, after: Sil.
Pregnancy, during Agg: Cp.
Pressure Agg: Cp; SIL.
Amel: NM.
Pulsating: Cp; NM; SIL.

Raising, Arm on Agg: Nm.
Up: NM.
Rest, During Agg: Kp; Sil.
Riding In Carriages, Agg: Cf;
SIL.
Rising, Bed, From Agg: NM;
Sil.
Sitting from: CP; CS; Fp;
Kp; Nm; SIL.
Stooping from: NM; SIL.
Room, Warm Agg: KS.
Rubbing Amel: Ns.
Sensitive: Mp.
Sexual Excess Agg: Nm; NP;
Sil.
Shivering: Nm.
Sitting while, Agg: Cf; Cs;
FP; Km; Kp; NM; Np; NS;
Sil.
Sleep, Before, Agg: Nm.
Sore, bruised: Cs; Kp; Ks;
NM; Np; NS.
Spasms (See Opisthotonos):
CP; NM; NS.
Spreads Like fan upwards:
Ns.
Standing while Agg: Fp; Km;
Kp; KS; Nm.
Stiffness: Cs; NP; KS; Nm;
Ns; SIL.
Chill, during: NS.
Sitting after: SIL.
Walking, amel: Cs.
Stitching, Shooting: Cs; Fp;
Km; KP; KS; MP; Nm;
Np; Ns; SIL.
Chest, front of, to: Ns.

Stool, after Agg: Nm; Sil.
Before, Agg: NM.
Stooping Agg: NM; SIL.
Prolonged from: NM.
Straightening up Agg: NM.
Amel: Nm.
Swallowing Agg: Cp; Nm.
Tearing: Cp; Fp; Kp; SIL.
Extending down: Ns.
Nape to, while walking: Ns.
Tension: NM.
Throbbing (pulsating): Cp;
NM; SIL.
Touched When Agg: Kp; NM;
SIL.
Turning, When Agg: Sil.
Head: Nm; NS.
Must sit up to turn over: Kp.
Turning Amel: Nm.
Bed in: Nm.
Frequent: Nm.
Twitching: Nm.
Urinating, With desire to: NS.
Before, Agg: NS.
After Amel: NS.
Urine, On retaining Agg: Ns.
Walking On Agg: Cp; Km; Sil.
While Agg: CP; Fp; Km; KP;
Ks; Ns.
Open air, in: Nm; SIL.
Warm, becoming when: SIL.
Walking, while Amel: Cf; KP;
Ks; Nm.
Wandering Pain: KS; MP.
Warts: Sil.

**Weak:** Nm; Sil.

Coition, after: Np.

**Windy** Weather Agg: Cp.

**Work,** During Amel: Nm.

**Yawning** Agg: Cp.

**BAD** News, Ailments from, Or Agg: Cp; Kp; Nm; Np.

**Parts,** Takes everything, in: Nm.

**Wildness,** At unpleasant news: Cp.

**BALD:** SIL.

Spots, In: Ks; Sil,

**Young** people In: Sil.

**BALL,** lump, Globus internally: Km; KP; Mp; Ns; Sil.

**BAND,** Hoop, As of a: MP; NM; **SIL.**

Bones, In: Nm; Sil.

**BANDAGED** feeling: Mp; Nm.

**BANDAGING** AMEL: MP; NS; Sil.

**BARBER'S** itch: Km; Mp; Ns; Sil.

**BARKING** (like a dog): KM.

**BASHFUL** (Timidity): **CS;** Kp; Nm; Np; Ns; Sil.

Appearing In Public: **SIL.**

**Night:** Nm.

**Undue** Sensitiveness, from: Kp.

**BATHING** Aversion to or Agg from: **CS;** Km; Ks; MP; Nm; Sil.

Cold Agg: **MP;** Sil.

Sea: Km; Nm.

**BATHING** Cold AMEL: Cs; NM.

**Face:** CS.

**Hot:** Mp.

**BATHING,** Desire for: Nm.

**BEADS** Like swelling etc.: NM.

**BED** Desire to remain in: KP.

**Driving** out of: **MP;** Ns.

**Hard,** Sensation: FP; NS; SIL.

**Heat** of Agg: KS.

**Lying** in Agg: Km; Kp; Ks; Nm; **SIL.**

Amel: **Nm; SIL.**

**Sinking** under him: Cp.

**Sliding** Down in: **NM.**

**Sores:** Sil.

**Turning** Over, in Agg: Nm. **SIL.**

Amel: Nm.

**Wetting:** Fp; Km; KP; **MP; NM; NP; SIL.**

Catheterization from: MP.

Children, weakly in: Mp.

Head, blow on, from: Sil.

Old men, in: Kp.

Prostate enlarged, with: Kp.

Typhoid in: Kp.

**BEES** stinging As if: Mp; Np.

Agg: Mp.

**BENDING** backwards Agg: Nm.

Sideways: **NM.**

**Turning Affected part: Nm.**

**BENDING** Forward (Doubling up) AMEL: Mp.

**Turning** Affected part: Np.

**BERI-BERI:** Km.

**BESIDES** himself.
Maddening Pain: Km; Mp; Nm.
**BEWILDERED:** Nm; Sil.
**BILE DUCTS:** NP.
**BILIOUS:** NS.
**BIRTH MARK,** Naevi: Cf.
**BITING** or chewing Agg: **NM;** Sil.
**BLACK:** Fp; Nm.
**BLADDER** (Urinary) Affections in general: CP; Fp; MP; Nm; **SIL.**
**Aching:** Cp.
To tip of penis: Fp.
**Atony** (Paralysis): Fp; Kp; Np; Ns; SIL.
Old people in: Kp.
**Burning:** Sil.
**Calculi:** Cp; Sil.
To prevent reformation: Cp.
**Cancer:** Cp; SIL.
**Catarrh** ( muco-pus): Cs; Km; Kp; Ks; Nm; SIL.
Gonorrhea, from suppressed: Ns; SIL.
**Constriction:** Cp.
Urination, After: NM.
**Crampy:** MP.
**Cutting,** Urination before: Cp; Mp.
**Emptiness,** Sensation, pain with: Cp.
**Haemorrhage:** Fp.
**Heaviness:** NM.

Compels him to bend forward when sitting: Nm.
**Inflammation** (cystitis)
Acute: FP; Km.
Chronic: Km.
**Pain:** Cf; **CP;** Fp.
Dragging, hold urine, attempting to: Cp.
Drawing upward: Cp; Sil.
Neck, in: CP; Fp.
Pressing: CP; Kp; KS; NM; Np; Sil.
deep, in left side: CP
neck: **CP.**
Sore, tender: CP.
neck: CP.
Squeezing: Nm.
Standing Agg: Fp.
Stitching, stinging: Kp; Ks; Nm.
neck: Cp.
penis tip of, with: CP.
Stool, before: NM.
Urging to urinate, on: CP; Fp.
Urination after: CP; NM.
before: Cp; KS; Np.
during: Cp; NM; SIL.
Urination Amel: Fp.
Walking, while: Nm.
**Paralysis:** Fp; Kp; Np; Ns; SIL.
Old people in: Kp.
**Plug:** SIL.
**Polypi:** Sil.

**Retention** of urine, in: C.; Km; **MP**; Sil.
Catheter, from: MP.
Children, in: Fp.
Fever in, acute illness from: Fp.
Painful: Cp.
Spasmodic: Mp.
Unable to pass urine in presence of others: **NM**.
**Spasm** of the neck: MP.
**Spasmodic** action: Cp.
**Tenesmus:** Fp; SIL.
**Urging** to urinate: See Urination, Desire.
**Urine** Remained in, as if: Sil.
**Weakness:** Np; Sil.
Sphincter of: Sil.
**BLEEDING** Agg: Nm.
**Amel:** Fp.
**Mental** symptoms, With: Km.
**BLINDNESS:** See under Vision.
**BLISTERS:** See under Eruptions.
**BLOATED:** Cs.
**BLOOD,** Boils: NM; SIL.
**Cannot** look at: Cp; Nm.
**Circulation,** Sluggish: CP; FP; Nm; Sil.
**Clots** quickly: Km.
Does not clot: Kp.
**Cold,** As if: Cp; Nm; Sil.
**Gushing:** Nm; NS.
**Streaked:** Sil.

**BLOOD SEPSIS** (Septic Conditions): Fever, etc: Fp; Km; **KP**; Sil.
**Adynamic: FP**; SIL.
**BLOOD VESSELS:** See Arteries, Veins, Lymphatics.
**BLOWING** nose AGG: Nm; Sil.
AMEL: Sil.
**BLOWS,** shocks, Electric like: CP; NM; Np.
**BLUISH,** purple Discharges, etc.: Fp; NM; Sil.
**Spots:** Sil.
**BOARD LIKE** Sensation: **FP; NS; SIL.**
**BOILS:** Cp; **CS; SIL.**
**Blood:** NM; SIL.
**Crops,** of: SIL.
**Large:** Sil.
**Maturing** slowly: Sil.
**Periodic:** Sil
**Small:** Nm.
**Stinging,** When touched: Sil.
**BOLDNES:** Sil.
**BONES: CF; CP; SIL.**
**Bare** become: Sil.
**Brittle,** Breaking: Cf; Cp; **SIL.**
**Caries:** Cf; Cs; Nm; **SIL.**
Periosteum: Sil.
**Cartilages:** Cp; Sil.
Rice-bodies, in: Cf.
**Crumbling:** Cp; Sil.
**Curvature: CP;** SIL.
**Cutting:** Km.
**Deep** in: Sil.

Development Tardy: Cf; CP;
Sil.
Exostoses: CF; SIL.
Fracture: Cf; Cp; SIL.
Inflammation: Sil.
Itching, In: Km.
Jerk, In: Sil.
Necrosis of: CF; Cp; SIL.
Non-Union of (slow repair):
Cf; CP; Sil.
Ossification, slow: CP.
Pains in: CP; Cs: Ks; Nm; Sil.
Periosteum, Inflammation: Cf;
Sil.
Skin, Adherent as if: Sil.
Softening of: Cf; CP; SIL.
Tearing Shattered as if: KS;
SIL.
Tuberculosis of: Cp; SIL.
BORBORYGMY: Nm; Ns; SIL.
BORING, Grinding: NM; SIL.
BORING Ears into: SIL.
Child by: SIL.
Sleep, during: SIL.
Nose, Into: NM; NP; SIL.
Till it bleeds: Sil.
BOUNDING internal: See Alive
sensation.
BOWELS: See Abdomen and
Intestines.
BRAIN: Cp; Fp; KP; NM; Ns;
SIL.
Bandaged, As if: Nm.
Bruised, As if: FP; Nm.
Concussion: Kp; Ns.

Congestion: CP; CS; FP;
Kp; Ks; NM; NP; NS; Sil.
Afternoon: Sil.
Alcoholic liquors from: Cs;
Sil.
Coughing, on: Cs; Kp; Ks;
Sil.
Evening: Np.
Face, heat of with: FP; Sil.
redness with: Sil.
Menses, after: Nm
during: Cp; Cs; FP; Nm.
suppressed, from: Cs.
Night: CS; Sil.
Sleep, during: Sil.
Warm room in: Cs; KS.
Crushed In vise, as if: NS.
Degeneration, softening: Kp;
Sil.
Fag, Weak tired: Kp; Sil.
Forced forward, as if: Sil.
Haemorrhage: Fp; NM.
Inflammation, meninges of
acute and chronic: CP;
Fp; NM; Ns; SIL.
Periosteum, of: SIL.
Traumatic: Ns; SIL.
Tubercular: CP; Nm; SIL.
Knocking Against skull, as if:
Nm; Sil.
Large and Heavy, as if: Mp.
Liquid, As if: Mp.
Loose, As if: Km; Ks; NM;
Ns.
Falling to temples: Ns.
Head shaking on: Nm.
Stooping, on: Ns.

**Pain,** Deep aching, in: N m; Sil.

Pressing as if bound up: **NM;** Sil.

outward: Nm.

would come out as though: SIL.

Pulsating, beating against skull: Nm.

hammers like little: Nm.

Sticking: Sil.

Sutures, along: **CP.**

Touch, from: NM.

**Paralysis,** Sensation, emissions after: Sil.

**Pressed** Against skull, as if: Cp.

**Sensitiveness,** Of: Kp; NM; SIL.

Brushing hair, from: **SIL.**

Jar, to the least: Fp; Kp; SIL.

**Softening:** Kp; Sil.

**Troubles,** In children: Mp.

Diarrhea, sudden cessation from: Mp.

**Tumours:** SIL.

**Vibrations,** with every step: Sil.

**Water-pipe,** Bursting, as if: Sil.

**BRANNY:** See Desquamation.

**BREAKFAST** Agg: Nm; Ns; Sil. AMEL: Nm; Ns.

**BREAKING,** Broken: Cp; Nm; Sil.

**BREATH** COLD:

Desire To take deep: Cp; Mp; NS; Sil.

Cannot: Cp.

**Holding** Agg: Cp.

Amel: Kp; Ns.

**Hot:** Nm.

**Mercury** of: Sil.

**Odour,** Foetor oris: Kp; Nm; SIL.

Sense of: Nm.

**Offensive:** Cs; **KP;** Ks; **NM; NS; SIL.**

Cheesy: Kp.

Eating, after: Sil.

Morning: Sil.

Putrid: Sil.

morning: Kp.

**Stops,** Children in, when lifted: Cp.

**BREATHE** Again cannot: Nm; Sil.

**BREATHING,** When Agg: Nm; Sil.

Deep, Agg: Cp; Fp; NM; SIL. Amel: Nm.

Wants to take deep: Mp; SIL.

**BRINY:** See Salty, Fishy.

**BRITTLE,** Broken feeling: Cp; Nm; Sil.

**BRONCHIECTASIS** (Dilatation of bronchi) with profuse, foetid, purulent sputum: SIL.

**BRONCHITIS** (Inflammation)

**Acute:** Cs; **FP;** KM; KP; **NM; NS; SIL.**

**Capillary:** FP; Km.
**Chronic** Winter catarrh: Ks; Nm; Ns; SIL.
**Irritation** of: Fp.
**Sensitive** to Cold air: SIL.
**BROWNISH:** Kp; Sil.
**BROWS:** Nm.
**Eruptions** About: NM; Sil.
**Hair** fall out: Sil.
**Itching:** Nm; Sil.
**Pain,** While reading: Fp.
**Perspiration:** Cp.
**Pimples** on: Sil.
**BRUISED:** See Pain, Sore.
**BRUNETTES: NM;** Sil.
**BUBBLES** sensation of: Nm.
**BUBO:** Km; SIL.
**Suppurating:** Sil.
**BULIMIA:** See Appetite Increased.
**BULLAE:** Ns; Sil.
**BUNIONS:** KM; **SIL.**
**BURNING** (See Heat): CS; Fp; NM; SIL.
**Bathing,** Washing Agg: CS.
**Fiery:** Nm.
**Internal:** Nm; SIL.
**Pepper** Like: Ns.
**Raw:** Fp.
**Stinging:** Sil.
**BURNS** and Scalds: Cs; KM; Ns.
**Blisters** from: Km.
**Suppuration,** with: Cs.
**X-ray:** Cf.

**BURNT,** Scalded as if: Cf; KM.
**BURROWING** (See Pain): NM; Sil.
**BURSAE:** Cp; NM; SIL.
**Cysts:** SIL.
**BURSTING:** Kp; **NM.**
**BUSINESS** Averse to: Ks.
**Worry:** Kp.
**BUSY** When Amel: Cp; Kp.
**BUTTOCKS** After-pains felt in: Sil.
**Emaciation:** Nm.
**Eruptions:** Nm.
**Boils:** Sil.
**Pimples:** NP.
**Scurfy:** Cp.
**Excoriation** (Rawness between) Nm.
**Itching:** CP; Sil.
**Numb:** Cp.
**Cold,** and: Cp.
**Rising** after, sitting on: Cp.
**Sitting,** while: CP.
**Pain:** Cp.
**Burning:** Cp.
**Drawing:** Nm; Sil.
**Sore,** bruised: CP; Nm.
**Stitching: CP.**
**small** spots: **CP.**
**Tension:** Sil.
**Tingling,** Prickling: Cp.
**BUZZING:** See Humming.
**CALCULI** (Urinary, Biliary): Mp; **NS; SIL.**
**Atheroma:** Cf; Np; Ns; Sil.
**CALF** (See Legs also): Cp; Np; Sil.

**2 F.A.**

**Bandaged:** Np.
**Blue** Spots: Kp.
**Boils:** SIL.
**Bruises:** Nm.
**Coldness:** See under Legs.
**Cramps:** CP; Fp; Kp; MP; NM; Np; **SIL.**
Cholera in: Kp; MP.
Pregnancy during: Mp.
Sleep, during: Nm.
Tailor: Mp.
Turning foot, sitting while: Nm.
Walking, on: CP; Nm.
**Emptiness,** Sensation: Nm.
**Eruptions:** See under Legs.
**Foot** Turning sitting while: Nm.
**Formication:** CP.
**Heat:** Cp; Ns.
**Heaviness:** Cp; Fp; NM; Np; Sil.
Ascending steps: **NM.**
Menses during: CP.
**Itching:** Nm.
**Numbnes:** Sil.
**Pulsation:** Nm.
**Sensitive:** NM; Sil.
**Short** As if: Sil.
**Swelling:** Sil.
**Tension:** NM; Np; Sil.
Cramp like: Sil.
Sitting, while: **NM.**
Walking, while: NM; NP; SIL.

**Trembling:** Nm.
**Weakness:** CP; Cs; NM; Sil.
**Weariness** (Palpitation, with): CP.
**CALLOSITIES CORNS: SIL.**
**Inflamed:** Sil.
**Shooting:** Nm.
**Sore:** Sil.
**Stinging:** Sil.
**Tearing:** Sil.
**CALLUS:** Cp; SIL.
**CALMNESS** (Tranquility): Nm; Np; Sil.
**CANCER:** Cp; **CS;** FP; Km; Kp; **KS;** Nm; **SIL.**
**Cachexia:** Sil.
**Encephaloma:** Kp; **SIL.**
**Epithelioma:** Cp; KS; **SIL.**
**Fungus,** Hematodes: Nm; **SIL.**
**Lupus:** Ks; Nm; **SIL.**
Vorax: Sil.
**Noma:** KP; Sil.
**Sarcoma:** Sil.
Osteo: Cf.
**Scirrhus: SIL.**
**Stomach** of: Cf; Mp; SIL.
**To Relieve** pain: Kp; Mp; Sil.
**To Remove** deposits: Kp.
**CANCRUM ORIS: KP; SIL.**
**CANTHI** (Eyes of): Nm; SIL.
**Burning:** Km; Nm; Sil.
Inner: Cs; Sil.
**Crack:** NM; Sil.
Outer: NM.

Discharge: Nm.
Morning: Cp.
Eye-gum: NM; Sil.
Inflammation: Cs.
Injected, Red: Np.
Itching: NM.
Inner and outer: NM.
Pain: Nm.
Inner: Nm; Np; NS.
left: Nm; NS.
Outer: Nm.
Pressing: Sil.
inner: Nm.
Stitching: Nm.
Tearing: Nm.
Pustules: Sil.
Red: Cs; NM; Sil.
Styes, inner: Nm.
Towards, Inner: NM; Sil.
Swollen: Sil.
Twitching, Inner: Km.
Outer: Nm.
CAP Sensation: Ks.
CAPRICIOUS: Cs; Sil.
CARBUNCLE: Cf; Km; Kp; SIL.
CARDIAC Dropsy: Cf.
CARE & Worry: See Anxiety
CARELESS( Heedless): NM.
CARESSES Agg: NM; KP; SIL.
CARIES (bones of): Cf; Cs; Nm;
SIL.
CARPHOLOGY, Picking at bed
clothes, nervous picking:
Nm.
CARRIED Wants to be: Kp.

CARRIES things from one place
to another and back again:
Mp.
CAR-SICKNESS: Fp; Nm; SIL.
Stomach, Felt in without nau-
sea: Kp.
CARTILAGES: Cp; Nm.
Rice Bodies, In: Cf.
CATALEPSY: Nm.
CATARACT: See Lens.
CATHETERISM: MP.
CAUTION: Kp; Sil.
CELIBACY: Kp.
CELLARS, vaulted places
Agg: Ns.
CELLULAR Tissue (cellulitis):
SIL.
Indurated: Sil.
Subacute: Sil.
CENSORIOUS: Cp; Nm; Sil.
CEPHAL-HEMATOMA: Cf; Sil.
CEREBRO-SPINAL axis: Kp;
Nm; Ns; SIL.
Fever (Meningitis): NM; NS.
Tubercular: Sil.
CERVIX (Uterus) Cancer: See
Uterus.
Erosion, of: Sil.
Induration: Sil.
Swollen: Cp; Nm.
CHAGRIN (Mortification):
Ailments, After: NM.
CHANCRE, Hard: Cf; Km; Sil.
CHANGE of position Agg: Sil.
Amel: Ns; Sil.

**Lying Long,** In one, after Agg: Ns.

**Temperature** or weather AGG: Cf; CP; Sil.

Cold to warm: **KS**; NM; NS.

**CHANGING MOODS:** CS; Sil.

**CHEEKS** Alternating: Np.

**Burning,** Glowing: Kp; Sil.

**Eruptions** herpes: Nm.

**Hot,** tooth-ache with: Fp.

**Itching:** Nm; Sil.

**Pain,** Aching: Km; Nm.

Burning: Kp.

Drawing, c' eek bones: Sil.

Sore, bruised: Nm.

Stitching: Sil.

ears to: Np.

Tearing, in: NS.

**Red** Discoloration: NM.

**Suppuration:** Cs.

**Swelling:** Cs; Km; Nm; SIL.

Hard: Cf.

Tooth-ache with: Cf.

**Ulcers:** Nm.

**CHEERFUL** (Gay, Contended, Happy): Cp; Fp; Nm; Np; Ns.

**Afternoon:** Cs.

**Alternating,** ill humour with: Nm.

Sadness with: Km; NM.

**Coition** after: Nm.

**Evening:** Nm.

**Forenoon:** NM; Ns.

**Irritability,** Followed by: Ns.

**Night:** Sil.

**Stools,** After: Ns.

**CHEST & LUNGS: CP; CS; FP; NM; NS; SIL.**

**Right:** Fp; NM; Np; Ns; Sil.

**Left:** CP; **NM;** Np; Ns; Sil.

Lower: KP.

**Sides:** Cp; Cs; Fp; KP; NM; NS; Sil.

**Abscess:** SIL.

**Aching:** CP; Nm; **Np.**

**Air,** open Amel: Nm.

**Alternating,** Rectal symptoms with: Cp; SIL.

**Anxiety,** In: Fp; Kp; KS; Nm; Np.

**Apprehension:** Nm.

**Arms,** Into: Nm.

**Backwards,** Extending: Nm; Sil.

Left: Nm.

**Band,** Around: Sil.

**Bending** Forward Agg: Nm.

**Boring:** Sil.

**Breath** At every Agg: NM.

**Breathing** Deep Agg: Np.

**Burning:** Cp; Cs; Kp; Ks; Np; NS; SIL.

External: Nm.

Throat to: Cp.

**Bursting:** Sil.

**Chilliness,** Left side: Nm.

**Cicatrices,** Suppuration: Sil.

**Clothes,** Sensitive to: Fp.

**Clucking** Sound: Nm.

**Coated** Sensation: **NM.**
**Coldness:** Nm; Np.
**Congestion:** Fp.
  Pregnancy during: NM.
**Constriction,** String tied with as if: Km.
**Constriction,** Tightness: CP; Cs; Fp; Kp; Ks; Mp; **Nm;** Np; **SIL.**
  Band as from: Nm; Sil.
  Cough, drying: MP.
  Exertion Agg: NM.
  Flatulence, from: Sil.
  Lying, while: Nm.
    Amel: CP.
  Spasmodic: Kp; Nm.
  Stretching Agg: Nm.
  Suppressed foot sweat from: **SIL.**
  Vapours of sulphur, as from: Km.
**Consumption:** See Consumption.
**Convulsions:** Ns.
**Costal** Cartilages: Cp.
**Cough,** During Agg: CP; Cs; Fp; Kp; NM; Np; NS; SIL.
  Standing when: Ns.
  When, desiring to: Sil.
**Cracking,** In: Cp.
**Cracking,** On motion: Nm.
**Cutting:** CP; Cs; NM; Np.
**Damp** Weather Agg: **NS;** Sil.
**Day** Only Agg: Cp.
**Dining** After Agg: Np.
**Distension,** Sense of: Sil.

**Dryness:** Nm; Sil.
**Dropsy:** NM; SIL.
**Elbow** to: Sil.
**Emaciation** about clavicles: NM.
**Emphysema:** CP; Nm.
**Emptiness,** Sensation of: Np; Ns.
  Cough, after: NS.
  Eating, after: Ni·
**Empyema: CS; KS;** Ns; **SIL.**
  Pleurisy, after: Sil.
**Eruptions:** Cs; Ks; Np; Ns; SIL.
  Crusts: Ns.
  Eczema: Cs; Ks.
  Pimples: Np.
  Pustules: Ks; SIL.
  Rash: Cs; SIL.
  Spring every, Agg: NS.
  Vesicles: Cs.
**Fluttering:** Cs; KP; **NM;** NS.
  Air, open Amel: **NM; NS.**
  Faintness, after: **NM; NS.**
  Lying, while: **NM.**
  on left side: NM.
**Foreign** Body, sternum behind: Nm.
**Fullness:** FP; Nm; Np.¹
  Evening, in bed: NS.
  Gurgling, rumbling in or right side of: Nm.
**Gangrene:** Sil.
**Gnawing:** Cp; Nm.
**Grasped** By hand as if sternum: Sil.

Hard, As if: Fp.
Heavy Load on: NS.
Hepatization: Cs; Km; Kp; Ks.
Hold, Must: Ns.
Inflammation (Pneumonitis): FP; KP; KM; KS; NM; NS; SIL.
Left: NS.
lower lobe: NS.
Aged persons in: FP; NS.
Neglected, lingering: SIL.
Results of: Cs.
Stage, consolidation of: Km.
resolution, of: Cs; Ks; Sil delayed: Ks; Ns.
Sycotic: NS.
Inspiration Agg: Cp; Cs; FP; Kp; NM; Ns; SIL.
Instrument, Passed through sternum as if: Cp.
Intercostal muscles, drawn in: Np.
'ntercostal Region: Fp; Mp; Nm; Sil.
Itching: Cp; Kp; Ks; Nm; Sil.
Jerking Pain: Cp.
Jerks: Sil.
Lifting Agg: Nm.
Lower Ribs: Sil.
Border of: Ns.
Lump, Sensation of: KM; Np.
Sternum, Under: Sil.
Motion Agg: KP; Nm.
Murmurs: NM.
Narrow as if too: Nm.

Oedema (Lungs): KP; NM.
Operation for fistula, after: Cp; Sil.
Oppression: Cs; Fp; KM; Kp; Ks; NM; NS; SIL.
Air, open Amel: NM.
Coughing, when: SIL.
Damp weather, in: Ns.
Deep breath desire to take: Mp.
Erect, after rising or sitting bent: Nm.
Fever, during: Nm.
Lying Amel: NS.
Morning: NS, Sil.
toward: Sil.
Motion Agg: Nm.
Palpitation, with: Km.
Respiration, on: Nm.
Sitting, when: NS.
Sneezing on: Sil.
Sunset, after: NS.
Walking on: NS.
while: Sil.
Warm room: Nm.
Orgasm of blood, heat flushes: Nm; SIL.
Pain: CP; CS; Fp; Kp; Ks; MP; Nm; Np; SIL.
Paralysis of diaphragm: Sil.
Paralysis of lungs: Fp; KS.
Perspiration: Sil.
Places Hand to head, Amel: Nm; Ns.
Pleurisy: FP; KM; KS; Kp; Nm; Ns; Sil.

Pneumonia: See Inflammation.
Pressing pain: Cp; Km; NM; NP; NS; SIL.
Pressure Agg: NM; Np. Amel: Nm; Ns.
Upwards: Nm.
Phthisis: See Consumption.
Pulsation: CP; Kp; SIL.
Quaking: Ns.
Quivering: Cp.
Rattling (See Respiration): Sil. Coarse: KS. Expectoration without: KS.
Rawness, Soreness: Cp; Cs; Fp; Km; Ks; Mp; NM; Np; Ns; SIL.
Respiration Agg: Cp; Km; KP; NM; Ns.
Deep: CP; Fp; NM; Np; Sil.
Rising on: Ns.
Sitting after: Sil.
Sensitiveness: Nm.
Sitting Upright Amel: NS.
Sneezing Agg: Sil.
Spasms: Fp; Kp; NS.
Spots, Blotches: Ns. Red: SIL.
Stabbing: Nm.
Standing Agg: Nm; NS.
Sternum: See Sternum.
Stinging: Nm.
Stitching: CP; Cs; Fp; Km; KP; KS; NM; Np; NS; SIL.

Stool, Before Agg: Cs.
Stooping Agg: Ns.
Swallowing Agg: CP.
Swelling: Sil. Ribs of, towards sternum: Ns.
Talking, While Agg: NM.
Tearing: KP; Mp; Nm; Sil. Inwards: Nm.
Thrusting: Nm.
Tight feeling: Nm; Sil.
Trembling: Cp; Np.
Tumours, (Intercostal muscles): Sil.
Twitching, muscles: Nm.
Walking while, Agg: Nm.
Warm room Agg: Nm; Sil.
Warmth, Sensation: Nm.
Weakness: Cs; Kp; Ks; Nm; Ns; Sil. Holding with both hands Amel: Ns. Sun, in: Nm. Walking in open air: Nm.
Yawning, Agg: Ns.
CHEWING (Biting) AGG: NM; SIL.
Motions: Nm.
CHICKEN POX: FP; Km; Nm; Ns; Sil.
CHILBLAINS: Fp; Km; Kp; Sil.
CHILDBED: See Pregnancy.
CHILDISH Foolish: Sil.
CHILDREN infants: CP; SIL. Afraid, Everything, of: CS; Kp; NM; Sil.

**Breath,** loses, angry when: Cp.

**Crawl** Nervously: Sil.

**Dragged,** Mother's arms on: Sil.

**Fontanelles,** Open: **CP; SIL.**

Re-opening of: CP.

**Lifting** Agg: Cp.

**Pale,** Running on: Sil.

**Scream** and cry always: CP.

**Suckling:** Cp.

**Talk,** Late: Cp; NM.

**Walk,** Late: Cp; SIL.

**CHILL:** Fp; Km; Kp; KS; MP; **NM;** Np; Ns; SIL.

**Affected** Part of: SIL.

**Air Open** Agg: Cp; Kp; Nm; SIL.

Cold or going into: Np; SIL.

Least draught of: CP; SIL.

Walking in: SIL.

Air Open Amel: Nm.

**Annual:** NM.

**Anticipating: NM.**

Every other day: Nm.

hour: Nm.

**Apyrexia,** During: Nm; Sil.

**Ascending:** CP; Ns.

**Autumnal: NM.**

**Bathing** Agg: Cs.

**Bearing** down, with: Sil.

**Bed** in, Agg: KP; Nm; Np; NS; **SIL.**

Putting hand out of: SIL.

Rising from: SIL.

Turning over in: Nm; Sil.

**Bed,** In Amel: NS.

**Begins** Back in: NM.

Body, right side: Nm.

Feet: Cs; **NM.**

Fingers and toes: **NM.**

Hands and feet: **NM.**

Head: Nm.

**Blue** Lips, nails with: Nm.

**Coition,** After: Nm.

**Cold** Air, Blowing around waist, as if: Sil.

Water dashed over, as if: Nm.

**Covers,** Agg: Cs.

**Creeping:** Cp; NM.

**Deficient,** Animal heat, with: Cp; SIL.

**Dinner** After Agg: Mp.

**Drinking** Agg: Cs; Nm; **SIL.**

Amel: SIL.

**Eating,** After: CS; KP; Nm; Np; Sil.

While: Sil.

**Emotions** From: Sil.

**Epileptic** Attacks, after: Sil.

**Evening** and Night: Mp.

**Exertion** Agg: Ks; Sil.

Mental: NM.

**Exposure,** After: Nm; NS.

Draught to, heated when: Sil.

Getting wet from: NS; Sil.

Living on water courses: NM; NS.

Malarial influence: NM; **NS.**

Rains during: Ns.

Sea-shore, residing at: NM; NS.

Sleeping in damp room: NS.

Soil, freshly turned up: NM.

Swamps: NM; **NS.**

Tropical Countries: NM; **NS.**

**External:** KP; Nm; Ns; Sil.

Hair, standing on end as if: SIL.

Spots in: Sil.

**Fright** From: Sil.

**Grasping** Cold object, Agg: Nm; SIL.

**Headache** During: **SIL.**

**Heated,** Overheated, during: Nm; Ns; **SIL.**

**Internal:** Kp; NM; Np; NS; SIL.

**Lying** Amel: Nm; Sil.

**Menses,** After Agg: Nm.

Before Agg: Nm; **SIL.**

During Agg: Nm; Np; NS; **SIL.**

**Mingled** With heat, then heat no sweat: Ks.

**Motion** During: NM; **SIL.**

**Motion** Amel: Sil.

**Nervousness** With: Nm.

**One sided:** Kp; NM; Np; SIL.

Left, before epilepsy: SIL.

Right: NM.

**Pain,** with: Cp; Nm; Sil.

**Pain** in limbs, bones soreness: Nm.

**Pains** During Agg: Cp; KP; Nm; Ns; Sil.

**Periodicity,** Regular and distinct: FP; NS.

**Perspiration** with and after: Nm.

**Quartan:** Nm.

**Quotidian:** Ks; **NM;** NS.

**Rising** after Agg: Cp; NS.

From bed Agg: Nm.

**Shaking,** Shivering, rigors: Cp; Cs; Fp; Ks; **NM;** Np; NS; SIL.

Hair standing on end with: Sil.

**Sleep,** After: Sil.

During: NM; Sil.

**Stool,** After: Mp.

Before: Nm.

During: Nm; SIL.

**Stretching,** With: Fp; NS.

**Suffocative** Feeling with: Mp.

**Summer:** Nm.

**Sun,** In: Nm.

**Tertian:** NM.

**Thirst,** With: NM.

**Thirstlessness:** NM.

**Touch** Agg: SIL.

**Trembling,** with: Sil.

**Uncovering,** Undressing Agg: Nm; **SIL.**

Amel: Cs.

**Urination,** After: Nm.

**Violent,** Delirium with: **NM.**

Unconsciousness with: **NM.**

**Vomiting,** Billious, with: Nm.

**Warmth,** Desire for, which does not relieve: Mp; NM; Sil.

**Warmth** of room or stove Agg: NM; SIL.
**Warmth** external Amel: Sil.
**Warm** Room Amel: Sil.
Stove Amel: Km.
**Warm** Weather Agg: Nm.
**Waves** In, along spine: MP.
**Wrapping** Amel, followed by severe fever and sweat: Sil.
**Yawning,** Sleepiness, accelerated breathing: Nm.
Stretching Amel: Ns.
**CHILLED from exposure to cold Agg: CP; KP; SIL.**
**While sweating,** or hot **Agg:** Fp; Ks; **SIL.**
**CHIN:** Sil.
  **Eruptions:** Fp; **NM;** Np; Ns; Sil.
  Blood boils: Sil.
  Burning, touching on: Ns.
  Crusty, scaly: Sil.
  Herpetic: NM; SIL.
  Itching: Nm.
  Pimples: Ns; Sil.
  Vesicles: NM; NS.
  **Heat:** Nm.
  **Itching:** Nm.
  **Red,** discolouration: Nm.
  **Stitching: SIL.**
  **Ulcers:** Nm.
**CHLOASMAE:** Kp.
  **Sun,** Exposure from: Nm.
**CHLOROFORM** Agg: Km; NM; Sil.

**CHLOROSIS: CP;** Fp; Kp; Ks; **NM;** Np.
**CHOKING:** Mp; Sil.
**CHOLELITHIASIS** (Gall Bladder stone): Mp; NS.
**CHOLERA:** KP; NM; Np.
**CHORDEE:** Cp; Km; Kp; Nm; Np; SIL.
  **Urethra,** Burning in, with: Cp.
**CHOREA:** Cp; Kp; MP; NM; Ns; SIL.
  **After-noon** Agg: **NS.**
  **Attacks** last for few minutes: Nm.
  Several times a day for several days: Nm.
  **Emotions,** From: Mp.
  **Facial:** Nm.
  **Fright,** From: Nm.
  **Jump** High: Nm.
  **One- sided:** Ns.
  Right: Ns.
  **Periodic:** NS.
  **Run** or **jump** must, cannot walk: Nm.
  **Scrofulous,** Tubercular: CP.
  **Stools** at Agg: Mp.
**CHOROID Inflammation: SIL.**
  Suppurative, iris with:
  Retina with: Km.
**CHRONICITY:** Ns; Sil.
  **To begin treatment:** Cp.
**CICATRICES:** Cf; Sil.
  **Break open:** Cp; NM; **SIL.**
  **Depressed:** Sil.

Nodular: Sil.
Painful: NM; **SIL.**
Red become: Nm; Sil.
Shining: Sil.
Sore become: **SIL.**
Stinging: SIL.
Ulcerate: Cp.
CIRCULATION: See Blood.
CLAIRVOYANCE: Sil.
CLAUSTROPHOBIA: Ns.
CLAVICLE: Cp; Nm.
 Below: Cp.
 Caries: Sil.
 Emaciation, About: Nm.
 Throat muscles to: Nm.
 Ulcers: CP.
 Wrists to: CP.
CLAVUS: See Plug.
CLERGYMAN'S sore throat: NM; **SIL.**
CLIMAXIS: Fp; Nm.
CLITORIS Erection, Urination after, sexual desire with: CP.
CLOTHING Disturbs, Cannot bear tight clothing: Cf; Cp; Fp; Nm; NS.
 Tight Amel: Nm.
CLOUDY weather Agg: Ns.
CLUMSINESS: NM; SIL.
CLUTCHING sensation: Nm; SIL.
COATED or furred as if: Nm.
COBWEB: Cp.

COCCYX: SIL.
 Eruptions, Scabs: SIL.
 Injuries: SIL.
 Pain, Aching: Cp; FP; NP; Sil.
 Bent back as if: Mp.
 Pressing: Cp.
 Sore, bruised: Nm; **SIL.**
 sitting, when: **SIL.**
 Stitching, shooting: Cp; Nm; **SIL.**
 startling: Cp.
 stinging: Sil.
 Tearing: CP; Ns; SIL.
 See back for Agg and Amel.
COITION Aversion To (females): Fp; Kp; Ks; **NM.**
 (Males): Nm.
 Enjoyment Absent: Nm.
 Extreme aversion (males): Nm.
 Menses after, aversion: Nm.
 Nauseating (females): Sil.
 Orgasm Painful during: Nm.
 Painful (females): Fp; NM.
 Prostration, followed, by (males): KP.
 Pollution and increased desire followed by (males): Nm.
COITION AGG: Kp; NM; Np; Sil.
COLD, frigid: Nm.
COLD AGG (Easily chilled, lack of vital heat): **CF; CP; Cs; KM; KP; MP; NM; NP; SIL.**

**Air:** CP; Fp; Km; Kp; **MP;** Nm; NP; **SIL.**
**Becoming:** CP; Fp; Km; Kp; Ks; MP; Nm; Np; **SIL.**
**Feet:** Mp; **SIL.**
**Parts** of the body, hands, head etc: **SIL.**
While sweating or hot: Fp; Ks; **SIL.**
**Damp** Weather: **SIL.**
**Dry** Weather: SIL.
**Heat,** and: NM; SIL.
**Place,** Entering a: Cp; Kp; **SIL.**
**Sitting** Or lying on ground: Sil.
**Wet** Weather: Cp; Cs; Km; Kp; **NS; SIL.**
**COLD** AMEL (feels too hot): Km; Ks; **NM; NS;** Sil.
**COLD Tendency** to take: **CP;** Cs; Fp; **KP;** Ks; **NM;** Np; **SIL.**
**Foot** through: SIL.
**Menses,** First Agg: Cp.
**COLDNESS:** Cp; Fp; Km; Kp; Ks; Nm; Np; **SIL.**
**Affected** Parts of: SIL.
**Bearing** Down with: Sil.
**Bed** in: Sil.
**Covers** Agg: Cs.
**Exertion** From: Sil.
**Extremities** of: Sil.
**Icy:** NM; **SIL.**
**Internal:** Nm; **SIL.**
**Left** side: SIL.
Before epilepsy: SIL.

**Menses** Before and during: SIL.
**One-Side:** Kp.
Convulsions during: Sil.
**Partial** or single parts: Nm; Sil.
**Spots** in: CP.
**COLDS:** See Coryza.
**Taking Agg: MP;** Nm; **SIL.**
Menses, first during: Cp.
**COLIC:** See Pain under abdomen.
**Biliary: NS.**
**Lead:** Ns.
**Renal:** Cp; Fp; Km; Kp; NM; Ns.
**COLITIS Mucous:** Kp.
**COLLAPSE,** (Rapid, Sudden prostration): Cp; Fp; **KP;** NP.
**Coition,** after: **KP; NP.**
**Diarrhea,** After: KP.
**Heart** of: Cf.
**Vomiting** After: Ns.
**COLLAR** (Pressure of clothes around neck): Cp; Nm; Ns.
**COLOURS Bright** AGG: Sil.
**COMA:** See Unconsciousness.
**COMPANY**
**Agg:** NM.
**Amel:** Fp; NM.
**Alone,** While, Agg: Kp; Sil.
**Aversion** To: CP; Cs; Fp; Kp; Ks; **NM;** Np.
Strangers to, urination during: **NM.**
**Desire,** For: Cp; **KP.**

**COMPLAINING** (See Lamenting): Sil.

**COMPREHENSION, Difficult:** See Dull.

**CONCENTRATION, Difficult:** Fp; Kp; NM; Np; SIL.

**Learns** with difficulty: Cp; Mp; Nm.

**CONCEPTION Difficult:** FP; NM; Np; SIL.

**Acrid,** secretion from vagina due to: Np.

Copious menses, from: NM.

**Easy:** Nm.

**CONCUSSION:** Fp; Kp; NS.

**CONDYLES:** See Under Bones.

**CONDYLOMATA: NS.**

**Anus,** Of: Km; Ns.

**Male** sexual organs: **NS.**

**Penis:** NS.

**Scrotum:** Ns.

**Vulva** and labia: **NS.**

Soft, red and fleshy: **NS.**

**CONFIDENCE, want** of self: Ks; Nm; SIL.

**CONFUSION** (Bewildered, Incoherence): CP; Cs; Fp; Kp; Ks; **NM;** Np; Ns; SIL.

**Calculating,** When: Nm.

**Cold Bath** Amel: CP.

**Concentrate** the mind, on attempting to: Nm.

**Conversation,** Agg: SIL.

**Hat,** Putting on Agg: Cp.

**Injury** to head after: **NS.**

**Intoxicated,** As after being: Nm.

As if: SIL.

**Know** Does not what he ought to say: Nm.

**Morning:** Cs; Ks.

Waking on: Cs; SIL.

**Motion,** From: Cp.

Amel: Fp.

**Night:** Sil.

**Stools** Amel: Ns.

**Washing** the face Amel: Cp; Fp.

**CONGESTION** Of Blood: Fp; **NM;** Ns; **SIL.**

**Brain,** Of: See under Brain.

**CONJUNCTIVA:** CS; Km; Nm.

**Discharge** (Mucus): **CS;** Fp; Kp; Ks; NM; Ns; SIL.

Bloody: Nm; Sil.

Clear: Km.

Creamy, profuse: Cs; NP; Ns.

Evening: Kp.

Morning: Sil.

Thick: SIL.

Yellow: CS; Ks; **SIL.**

Yellowish green, purulent: Km.

**Inflamed** (Conjunctivitis): **CP; CS;** FP; Km; Kp; Np; NS.

Granular: Nm; Np; Ns; SIL.

Neonatorum: Cs; Ks.

Phlyctenular: Sil.

Sympathetic: Sil.

Trachomatous: Km.

**Injected,** full of dark vessels: CP; Kp; Ks; **NM; SIL.**

**Pannus:** Sil.

**Swollen,** Dermoid: NM.

**Yellow:** Fp; Np; NS.

**CONSOLATION** Agg: Ks; NM; SIL.

**CONSTIPATION** Agg: Nm; **SIL.** Amel: Nm.

**CONSTIPATION:** Cf; CP; CS; Fp; Km; Kp; KS; **NM;** Np; Ns; **SIL.**

**Alternate** Days, on: · **NM.**

**Children,** Infants, in: Cp; Mp; Sil.

**Constant** Desire: Np; Sil.

**Consumption,** During: Cs.

**Diarrhea,** Alternating with: Ns.

**Feces,** Hard, From: Mp; **NM; SIL.**

**Habitual:** Cs; Fp; Ks; **NM;** Np; Sil.

**Haemorrhoidal:** Nm.

**Hectic** fever, in: Cs.

**Inactivity** from, difficult stools: Nm; Sil.

**Liver** symptoms with: NS.

**Menses** before: Nm; Ns; Sil. During: Ks; **NM;** NS; SIL.

**Obstinate:** Ks; NP.

**Old** people, in: CP.

**Painful:** Nm.

**Pregnancy,** During: **NS.**

**Rheumatic** subject, with flatulence and indigestion: MP.

**Spinal** Affections,· with: Sil.

**Stool,** Difficult though soft: Sil.

Recedes: SIL.

menses During: Sil.

Removed must be: NM; Sil.

**Strain** Must: Sil.

**Travelling** When: Sil.

**Unsatisfactory,** Insufficient stools from: Nm.

**Urging,** Abortive: NM; Sil.

Coition, after: Np.

Irresistible: Np; Sil.

Passes flatus only: NS.

**With** no desire: Kp.

**Women:** NM; Sil.

**CONSTRICTION, band,** etc: CP; MP; Nm; Sil.

**Internally:** MP; **NM;** Sil.

**Bones** of: SIL.

**Orifices,** Of: Cs; Km; Nm; SIL.

**Stomach,** of: Cs; Km; Nm; Kp; Ks; Nm; Sil.

Convulsive: Nm.

**CONSUMPTION, Tuberculosis:** CP; CS; Km; Kp; **KS;** NM; **SIL.**

**Acute: FP;** Nm; **SIL.**

**Fever, In:** Fp.

**Florida:** Fp; Np.

**Incipient: CP;** Fp; KP; NS; **SIL.**

**Old** People, in: Ns.

**Pitutious: FP;** NS; SIL.

**Purulent** and Ulcerative: Kp; Nm; SIL.

**Relapsing:** Fp.

Stone cutters: SIL.
Sycotic: FP; NS; SIL.
CONTEMPT, Scorn: Nm.
Ailments, from: NM.
CONTINENCE Agg: Kp.
CONTORTIONS, Distortions: Sil.
CONTRACTIONS General Sense of: Km; NM.
Muscles of, Congenital: Nm.
Strictures, Stenosis: Nm.
CONTRADICT Disposition, to: Nm; Sil.
CONTRADICTION, Has to re-strain himself, to keep from violence: Sil.
Intolerant of: Cp; SIL.
CONTRADICTORY and alternating states: NM.
CONTROL LACKS: Cp; KP.
CONVALESCENCE: CP; KP; Nm.
CONVERSATION AGG: NM; Sil.
CONVULSIONS: Km; MP; NM; Ns; SIL.
Left-sided: CP; Nm.
One sided: CP.
Children, In: CP; KP; MP; SIL.
Dentition during: Mp.
fever with: Cp.
Clonic: CP; Km; MP; NM; SIL.
Consciousness with: NM; Sil.
without: CS; Nm; Sil.
Diarrhea, After: Mp.
Dysmenorrhea with: Nm.

Emissions, During: NP.
Epileptic: See Epilepsy.
Epileptiform: Cs; Km; Ks; NM; SIL.
Exertion, after: Nm.
Falling, with: CP; SIL.
forward: Sil.
Fever With: Fp.
Without: MP.
Grief, After: Nm.
Hysterical: Cs; Kp; NM.
Injuries, From: NS.
Menses, During: NM.
Suppressed from: CP.
Morning: Cp; Mp.
Night: Sil.
Sleep, during: SIL.
Odours, strong from: Sil.
Onanism, After: Sil.
Periodic: Nm.
Every seventh day: Nm.
Pregnancy During, Puerperal: Mp; Nm.
Sleep, during: SIL.
Sleeplessness And: Sil.
Suppressed Foot-sweat, after: SIL.
Tetanic Rigidity: MP.
Tonic: Mp; Nm; Sil.
Twitching Of arms and legs preceded by: Nm.
Uremic: KS.
Vaccination, After: Km; SIL.
Warm Bath Agg: Nm.
Worms, From: Sil.

**CO-ORDINATION** disturbed: Kp; SIL.
**CORNEA Abscess:** Cs; Fp; Km; Ks; Sil.
**Ectasia:** Cp.
**Fistula:** Sil.
**Inflammation** Keratitis: Cp; Km.
Herpetic, vesicular: Cp.
Parenchymatous, Syphilitic: Cp; Km.
Phlyctenular: Cf; Cp.
**Opacity:** Cf; Cp; Ks; SIL.
Right: Sil.
Small-pox vaccination after: Sil.
Spots in: Cf.
**Painful:** SIL.
**Pustules:** Km.
**Rough:** Sil.
**Smoky:** Sil.
**Spots** or specks, on: CF; CP; Km; Ks; NM; Ns; Sil.
Dark: Mp.
Scar like: Sil.
White: Nm.
**Staphyloma:** Sil.
**Thickening:** Sil.
Mass of hypertrophied tissue, as if: Sil.
**Ulcers:** Cf; CP; CS; KM; Ks; NM; SIL.
Deep: Cp; Cs; Nm; Sil.
Flat: Km.
Indolent: Sil.
Scars, from: Sil.
Vascular: Sil.

**Vesicles:** Km; NM.
**CORNS:** Cs; NM; SIL.
**Aching:** Sil.
**Boring:** NM; SIL.
**Burning:** Cs; NM; Sil.
**Inflamed:** SIL.
**Painful:** Cs; Nm; Sil.
**Pressing:** Cs; Sil.
**Pulsating:** Sil.
**Shooting:** NM.
**Soft:** SIL.
**Stinging:** CS; NM; Np; SIL.
**Tearing:** Cs; SIL.
**Tender:** NS; Sil.
**CORPULENCE:** See Obesity.
**CORRODING:** See Secretions Acrid.
**CORYZA:** Cf; CP; CS; FP; Kp; KS; NM; Np; NS; SIL.
**Left:** Ks.
**Right:** Cs.
After a bath: Cs.
**Aching** in limbs with: Nm.
**Air** Open, in Agg: Cp; Cs.
Amel: Cs.
**Asthmatic** Breathing with: NS; Sil.
**Bloody,** infants in: Cs.
**Chest,** Bursting pain with: Sil.
**Chilliness** With: Cp; Sil.
**Chronic:** Cp; Nm; SIL.
Asthma, causing: Sil.
Dry: NM; SIL.
**Cold** Bathing Amel: Cs.
**Cold** Room, Agg: CP.

**Cough,** With: FP; Km; NM; Sil.
**Drinks,** Warm Agg: Fp.
**Epistaxis** With: Sil.
Infants, in: Cs.
**Fluent,** Indoors: Cp.
Dry and alternately: Nm.
**Frontal** Sinus, to: Cp; **SIL.**
**Hay Fever,** Annual: Kp; Nm; Sil.
**Indoors,** Agg: Cs.
**Inflammation** of Larynx with: CP; Cs; Fp; Nm.
**Mercury,** Abuse of: Km.
**Nervous:** Kp; Sil.
**Night:** Ns.
**Over-Heated,** From becoming: Sil.
**Periodical:** Nm; Sil.
Weekly: KS.
**Perspiration,** After Amel: Nm.
**Recurrent:** Sil.
Easily: **SIL.**
**Salivation,** With: **CP.**
**Sore** throat, with: CP.
**Suppressed:** NM; Ns; SIL.
**Taste,** Loss of with: **NM.**
**Uncovering** the Head, from: NM.
**Unilateral:** Nm.
**Urging** to cough, with, in throat: Sil.
**Violent** Attacks: Sil.
**Warm,** Room Amel: Cp.
**Washing,** Cold water, with Amel: Cs.

**COUGH:** Cf; CP; CS; FP; Km; Kp; **KS;** MP; NM; Np; **NS; SIL.**
**Abdomen** or Epigastrium, from: KM; Nm.
**Air,** Cold, Agg: Fp; Kp; Ns; SIL.
Damp, cold: Sil.
Hot: Ks.
Open: Fp; Sil.
**Air,** Cold Amel: CS; Ks; Mp.
Open: Cs; KS; **MP;** NS.
**Anger,** From: NM.
**Asthmatic:** Cs; FP; Kp; Nm; SIL.
**Auditory** Canal touching, Agg: Sil.
**Barking:** Km.
**Bathing** Agg: Cf; CS.
**Bed** in, or becoming warm: Nm.
**Bending** Head backwards Agg: SIL.
Downwards: FP.
**Brain** complaints in: Kp.
**Breathing** Agg: **NM;** Ns.
Deep: Fp; Kp; Nm; Sil.
**Bouts:** See Paroxysms.
**Cervical** Glands, pain with: Nm.
**Chill,** During Agg: Cp; Kp; Np; Sil.
**Choking:** Mp; Nm.
**Chronic:** Nm; Sil.
**Cold,** Becoming, Agg: CP; **SIL.**

Drinks: SIL.
Food: SIL.
**Constant:** Fp; Nm; Np.
Day and night: Nm.
**Constriction** of Larynx, from: SIL.
Trachea of: Nm.
**Coryza,** With: Km.
**Crawling,** Larynx in: Cp.
**Croupy:** Cf; Cp; CS; KM; Kp; Ks.
Morning: Cs.
Walking, only after: **CS.**
**Crying** Agg: Sil.
**Cutting** Pain in chest, with: Nm.
**Deep:** Sil.
**Day** Only: Km; Ns.
**Dentition,** During: Cp.
**Dinner,** After: Cf; Kp; Sil.
**Drinking** After: Nm; Np; Sil.
Cold things: Cp; Sil.
Hurriedly: Sil.
**Drinks** Cold amel: Ks.
Warm: **SIL.**
**Dry:** Cp; **CS;** FP; Ks; **MP;** NM; Np; Ns; SIL.
Day and night: NM.
Evening: Nm; Np.
loose, in morning: Nm; SIL.
Morning and evening: Fp.
Night: Cs; Kp; Nm; Ns; SIL.
loose by day: Sil.
Spot in larynx from: Nm.

**Dust,** As from: Cs.
Inhaling Agg: Nm.
**Ears,** Stopped with: Sil.
Ringing Agg: Nm.
**Eating** Agg: Cf; Fp; KP; Ks; Nm; Sil.
After: Km; SIL.
Cold things: Sil.
Hastily: Sil.
**Evening: NM.**
8 p.m. TO 11 p.m.: NM.
9 p.m.: Sil.
Lying down on: Km.
**Excoriative** Soreness in chest with: SIL.
**Exertion** Agg: Nm; SIL.
**Exhausting:** Sil.
**Eye** Symptoms with: Nm.
**Fever** During Agg: Fp; Kp; KS; **NM;** Sil.
Intermittent, after: Nm.
**Filling** Up Sensation as of, in throat, from: Sil.
**Foreign** Body in larynx, as if from: Sil.
**Gagging:** Sil.
**Hacking:** Cf; Cp; Cs; Fp; Kp; Ks; **NM;** Np; SIL.
Evening: Fp.
Morning: Fp.
3 to 4 P.M.: Cf.
**Hair** in trachea or tongue, as if from: SIL.
**Harsh:** Km.
**Head,** Bursting pain in with: Nm.

**Heated,** Or becoming Agg: Sil.

**Hectic** (Chronic phthisical): Cf; Cp; SIL.

**Hernia,** Pain in with: Sil.

**Hoarse:** Cs; Ks; Nm; SIL.

**Holding,** Chest, Amel: NS.

Must with both hands: Nm; Ns.

**Hollow:** Nm; Np; Sil.

**Hot,** Application Amel: Sil.

Abdomen, to: Sil.

**Hypogastrium,** Pain in, with: Sil.

Thrusts in, with: **NM.**

**Inability** to: Ns.

Pain, from: Ns.

To speak with: Mp.

**Influenzal:** Ks.

**Inguinal** Region, pain in, with: Nm; Sil.

**Inspiration** Deep Agg: Fp; Kp; Nm; Sil.

**Irritation** in air passages from: Fp; Ns.

Chest in from: FP; Np.

Epigastrium in from: Nm.

Larynx in, from: Cf; Kp; **NM;** Np; SIL.

Throat pit in, from: Nm; SIL.

Trachea in, from: Kp; **SIL.**

**Lachrymation,** with: Nm; Sil.

**Larynx,** Burning in with: Nm.

Itching in from: Cf; Sil.

Rawness in from: SIL.

Roughness in from: Ns.

Scraping in from: Sil.

Spot, dry, from: NM.

Stitching in from: SIL.

Tickling in from: **CF;** Kp; Ks; **NM.**

Touching on: Fp; Np; Ns; SIL.

**Laughing** Agg: Sil.

**Loose:** Cs; Fp; Km; Kp; Ks; NS; SIL.

But, violent: Ns.

Day, during: Sil.

Expectoration without: KS.

Morning: Km; Nm.

awakening, on: SIL.

worse toward: **SIL.**

**Lower** and Lower, coming from: SIL.

**Lying** Agg: Cf; Cs; Fp; Kp; KS; Mp; Nm; Ns; SIL.

Back on: NM; Ns; Sil.

Bed in: Fp; Ks; **NM;** SIL.

Evening: Km.

Right side: Sil.

**Lying** Amel: CP.

**Manual** labour from: Nm.

**Menses,** During: CP; Nm.

**Mental** Disturbances, Agg: NM.

**Morning** and Evening: Nm; SIL.

6 A.M. to 6 P.M.: Cp.

**Motion** Agg: Nm; Ns; SIL.

Arms of: **NM.**

Chest of: Nm; Sil.

Rapid: **NM.**

**Motion** Amel: Sil.
**Move** On beginning to: Sil.
**Mucus** in chest from: NM.
**New moon:** Sil.
**Night** Agg: Km; Nm; Sil.
3 A.M.: **KM.**
3 to 4 A.M.: **NS.**
Until, 4 A.M.: Sil.
**Nose,** Bleed with: Fp.
Discharge, with: Sil.
**Painful:** Cp; Fp; **NM;** Ns.
**Paroxysmal:** Cf; Fp; KP; Ks; Mp; Nm; Sil.
**Pregnancy,** During: Fp; Nm.
**Pressure** in affected parts with: Sil.
**Racking:** Cs; Km; KP; Ks; Nm; Np; Sil.
**Rattling:** CS; Kp; **KS;** NM; **NS; SIL.**
Hoarseness, without: KS.
**Retching:** Fp; Ks; Mp; Nm; Sil.
**Retiring** after: SIL.
**Rising on:** Cs; Fp; Ns.
Bed from: Cs; Fp; Ns.
**Room,** in: Nm.
Entering, open air, from: NM.
Warm: KS; Mp.
**Rough:** Sil.
**Running** Agg: Sil.
**Saliva** Accumulation, with: Nm.
**Scapula,** Stitches in with: Sil.
**Scraping:** Sil.
**Shaking:** SIL.

**Sharp:** Cs.
**Short:** Cs; Fp; Km; KP; NM; KP.
**Singing** Agg: Fp; Sil.
**Sit up** Must: Ns.
**Sitting** Agg: Np; Ns.
Erect: Nm.
**Sleep,** during Agg: Sil.
Day-time: Fp.
**Sneezing,** Before: Nm.
With: Nm; Sil.
**Snoring with:** NM.
**Spasmodic:** Cp; Cs; Fp; Km; Kp; MP; NM; SIL.
**Standing** Agg: Nm; NS.
Erect while: Nm.
**Sternum,** Pain at, with: Sil.
**Stooping** Agg: Sil.
**Sudden:** Kp; Mp.
**Suffocating:** Ks; MP; NM; SIL.
Children, In lying down, Amel: Cp.
Lifting up from craddle Agg: Cp.
**Swallowing** Agg: NM.
Empty: NM.
**Sweat,** After: Sil.
**Sympathetic,** Reflex: Kp.
**Talking** Agg: CS; Fp; Mp; Nm; SIL.
**Temperature,** Change of: Sil.
**Throat,** Dryness with: Cp.
Sore: Cp.
**Thunderstorm:** Sil.

**Tickling:** Cp; Fp; Kp; Ks; NM; Np; Sil.
Chest, to: Sil.
**Tight:** Cs; MP.
**Tormenting:** Fp; NM.
**Uncovering:** Sil.
Feet or head: **SIL.**
Hands: Sil.
**Violent:** Km; MP; Np; SIL.
**Vomiting, With:** Fp; Nm.
Viscid mucus, with: Sil.
**Waking,** From sleep: SIL.
**Waking,** On: Fp; Sil.
**Walking,** From: Nm.
Fast: Nm; Sil.
**Weather,** Change of: See Temperature.
Damp: NS; Sil.
Stormy: Sil.
**Wet** Getting: CS.
**Whistling:** Kp.
**Whooping** (pertussis): CP; Fp; KM; KP; **KS;** MP; NM; SIL.
Body, stiff, rigid, cyanosis with: Mp.
Flow of tears,with: Nm.
Obstinate: Cp.
**Winter** Agg: Km; Nm.
**Yawning,** Agg: Ns.
**Yawning** and Consecutively: NM.
**COUGHING** AGG: **NM;** Sil.
**COUNTS,** Continuously: Sil.
**COVERS** AGG: Ks.
Amel: Sil.

**COWARDICE:** Cs; Kp; Nm; SIL.
**COWPERITIS:** Sil.
**COXALGIA:** See Pain in Hip joint.
**CRACKING** in joints: KS; KM; Np; NS.
**CRACKS, Fissures** Chaps (See also Skin): Cf; SIL.
**CRAMP:** See Pain Crampy.
Writer's: MP.
**CRASH** (Blows): NM; Sil.
**CRAVINGS:** See also Desires.
**Beer:** Np.
**Bacon:** Cp.
**Bitter** things: Nm.
**Coarse,** Raw food: Cp.
**Cold** Things: Ns.
**Condiments:** Cp.
**Eggs:** Np.
**Farinacious** Food: NM.
**Fats,** fatty things: Cp.
**Fish:** Nm.
Fried: Np.
**Green** Things: Cs.
**Ice-cream:** Sil.
Water: Sil.
**Indigestible** Things: Cp.
**Lime,** Chalks, clay: **SIL.**
**Pregnancy,** During: Cp.
**Salty** Things: **NM.**
**Sand:** Sil.
**Sweet** things: KP.
**Tobacco** Smoking: Cp.
**Vinegar:** Kp.
**CRAWLING:** See Formication.
**CRAZY:** See Insanity.

CREEPING, Running as of a mouse, etc.: Sil.
CREPITATION synovial: Np.
CRETINISM: CP.
CRIES, Shrieks Screams: Mp.
Anger From: Kp.
Convulsions Before: Sil.
Kindly Spoken to when: Sil.
Pain, with: Mp.
Sleep, During: Cp; Nm; Sil.
CRITICAL, Exacting: Sil.
CROSSNESS (See Anger): Cp; NM; SIL.
CROUP: KS.
CROWD: See Company.
Fear of: Fp; Kp; NM; Ns.
Room in Agg: Ks.
CRUELTY: Kp; Sil.
CRUMBLING of Bones: Cp; SIL.
CRUSHING: See Pain Squeezing.
CRUSTA LACTEA: Cs; Km; Sil.
CRUSTS Scabs: CS; KM; Kp; Ks; NM; Np; SIL.
Moist: KS; SIL.
Suppurating: Sil.
Yellow: Cs; Np.
CURSING: Nm.
CURVATURE: See Bones, Spine.
CUTTING: See under Pain.
CYANOSIS: Nm; Sil.
CYSTITIS: See Bladder Inflamed.

CYSTS: SIL.
Eye-lids: Fp.
Ovarian: Ns.
DAMP COLD Agg: CP; CS; Km; Kp; Nm; NS; SIL.
DAMPNESS Agg: Cp; Mp; NS; SIL.
Damp Dwelling, Being in: Km; NS; Sil.
Washing With water: MP; NS; Sil.
Water, Use of, in any form: Ns.
Weather: Cf; SIL.
Warm wet: NS; SIL.
Wet: CP; CS; MP; NS; SIL.
Wet Applications: Sil.
Getting: Cp; Cs; KM.
drenched: NM; NS.
feet: NM; SIL.
DANCING: Nm.
Agg: NM.
Amel: Nm; SIL.
DANDRUFF: CS; KM; Kp; KS; Mp; NM.
White: Km; NM.
Yellow: KS.
DARK (See Black): Fp; Nm.
DARKNESS Agg: Km; Nm; Sil.
Amel: FP; Kp; NM; Np; NS; SIL.
DARTING Pain: Km; MP.
DAY Alternate on, Agg: NM.
Every seventh (Weekly): Sil.
DAY Blindness: SIL.
Hot, with Cold night Agg:
Time only Agg: NM.

DAZED (Bewildered): NM; SIL.
DEAD LOOK: Fp.
DEAD, Thinks, He is: Nm; Sil.
DEAFNESS: See Hearing Bad.
DEATH Agony: Fp.
Desires: Cs; Km; Kp; NM; NS; SIL.
Must restrain herself to prevent doing injury to herself: NS.
Fear of: Cs; FP; Kp; Ks; Nm.
Near seems: Nm.
Sensation of: Sil.
DEBAUCHERY: Ns.
DEBILITY: See Weakness.
DECOMPOSITION: Kp.
DECUBITUS: See Bed Sores.
DEFIANT: Sil.
DEGENERATION, Fatty: Ks.
Muscles of: Kp.
DEJECTED: See Despair, Sadness.
DELICATE: Cp; Kp; Sil.
DELIRIUM: Fp; Kp; Nm; Sil.
Anxious: Sil.
Convulsions After: Km.
Fantastic: Sil.
Frantic: Sil.
Frightful: SIL.
Hallucinations, with: Sil.
Maniacal: Nm.
Muttering: Nm.
Raging, Raving: Nm.
Sleepiness, With: Cp.
Tremens: Nm.

Very talkative, Being wide awake: Fp; NM.
DELTOID: FP.
DELUSIONS (Imaginations, hallucinations, illusions): Cs; Kp; Nm; SIL.
Auditory, Bells, Music, etc. Ns.
Bed, Lying when, did not touch: Nm.
Sinking, as if: Cp.
Body Divided: Sil.
Criminals, About: Sil.
Dead Persons, Sees: Kp; Nm; Sil.
Die, She would, as if: Sil.
Dogs, Sees: Sil.
Drawing Her to right, something were, when walking: Sil.
Every-One who looks at him, pities him, because of his misfortune: Nm.
Faces, Stopping when: Nm.
Fail, Everything will: Sil.
Figures See: Kp.
Fire, Visions, of: Cp; NM.
Foot-steps, Hears, in next room: Np.
Furniture to be persons, night on waking : Np.
Half left, does not belong to him: Sil.
Head Belongs to another: Ns.
Home, Away from, Must get there: Cp

**House** is full of people: Nm; Sil.

**Images,** phantoms, sees: Cs; Kp; NM; Np; Sil.

Dwells upon: Sil.

Eyes closing on: Sil.

Frightful: Cs; KP; Np; Sil.

Night while trying to sleep: Cs.

Sees all over: SIL.

**Inanimate** objects are persons: Np.

**Injury,** is about to receive: Sil.

**Insane,** that he will become: Nm.

**Journey,** that he is on: Sil.

**Misfortune,** Impending: Kp.

**Movement,** loss of, as if: Mp

**Needles,** Sees: Sil.

**Objects** Appear different: Nm.

**People,** Sees: Nm.

Behind Him: Sil.

**Pins,** about: **SIL.**

**Places,** of being in two at the same time: **SIL.**

**Poor** thinks he is : Cf.

**Pursued** by enemies: Sil.

**Raised up,** he were being: Sil.

**Rocked,** one were being: Nm.

Lying down and closing eyes on: Nm.

**Sick,** Imagine himself: Nm.

That he were going to be: Np.

**Spectres,** Ghosts, spirits, sees: NM; Sil.

**Starve,** He must: Km; Nm.

**Stepping,** on air: Nm.

**Stones,** were sinking under him, when crossing the bridge: Nm.

**Strange,** Familiar things seem: Kp.

**Talking,** Dead people with, fancies herself: Ns.

**Thieves,** Sees: NM; Sil.

Dream, after will not believe the contrary till the search is made: Nm.

House in: NM; Sil.

**Typhoid** fever, that he will have: Np.

**Vermin** sees, crawl about: Sil.

**Visions,** Images: Cs; NM; SIL.

Horrible: Sil.

**Voices,** Hears: Nm.

Dead people of: Nm.

Distant: Nm.

**Water:** Sil.

**Worms** Creeping as if: SIL.

**DEMENTIA:** Cp.

**Epileptic:** SIL.

**Masturbation,** from: Cp.

**Senile:** Cp.

**DENTITION Difficult: CP; SIL.**

**Diarrhea** with: CP; Fp; SIL.

**Slow: CP; SIL.**

**DEPRAVITY** (Moral Perversions):

**DERMOID:** Nm.
**DESCENDING** AGG: Nm; Sil.
**DESIRES:** See also Cravings.
**Abnormal:** Cp.
**Alcoholic Drink:** Cs; Fp; Np.
**Ale:** Fp.
**Bacon:** Cp.
**Beer:** NM; Np; NS.
**Bitter** Food and drinks: Nm.
**Bread:** NM; Sil.
**Claret:** Cs.
**Coarse** or Raw food: CP; Sil.
**Coffee:** Cp; Nm.
**Cold drinks:** Cs; Km; KP; KS; Nm; NP; NS.
Food: Fp; Kp; KS; Nm; NS; SIL.
Icy: NM.
**Eggs:** Np.
Fried: Np.
**Farinaceous food:** CP; NM.
**Fish:** NM; Np.
Fried: Np.
**Fruit:** Cs; Nm.
Acid: CS.
Green: CS.
**Garlic:** Nm.
**Green Things:** Cs.
**Ham:** Cp.
**Ham Rind:** Cp.
**Ice** or **Ice cold water:** KP; NS; Sil.
**Indigestible** things: Cp.
**Indistinct,** Knows not for what: Sil.

**Lime,** Slate clay etc.: NM; SIL.
**Meat:** Cp; Nm.
Salted: **Cp.**
Smoked: CP; Cs.
**Milk:** NM; Sil.
Boiled: Ns.
**Mucilaginous** things: Nm.
**Oysters:** NM.
**Pickles:** Nm.
**Piquant** Things, Condiments: Cp; Nm; NP.
**Pork:** Cp.
**Potatoes:** CP.
**Pregnancy,** During: Cp.
**Preserves:** Sil.
**Pungent** Things: Cs.
**Salty** things: Cp; Cs; **NM.**
Pregnancy, During: Nm.
**Sand:** Sil.
**Smoked** Things: Cp.
**Sour,** Acids: Cs; Fp; Kp; Ks; NM.
Headache, after: Ns.
**Stimulants:** Fp.
**Strange** things: Cp.
**Sweets:** CS; Kp; Ks; Mp; Nm; Sil.
**Tea:** Cs.
**Tobacco** Smoking: Cp.
**Uncooked** Food: Sil.
**Vegetables:** Cs.
Green and sour: Cs.
**Vinegar:** Kp.
**Warm food:** Sil.
Soup: Nm.

**Wine:** Nm.
**DESIRES Activity:** Cp; Ns.
**Coition after:** CP.
**Get** out of bed and run: **Fp.**
**DESIRES death:** See Death
desire.
**DESPAIR hopelessness:** Cs;
NM; Ns; Sil.
**Recovery** of: Cs; Ns; Sil.
**Salvation, Religious: KP;** Nm.
**DESQUAMATION:** Fp; Km; **KS;**
Nm; Np; Sil.
**DESTRUCTIVE:** Ns.
**DETERMINED:** See obstinate,
Stubborn.
**DIABETES, Insipidus:** See
Urine, Copious
**Mellitus:** CP; Km; KP; NM;
NS; SIL.
Boils successive with: Np.
Gouty symptoms with: Ns.
Liver derangement with: Km.
Lung involvement with: Cp.
**DIARRHEA:** CP; Cs; FP; Kp;
KS; **NM; NP; NS; SIL.**
After-noon Agg: Fp.
Aged People: Ns.
Air, Cold in: Ns; Sil.
Currents of Agg: Sil.
Night Agg: Ns.
**Amel:** Ns.
**Anger** After: CP.
**Anxiety** After: SIL.
**Asthma,** Then: Ks.
**Children** in: Cp; **CS;** Nm;
SIL.

Scrofulous: **SIL.**
**Cholera** infantum: Nm; SIL.
**Chronic:** Cp; Fp; Nm; NS;
SIL.
Cider, After: CP.
**Coffee,** After: Nm.
**Cold,** Drinks, or food from:
NS; SIL.
Summer in: NS.
Taking, after: Ns; Sil.
Weather: Ns.
**Cramps** in calves of legs,
with: Kp; Mp.
**Damp,** weather: Ns.
**Day,** Time only: Km; **NM;** Ns.
Night, and: Cp; Sil.
**Dentition,** During: CP; **SIL.**
**Eating,** After: Cs; Fp; Kp; Np;
NS.
While: Kp.
**Emaciated,** People, in: CP;
Nm; **SIL.**
**Eruptions,** Alternating, with:
Cp.
**Excitement,** From: Kp.
**Exertion,** Physical: Ns.
Mental, Amel: Kp.
**Farinaceous** Food: **NM; NS.**
**Fats:** Km; NP.
**Food,** Cold: NS.
**Fright,** emotions: Cp; KP.
**Fruits:** Cp; **NS.**
**Grief:** Cp.
**Gushing:** Nm.
**Hot** weather: Fp; NM; Np; Sil.

Ice cream: Cp; Ns.
Indiscretion In eating, slightest: Nm.
Jaundice during: Np; NS.
Menses, After: Nm.
Before: Ns; Sil.
During: Kp; Ks; NP; Ns; Sil.
Milk, After: Sil.
Boiled: Ns.
Mid night, After 3 a.m. to 11 a.m.: Nm.
Morning: Fp; NS.
Bed, driving out of: Ns; SIL.
Consumption, in: Cp.
Rising after and moving about: NM; NS.
6 a.m.: Kp.
Nervous: Kp.
Night: Fp; Km; KP; MP; Nm; NS; Sil.
Children: Cp; MP; Nm; Sil.
Involuntary: NS.
3 A.M. to 4 A.M.: Km.
Opium after: NM.
Painless: Cs; FP; Kp; Ks; NM; NP; IIS; SIL.
Pastry, After: Km; NS.
Perspiration, Checked: Fp.
Preceded by Pain in groins and hypogastrium: Ns.
Rumbling, gurgling: Nm.
Quinine, After: Nm.
Raising up, after: Ns.
Rich food: NS.
Rising, After: Cp; Ns.
School girls, In: CP.

Scratching Agg: Nm.
Sequelae of: Nm.
Starchy food: Ns.
Stoppage, Suddenly from Agg: Mp.
Sugar Maple, sweets: Cs.
Summer Agg: Fp.
Thin Persons in: Cp; Nm; SIL.
Urination, During: Nm.
Vaccination Agg: Km; Sil.
Vegetables, Agg: NM; NS.
Vexation, From: CP.
Walking, Motion, Agg: NM; NS.
Warmth of bed, wrapping Amel: SIL.
Winter: Ns.
DIGESTION Affected (Indigestion): CS; Fp; Kp; Ks; NM; NP; NS.
Atonic: Kp.
Bread, After: Nm.
Debauchery In general: Nm; Ns.
Every Bite hurts: Cp.
Fatigue, Brain fag, in children: Cf.
Farinaceous Food, from: NM; NS.
Fat, Food, after: Km; Np.
Ice cream: CP.
Meat, After: Np.
Pastry: Km.
Pregnancy, During: Nm.
Wine, Liquors: Ns.

**DIGGING:** See Pain Boring.
**DINNER** Agg: Np.
**Amel:** Ns.
**DIPHTHERIA:** Cp; KM; Kp; NM.
**DIPLOPIA** (Double Vision): Kp.
Mp; **NM.**
**DIPSOMANIA:** Cs; Fp; Kp; Np;
NM.
**DIPTHERIA:** Cp; KM; Kp; NM.
**Croup** with: Km.
**Tonsils,** Extending, to: Kp.
**Trachea,** Involving: Cf.
**Yellow** Membrane: **NP.**
**DIRECTION of symptoms:**
**Alternating** States, Sides etc.
Cp; Fp; Nm.
Contradictory: Nm.
**Appear** on one side go to
other side and there Agg:
Nm.
**Ascending:** Fp; Nm; SIL.
**Backward:** Nm.
**Crosswise,** Across: Nm; Sil.
**Diagonal:** Nm; Sil.
**Downward:** Nm; Sil.
**Forward:** Sil.
**Here** And **There:** MP.
**Increase gradually,** And **De-**
**crease gradually:** Nm.
And decrease suddenly: MP.
With the sun: NM.
**Outward:** Km; Sil.
**Radiating,** Spreading: Mp; Sil.
**Side,** Lain on goes to: Nm; Sil.
Left: Cf; Fp; Ns; SIL.
Right: Cp; Fp; Mp; Sil.

One sided: Kp; Nm; Sil.
Right to left: Cp; Sil.
Left does not belong to her:
Sil.
**Up** And **Down: SIL.**
**DIRTY:** Nm; Sil.
**DISAPPOINTMENT:** Nm.
**DISCHARGES** (Loss of Vital
fluids): See Secretions.
**Agg:** Cp; Kp; Np.
**Amel:** SIL.
**DISCONTENT,** (Displeased, dis-
satisfied): **CP;** Cs; Fp;
Km; Kp; KS; **NM;** SIL.
**Everything** with: Kp; Nm.
**Wants** this and that: Cp.
**DISCORDANT:** See Confusion,
Co-ordination disturbed.
**DISCOURAGED:** Km; Sil.
**DISGUST:** Nm.
**DISLOCATED, Sprained,** As if:
See Sprains.
**Tendency** to: Nm; SIL.
**DISLOCATION Easy:** Cf.
**DISOBEDIENCE:** Sil.
**DISPLEASURE Reserved:** Nm.
**DISSATISFIED:** See Discon-
tent.
**DISTENSION, Feeling** of: Cp;
Mp.
**DISTORTION:** Sil.
**Joints** of: SIL.
**DISTRACTION:** Kp; NM; SIL.
**DISTRUSTFUL:** CP; Kp; NS.
**DIVERSION amel:** Fp; Ns.

**DIZZINESS:** See Vertigo.

**DOMINEERING:**

**DOUBLING Up** Amel: Mp.

**DOUBTING People;** See Suspicious.

**DOWNWARD:** Cp; Nm.

**DRAFT Agg:** Cp. (See also wind).

**DRAGGING, sensation:** Nm; Ns.

**DRAWING up:** Nm.

**DRAWN back:** Nm; Sil.

**Together:** Nm.

**DREAMINESS, Revery, ecstasy:** Nm; Sil.

**DREAMS:** NM; SIL.

**Accidents:** Ns.

**Agreeable:** See Pleasant.

**Amorous:** Cp; Km; Kp; Nm; Np; Sil.

**Animals** of: Sil.

**Anxious:** Cp; Cs; FP; KM; KS; **NM;** Np; NS; **SIL.**

Asleep, on falling: Nm.

Menses, during: Nm.

**Assassins:** Sil.

**Awake,** While: SIL.

**Battles:** Sil.

**Blood,** of: See Fire.

**Business:** Nm; Sil.

Neglected: Sil.

Day, of the: Cf; Sil.

**Carousing:** Nm; Sil.

**Cats:** Cp.

**Choking** Her, something: Sil.

**Confused:** Cf; Fp; Nm; Sil.

**Continued,** After waking: Nm.

**Crimes:** Nm; Ns.

That he had committed: NS.

**Cruelty:** Nm; Sil.

**Cutting:** Cf.

Woman of, for salting: Cf.

**Danger:** Cf; Cp.

**Day's** work, Difficulties: Cf.

**Dead,** of the: Cf; Sil.

Bodies: Np.

**Death** of: Cf; Km; KS; Nm; SIL.

Approaching: Sil.

Relatives: CF.

That he is to die: Sil.

**Disconnected:** Sil.

**Disease:** Ks; Ns; Sil.

Apoplexy, daughter has: Ns.

Epilepsy: Sil.

**Disgusting:** Nm.

**Dogs:** Sil.

Large one following him: Sil.

**Drinking:** Nm.

**Drowning:** Sil.

**Earthquake:** Sil.

**Events,** Previous: Cf; Ks; Np; **SIL.**

Long past: **SIL.**

Previous day of: Cf; Sil.

**Exciting:** Nm.

**Falling** of: Fp; Kp; NS.

**Fantastic:** NM; NS; Sil.

**Fights:** NM; Ns; Sil.

Fire, Blood, vivid: CP; NM; Np; Ns; Sil.

Fit, That he has: Sil.

Flowers: Ns.

Flying: NS.

Frightful: CF; CP; CS; Km; Kp; KS; **NM;** Np; NS; SIL. Sleep, falling to, on: SIL.

Ghosts, Specters: Ks; Nm; SIL. Pursued, by: Sil.

Heavy, Laborious day work: NM.

Historical: SIL.

Humiliation: SIL.

Injuries: Ns.

Insane, Becoming: Fp.

Insults: Nm.

Journey: Cf; CP; Nm; SIL.

Jumping out of bed, as if: Cf.

Lascivious: Nm; NP; Sil. Emission, with: Sil.

Love, of: Nm; SIL.

Many: Nm; SIL.

Menses, During: NM.

Mental Exertion: NM.

Mind, Affecting: Nm.

Misfortune, of: Km; Kp; KS.

Murder: NM; SIL. Of being murdered: Sil.

Naked, of being: Kp.

New scenes, places of: Cf. Danger, sense of impending, with: Cf.

Night mare: Fp; Kp; Nm; Np; SIL.

Persistent: SIL. Continuing, after waking: NM; SIL.

Pleasant: Km; Kp; NM; NP; SIL.

Poisoned, of being: Nm.

Prisoner, of being taken, a: Nm.

Pursued, of being: SIL. Cats or dogs, by: Sil. Ghosts: Sil. Wild beasts: Sil.

Quarrels: Fp; Nm; Ns; Sil. Changing suddenly to happy conversation: Fp.

Repeating: Nm.

Riots: Nm.

Robbers: Kp; **NM;** SIL. And cannot sleep till house is searched: **NM.** Menses during: NM. Fighting with: Sil.

Sad: Nm.

Sailing: Ns.

Sexual: See Lascivious.

Sleep, First: Sil.

Snakes: Sil.

Sorrowful: Nm.

Storms: SIL. At sea: Sil.

Strangled of being: Sil.

Teeth, pulled out: Nm.

Thirsty: **NM.**

True, seem on waking: Nm.

Unimportant: **NM; SIL.**

Unpleasant: Nm.
Unremembered: NM; Ns.
Unsuccessful Efforts to do various things: Cf.
Vertigo: Sil.
Vexation: Km; NM; Np; NS; SIL.
Disgusting: Nm.
Visionary: NM; SIL.
Vivid (See Fire): Cf; CP; Fp; Km; Kp; Ks; NM; NP; SIL.
Voyages: Sil.
Water: Nm; Ns; SIL.
Boat, foundering: Sil.
Daughter is in, crying for help: Ns.
Flood: Sil.
Wedding: Ns.
Weeping: Cf; Cp; Nm; Sil.
Window, Trying to get out of: Cf.
DRINKING AGG: SIL.
After: NM; SIL.
Cold: KM; SIL.
Rapidly: NM; SIL.
DRINKING AMEL: Sil.
DRINKS cold AGG And AMEL: See under Food.
Desire for: See Thirst.
Little, Eats much: Nm.
Much, Eats little:
Thirst without:
Warm seem: Nm.
DRIVING Agg: Cp; Nm; SIL.
After Agg: Nm.
Amel: Nm.

DROPPING like Water: See Trickling.
DROPS Things (See Awkward): Cs; NM; Sil.
DROPSY: Fp; Km; Kp; Ks; NM; NS; Sil.
Fever, From: Km.
Heart, Disease from: Cp; Fp; Km.
Kidney Disease from: Cp; Fp; Km.
Loss of blood from: Cp; Fp
Morning Agg: Sil.
DROWSINESS: See Sleepiness
DRUGS, Abuse of, in general: Nm.
Anaesthetic Vapours: Km; NM; Sil.
Aspirin and similar: Mp.
Mercury: Ns.
Narcotics: Nm; Np.
Opium: Nm.
Purgatives: Mp.
Quinine: Nm.
Tetanus Anti-toxin: Mp.
DRUNK As if: Cs; Kp; Np; Sil.
DRY CLEAR or COLD Weather: See Weather.
DRYNESS: NM; Ns.
Internal: Nm; SIL.
Partial: NM.
Profuse, Secretion with: Nm.
DUALITY, Separated As if: Cp; Nm; Sil.
As if divided into half, and left side does not belong to her: Sil.

**DULL** (Sluggish, Difficult Comprehension): **CP; CS;** Kp; KS; **NM;** NP; NS; **SIL**..
**Afternoon:** Sil.
**Children, In: CP;** Sil.
**Dream,** After: Sil.
**Eating** Amel: Sil.
**Evening** Amel: Sil.
**Forenoon:** Sil.
**Morning:** Kp; Sil.
**DUSKY COLOUR** (Pale): Cf; Fp; NM; **SIL.**
**DUST, Feathers,** as of: Cs.
**Fine,** Air, In Agg: Cs.
**DWARFISH: CP;** Sil.
**DWELLS** on past disagreeable occurrences: NM.
**DYSENTERY:** Fp; Km; Kp; MP.
**Blood** only: Km; Kp.
With: Kp.
**Fever,** with: Kp.
**Very** Painful: Mp.
**DYSMENORRHEA:** See Menses Painful.
**DYSPHAGIA:** See Swallowing Difficult.
**DYSPEPSIA:** See Digestion affected.
**DYSPNOEA:** See Respiration Difficult and Asthma.
**DYSURIA:** See Urination Difficult.
**EARS: FP; SIL.**
**Right:** Sil.
**Left:** Nm.
**Alternating:** Fp.

**Behind** And Mastoid: Sil.
**Abscess: SIL.**
Caries, Mastoid: **SIL.**
Eruptions: Cs; Ks; Nm; **SIL.**
eczema: Km.
Inflammation (Mastoiditis) Cp; Fp; Km; Mp; Sil.
Itching: **NM.**
burning, followed by: Sil.
Moisture: Sil.
Pain: CP; CS; KP; Nm; Ns; SIL.
aching: Nm.
boring: CP.
right: Cp; Nm.
burning: Cp.
drawing: Sil.
jerking: Sil.
**External:**
Boils: Sil.
Coldness and aching: Sil.
Deposit thin on: Np.
Eruptions: Cp; Kp; Ks; Nm; Np.
crusts on concha: Np.
eczema: Km; KS.
pimples: Ks; Nm.
scaly: Np; Sil.
scurfy: Sil.
Formication: Nm.
Heat: CP; Kp; NM; Np; Ns; Sil.
afternoon, after coffee: Nm.
Inside: Cp.

one-sided: Np.
right: Np.
Inflammation:
 erysipelatous: Cp; **FP;** Km;
 Sil.
 concha of: Nm; Sil.
 inside: **CS;** FP; NS; SIL.
 margins, of: Sil.
Itching: Cp; Cs; Nm; Np.
 red hot: Np.
 burning: Cp; Np.
Moisture: Sil.
Soreness: CP; Km.
Swelling: CP; Kp; NM; SIL.
 glands, of: Cp; Km.
 sudden: Cp.
Twitching: Cp; Kp; Nm; Sil.
 left: Sil.
 right: Nm.
Ulceration: Cp.
 inside: Sil.
 low form: Kp.
**External auditory canal:**
Abscess: **CS; SIL.**
Boils, pimples: Kp; Nm; SIL.
Boring, fingers in: SIL.
 amel: Sil.
 child by: SIL.
 sleep, during: SIL.
Dryness: Sil.
Granulations: KM.
Inflammation: **CS;** FP; KM;
 NM; **SIL.**
Itching: CS; KP; KS; Nm;
 Np; Ns; SIL.

burning: Cp; Np.
 warm room, in: Cp.
 left: Ns.
 lying: Kp.
 riding, after: Cp.
 scratch must, till it
 bleeds: Np.
 touch, amel: Nm.
Pain: CP; Fp; KM; NM; Np;
 Ns.
Polypus: Cp; KM; KS; Sil.
Sensitive to air, or touch:
 FP.
Swelling: Cp; Kp; NM; SIL.
**Glands,** Abscess: Sil.
Swelling: Cp; Km.
**Internal** Hypersensitive: Fp;
 SIL.
Noises: See Hearing.
**Lobules,** Boils: Sil.
Cysts: Sil.
Itching: Nm; Np.
Ulceration of ring hole: Km.
**Ossicles,** Caries of: Cf; Cs;
 Nm; **SIL.**
**Tympanic** Membrane: Km.
Calcareous deposit, on: CF.
Dark, beefy red: Fp.
Granular: Km.
Perforation: Sil.
Red, bulging: Fp.
Retracted: Km.
Thickened: Fp.
Ulceration: KP; SIL.
**Abscess: SIL.**

3 F.A.

**Aching:** See Pain.
**Air,** As if in: Nm.
Rushing out: Sil.
**Boring** Fingers, in amel: Sil.
Tendency: Sil.
children in: Sil.
**Chewing Agg:** Km; **KS;** NM; Sil.
**Cold Agg:** Sil.
**Colds,** Agg: Fp; Km.
**Cold,** As if: Cp.
**Coughing,** Agg: CS; FP; **NM;** SIL.
**Crawling:** Nm.
**Crusts:** Np.
**Discharge,** From: Cf; **CP;** CS; Fp; Kp; **KS;** NM; NS; **SIL.**
Bloody: CS; Fp; Kp; Ks; **SIL.**
Brownish: KS.
Caries, threatening: CF; CS; Nm; **SIL.**
Cheesy: **SIL.**
Ear wax: Nm.
Excoriating: CP; NM.
Gluey: Nm.
Ichorous: Cp; SIL.
Milk white mucus: Km.
Offensive: Cs; Kp; Ks; SIL.
putrid, meat-like: **KP.**
Painful: CS; Fp.
Polypus, with: Ks.
Purulent: **CS;** KP; **KS;** NM; **SIL.**

mercury, after abuse of: SIL.
Sensation of: Nm; Sil.
Thick: CS; Nm; SIL.
Thin water: **KS;** SIL.
White: Km; NM.
Yellow: CS; **KS;** NS; SIL.
Yellow green: KS.
**Foetor,** from: Kp; Sil.
**Head,** Turning Agg: Mp.
**Hot:** Np.
**Inflamed: FP.**
Slap, after: Cs.
**Itching:** Sil.
Scratch must, till it bleeds: Np.
**Pain** (Otalgia): CP; CS; FP; KP; **KS;** NM; NS; SIL.
Left: Nm.
Right: NS.
Aching: FP; Cp; **KS;** Sil.
left: Nm; Sil.
to right: Cp.
right: Np.
Air bubble, in: NM.
rushed through eustachian tube, in middle with tingling: Sil.
Alive, as if, something in: Sil.
Blow, as from: Nm.
Blowing nose Agg: Sil.
Burning: **NM;** Np.
right: Nm; Np.
spots: Cp.

3 F.B.

Cold, air agg: Cp; Km; Mp.
application, agg: SIL.
Cold feeling, followed by heat and throbbing: CP.
Cramp in: Kp; Nm; SIL.
left: Nm.
Cutting: Ks.
Day time agg: Nm.
Digging: Nm.
Drawing: Fp; Kp; NM; SIL.
right: Nm; Sil.
Ear, above: Nm; Sil.
below: Np; Sil.
front of: Cp; Np.
inward: Ns.
left to right: Cp.
neck to: Nm; Sil.
side of: MP; NM.
shoulder to: NM.
left: NM.
Evening Agg: Ks; Nm.
8 P.M.: Ns.
Flowing, something, from: Sil.
Forced outward, as if: Ns.
Forenoon Agg: Nm.
9 A.M.: NS.
Full moon, during: Sil.
Fullness: Kp; Np; Ns.
Hammering: FP.
throbbing, beating: SIL.
Head, turning Agg: MP.
Intermittently: Mp; Nm.
Jerking: Cp; Sil.

Lying Agg: Fp; Nm.
bed in agg: KP.
Morning Agg: NS.
Motion Agg: SIL.
Amel: Sil.
Night Agg: Cp; Fp; SIL.
1 A.M.: Sil.
Noises Agg: Kp; SIL.
Opening and closing like a valve: NS.
Periodical: Nm.
Pressing out, as if:
something must be torn from within: Ns.
Pricking: Sil.
Rising from a seat: SIL.
Sitting after long, Agg: SIL.
while: Nm.
Soreness: CP; SIL.
ear, about: Cp.
Stinging, shooting: CP; Cs; Fp; Kp; KS; NM; Np; NS; SIL.
evening on going to bed: Fp.
leaning: **SIL.**
left: Kp; Sil.
right: Fp; Nm; NS.
**Periostitis,** Mastoid of: Cf.
**Pulsations:** Cp; CS; Fp; Kp; Ks; Nm; Np; SIL.
Behind: Cp.
Lying on the ear: Sil.
Night: Sil.
**Redness:** Cp; NM; Np.
Concha of: Nm.

**Slap,** After Agg: Cs.
**Stopped:** Cs; KM; KP; Ks; Nm; Np; Ns; **SIL.**
Loud reports, ear open: SIL.
Plug, as from: Km.
Right: Ns.
Swallowing, Amel: SIL.
Valve, as if, by: Nm.
Yawning Amel: Nm; Sil.
**Stuffy:** Km.
**Surging,** in: Kp.
**Swallowing** Agg: Nm.
**Tearing,** About: Cp; Fp; Kp; Ks; NP; SIL.
Ear, about: NS.
**Tingling:** Km; Nm.
**Torn out,** as if: Nm.
**Touch** Agg: Cp; Fp; Sil.
**Twitched** Out of ear, with hook, something were: Nm.
**Vision,** Exertion, Agg: Sil.
**Warm** Room Agg: Sil.
Entering in, from cold air: Ns.
**Warmth** Agg: Cp.
**Warmth** of bed and wrapping Amel: MP.
**Water** Dropping, as from a height, into a long thin narrow vessel: NP.
**Waves,** In: Kp.
**Wax** (Cerumen), Brown and dark: Cs.
Dark flowing: Cs.
Increased: Sil.

Soft: Sil.
Thin: SIL.
**Weather,** Changing Agg: Sil.
Damp, Agg: CP; NS; SIL.
**Wind,** blowing into, as if: Nm.
puffed out of ear: Sil.
**Middle ear**
Acute Catarrh: FP; KM; Sil.
Chronic: KM; Sil.
Suppuration, Acute: Cs; Fp; Km; Sil.
Chronic: Cf; **CS;** Km; Kp; KS; Nm; **SIL.**
**EAT Aversion** or Refuses to: Kp.
**Chokes** On attempting to: Sil.
**Everything** And anything: Np.
**Excreta,** His own: Sil.
**Little** is sufficient: Nm; Sil.
**Neither** Drink, for weeks:
**TOO** tired to: Kp.
**EATING Agg: CP;** Fp; Km; Kp; Ks; **NM;** Ns; **SIL.**
**A** little: Np.
**Before:** Fp; Np; Sil.
**Fatigue:** Nm.
**Hastily:** Sil.
**Long,** After: Nm.
**Over:** Nm; Sil.
**Too** Much: Np.
**While:** Cp; Kp; NM; Sil.
**EATING Amel:** Cp; KP; Nm; Sil.
**After:** CS; Kp; Ks; Nm; SIL.
**EBULITION:** Nm; Sil.

**ECCHYMOSES, Petechiae**
purpura: Nm; Sil.
**ECLAMPSIA:** CP; NM; Sil.
**ECSTASY:** Sil.
**ECTASIA** (Bulging of Cornea):
Cp.
**ECTHYMA:** Sil.
**ECTROPION** (Eyelids turned
up): NM; Sil.
**Nitrate** of Silver after: Nm.
**ECZEMA:** CS; Km; KS; Nm;
Np; **SIL.**
**Dry,** Children in: Cs.
**Neurotic:** Kp.
**Sun,** Exposure from: Nm.
**EDGE** On, as if: NM; Sil.
**EFFECTS** Single: Nm; Sil.
**EFFUSION deposit:** CP; Fp;
KM; Kp; KS; NM; **SIL.**
**EGG Albumin** Dried on as if:
Nm.
**EGOTISM** (Pompous): SIL.
**Ailments,** from: Sil.
**ELBOWS Ankylosis:** Sil.
**Compression:** Ns.
**Cracking:** Nm.
**Eruptions:** KS.
Bend of: Nm.
herpes: **NM.**
warts: Cf.
Psoriasis: KS.
Scabs: KS.
Vesicles: Np.
**Inflammation:** Sil.
**Itching:** Np.

**Jerking:** Nm.
**Numbness:** NS.
**Pain:** Cp; Cs; Ns; SIL.
Boring: Ns.
Burning: Cp.
Drawing: Ns; Sil.
bone, in: Sil.
Left: Km.
then right: CP.
Motion Agg: Sil.
Pressing: NS.
Shooting: CP.
Sore, bruised: Cp; Ns.
Stitching: Cp; Cs; Sil.
olecranon in: Nm.
Tearing: Kp; Np; NS; Sil.
bend of: Ns.
Touched when agg: Cp; Sil.
**Sprain** of: Fp.
**Swelling:** Cf; Sil.
Condyles: CP.
Sprain, from: Fp.
**Tension,** bend of: Nm.
**Twitching:** Nm.
**Ulcers:** Ns.
**Weakness:** Km; Ns.
Paralytic: Sil.
**ELECTRIC SHOCK** Agg:
**Sparks** Sensation: CP; Nm.
**ELECTRICITY** Amel: Sil.
**ELEPHANTIASIS:** Sil.
**ELEVATING Limbs** Amel: Mp;
Nm.
**ELONGATED As** if: Nm; Ns;
**SIL.**

EMACIATION Atrophy: **CP**; KP; Ks; **NM**; NP; NS; **SIL.**
**Affected parts** of: Nm; Sil.
**Appetite** good with: Nm.
**Children** (Marasmus): CP; **NM; SIL.**
**Downwards** Spreads: Nm.
**Insanity** with: Nm; Sil.
**Pining Boys: NM.**
**EMBOLISM**: Km.
**EMISSIONS:** See Seminal emissions and prostate.
**EMOTIONAL** (See Excitement): KP; NM.
**EMOTIONS,** Mental Excitement
•   Agg: **CP**; CS; **KP**; Ks; **NM**; NP; NS; **SIL.**
**Pleasurable** Amel: KP.
**EMPHYSEMA: CP**; **NM.**
**IN PROSTHOTONUS: CP**; MP; NS.
**EMPTY, Hollow,** Sinking: Nm.
**EMPYEMA: CA; KS;** Ns; **SIL.**
**EMPYOCELE: KS; SIL.**
**ENAMEL, Thin:** CF; Sil.
**ENERVATED, Delicate:** CP; Kp; Sil.
**ENLARGED,** Swelled, as if: CP; Sil.
**ENTROPION** (Eye-lids turned in): Nm; Sil.
**ENURESIS:** See Urination, Involuntary.
**ENVY:** Cp; CS.
**EPHELIS,** Sunburn, freckles: Cp; Np; Sil.

**EPIDIDYMITIS:** Fp.
**EPIGASTRIUM Above: Nm.**
**Aching:** Sil.
**Anxiety,** Emotions felt in: CP; NM.
**Beaten,** Bruised, as if: **NM.**
**Boring:** Nm.
**Burning:** NM; **SIL.**
**Constriction:** Nm.
**Contraction:** Nm.
**Foreign Body,** as if: **NM.**
**Lump,** Above, as if: Nm.
**Pain,** Constant, in: Kp; Sil.
Crampy, pinching: Sil.
**Pressure,** Sense of: Nm.
**Pricking:** Nm.
**Pulsation:** Nm.
**Pustules, on:** Nm.
**Red** Spots, on: Nm.
**Sensitive: NM.**
**Suppurative,** Festering pain: **NM.**
**Swollen,** Distended: **NM.**
**Tender,** To touch: Fp; NM.
**Throat,** to upward: Nm.
**Throbbing:** Nm.
**Tremulous,** Sensation, in: Ns.
**EPILEPSY** (Convulsions): CP; CS; Km; Ks: MP: NM, Ns; **SIL.**
**Coldness** of left side before: SIL.
**Eye-balls,** Bulging of with: KM.
**General** Nervous feeling before: Nm.

Injury to Head, from: Ns.
Menses, Suppressed, from: Cp.
Mouse, Running up, sensation like: SIL.
Nervous Children, with dyspepsia and urticaria: Km.
Solar Plexus, from: SIL.
Stiffness, Rigidity, with: Sil.
Suppression of eruptions from: Km.
Twitching of Arms and legs with: Nm.
Unconsciousness, with: Nm; Sil.
EPIPHORA: Nm; Sil.
EPISTAXIS: CP; CS; FP; Km; Ks; Nm; NP; Ns; SIL.
Acrid: Sil.
Afternoon: Cp.
Anemic persons: Cp; Fp.
Blowing Nose, from: Cp; Fp; Kp; Ks; NM; Np; Ns; Sil.
Bright: Fp; Ns; Sil.
Children, in: FP.
Scrofulous: Sil.
Chill, In place of: Nm.
Clotted: NM.
Coryza, with: Sil.
Coughing, from: Fp; Nm; Sil.
Night, at: Nm.
Face Washing, When: Km.
After: CS.
Fever, During: Fp.
Typhoid: Fp; Kp.

Headache, During: Fp.
Heaviness with: Ns.
Infants in: Sil.
Menses Absent: Sil.
Before: Ns.
During: Nm; Ns.
Morning: Nm.
9 A.M.: Km.
Night: Km.
Coughing, on: NM.
Nose, Blowing: See Blowing, Nose.
Old People, in: Fp.
Periodic: Km
Posteriorly: Fp.
Predisposition, To: FP; Kp; SIL.
Puberty, At: Fp; Nm; Sil.
Scrofula, with: Cs; Sil.
Stooping Agg: Nm.
Vicarious: Ns.
EPITHELIOMA: Cp; Ks; Sil.
EPULIS: NM.
ERECTIONS (of Penis)
Continued: NM; Np; Sil.
Excessive: Sil.
Frequent: Nm.
Incomplete: Cs; NM; NP.
Itching of Scrotum with: Km.
Morning, Sexual desire with: Ns.
Night: KP; Nm; Sil.
Painful, (Chordee, priapism) : Cp; Km; Kp; Mp; Nm; Np; SIL.

**Riding** while: CP.

**Sexual** Desire, without: CP; Kp; NM; Np; Sil.

**Stools,** After: Nm.

**Troublesome:** Fp; Km; NM; Np; SIL.

**Violent:** Nm; Np; SIL.

Day time: Sil.

Morning: KP.

**Wanting** (Impotency): CS; Kp; Ks; NM; NP; Sil.

Evening and night: Kp.

**ERETHISM false:** Kp; Nm.

**EROTIC** (Amcrous): Cs; Nm; SIL.

**EROTOMANIA: CP;** Fp; Kp; **NM; NP; NS; SIL.**

**ERRATIC Complaints:** Ks; Nm; Mp; Sil.

**RRORS,** Diet, in: Np.

**ERUCTATIONS:** Cs; Fp; Kp; Ks; **NM;** NP; NS; SIL.

**Agg:** Sil.

**Amel:** Kp; KS; Nm; Sil.

**Abortive:** CS; Nm.

**Acrid:** CS; Nm.

Eating, Agg: Nm.

**After-Noon** 4 p.m.: Nm.

**Alternating** With Pain in chest and abdomen: Km.

**Bitter:** CS; Fp; Km; Ks; **NS;** Sil.

Eating, After: Kp.

Food comes up: Ns.

Night, at: NM; NS.

**Burning:** Nm; Sil.

Eating Agg: Nm.

**Chilliness,** with: Nm.

**Difficult:** Cp.

**Disagreeable: NM;** NS.

**Drinking,** after: Cp; NM.

Water, after: NM.

**Empty** (Tasteless): Cs; Fp; Kp; KS; **NM;** Np; Ns; SIL.

**Evening:** Sil.

**Food** of (Regurgitation): CS; **FP;** Km; Kp; Ks; MP, NM.

Afternoon: Np.

Bitter: Ns.

Dinner, after: Np.

Eating, immediately, after: MP.

after: Mp; NM.

mouthful: Np.

vexation, after: Fp.

while: Mp.

**Forenoon:** CP.

**Foul:** Cs; Fp; Nm; Ns.

Milk, after: Nm.

**Greasy:** Fp.

**Headache,** During: Sil.

**Hot:** Sil.

Drinks, from: Km.

**Ineffectual,** incomplete: Km; Kp; **NM.**

Forenoon: Sil.

Menses, before: NM; Ns.

Milk, after: NM; Ns.

Rich food, after: Nm.

Stools, after: Sil.

**Ingesta,** Tasting of: NM; **SIL.**
**Loud:** NM; **SIL.**
Stomach, pain in, with: Sil.
Uncontrollable: SIL.
**Menses,** Before: Nm.
**Milk,** after: Nm.
**Morning:** Nm.
**Nauseous:** Cs; Km; Nm; Sil.
**Night:** Nm.
**Repulsive:** Cs; Km; Nm; **NP.**
**Rich** food after: Nm.
**Salty:** Nm.
**Sour:** CP; CS; FP; Kp; **KS;**
**NM; NP; NS;** SIL.
Eating, After: Km; NM; SIL.
**Stool,** after: Nm.
**Sweetish,** Menses, before:
Nm.
Pregnancy, During: Nm.
**Supper,** After: Sil.
**Water,** of: Ns; Sil.
**ERUPTIONS: CS;** Kp; **KS; NM;**
Np; **SIL.**
**Acne:** See Pimples.
**Acuminate,** Conical: SIL.
**Alternating,** Diarrhea, with:
Cp.
stomach and menstrual
complaints: Km.
**Areola,** Red: Nm.
**Biting:** Nm; Sil.
**Black** Head with: CS.
**Blisters:** Ks; Nm; Np; **SIL.**
Inflamed: **SIL.**
**Blotches:** Nm.

**Boils** (Furuncles): Cp; CS;
Sil.
**Blood:** NM; SIL.
**Large:** Sil.
**Maturing,** slowly: Sil.
**Periodic:** Sil.
**Recurring:** Cp.
**Small:** Nm.
**Stinging,** when touched: Sil.
**Burning:** CS; Ks; Nm; Np;
SIL.
**Carbuncle:** Cf; Km; Kp; **SIL.**
**Clustered:** Nm.
**Crusty:** See Crusts.
**Desquamating:** Fp; Km; **KS;**
Nm; Np; Ns; SIL.
**Discharging** (Moist): CS; Kp;
KS; **NM;** Np; NS; **SIL.**
Corrosive: NM.
Destroys hair: NM.
Glutinous: NM.
Pus: Nm; SIL.
Thin: **NM.**
White: NM; **SIL.**
Yellow: NM; Np; **NS; SIL.**
**Dry:** CS; Km; Ks; Nm; Np;
**SIL.**
**Ecthyma:** Sil.
**Eczema:** See Eczema.
**Elevated:** Nm.
**Excoriated:** NM.
**Fetid:** Sil.
**Fine:** Nm.
**Fish,** after: Nm; Ns.
**Flat:** Sil.

Granular: NM.
Gritty: Nm.
Groups, In: Nm.
Gummata, Nodes: CF; SIL.
Hairy Parts, on: Nm.
Hard: Sil.
Heated, When; NM.
Herpetic: CS; Km; Kp; KS; NM; Np; NS; SIL.
Burning: Nm; Sil.
Chapping; Nm; SIl.
Circinate: NM.
Corrosive: SIL.
Crusty: Nm; SIL.
Itching: Nm; SIL.
Patches: Nm; Sil.
Scaly: Nm; Sil.
dry, mealy: Sil.
Tearing: SIL.
Zoster: Km; NM; SIL.
Horny: Sil.
Hot water, Amel: Sil.
Impetigo: Nm; SIL.
Itching: CP; CS; Kp; KS; NM; SIL.
Jerking Pain with: Sil.
Joints, on: CS; Cp; NM; Np.
Leprosy: Nm; SIL.
Lichen: Nm.
Lumps, Hard, bluish: CP.
Mealy: SIL.
White: Sil.
Menses, before: Nm.
Miliary: Nm.
Moist: Nm; Sil.

Nodular: NS; Sil.
Painful: Ks; Np; SIL.
Papular: Ks; Sil.
Pearly: Nm.
Pemphigus: NM; NS; SIL.
Petechiae: Nm; Sil.
Phagedenic: Nm; NS; SIL.
Pimples: CP; CS; Km; Kp; Ks; NM; NP; NS; SIL.
Burning: Ns.
Depressed, black head: Cs.
Flea bites, like all over: Np.
Inflamed: Cs.
Itching: Nm; NS; SIL.
Sensitive: CS.
Stinging: Cp.
Tensive: NS.
Pocks: Sil.
Psoriasis: CS; Kp; Ks; Nm; SIL.
Inveterate: SIL.
Pustules: CP; CS; Ks; NM; SIL.
Malignant: Kp; SIL.
Ulcerated: Sil.
Rash: CS; KS; Mp; NM; SIL.
Biting, stinging: Nm.
Receding: Km.
Red: Ks; Sil.
Ring worm: See Herpetic
Rhus Poisoning, from: Ks.
Roseola: Np.
Rubella: Nm.
Rupia: NM; NS; Sil.
Scabies: KS; SIL.

Dry: **SIL.**
Moist: Sil.
Suppressed: Nm; Sil.
mercury and sulphur with: Sil.
**Scabs: KS; SIL.**
**Scaly:** CS; Km; KS; SIL.
Bran like: Km; Nm; SIL.
Ichthyosis: Sil.
Spots: Sil.
Yellow: **KS.**
**Smarting:** KS; NM; Sil.
**Spring,** Agg: NS.
**Stinging:** NM; SIL.
**Suppressed:** KS; Sil.
**Suppurating:** Cs; Ks; Nm; Np; SIL.
**Swelling,** with: Nm; Sil.
**Syphilitic:** SIL.
**Tearing** Pain, with: **SIL.**
**Tet'ery:** NM.
**Touch** Agg: Kp; Nm; Sil.
**Tubercles:** Cp; Cs; Ks; NM; Sil.
Miliary: Nm.
Red: Nm.
Syphilitic: Sil.
Tuberous: Sil.
Ulcerative pain, with: **SIL.**
**Urticaria:** See Urticaria.
**Vesicles:** Cp; CS; KM; KS; **NM;** Ns; SIL.
Bloody: Kp; NM.
Burning Nm; SIl.
Gangrenous: Sil.

Hard: Sil.
Itching: Sil.
Phagedenic: NM; Sil.
Red: NM; Sil.
areola: Sil.
Scurfy: Nm; Sil.
Small: Nm.
Smarting: Sil.
Sudamina: **NM.**
Whitish: Cs; NS.
Yellow: Cp; NS.
**Zoster:** Km; NM; SIL.
**ERYSIPELAS:** Km; KP; Ks; Nm; Np; Ns; SIL.
**Gangrenous:** Sil.
**Occasional:** Cf.
**Phlegmonous:** SIL.
**Recurrent,** Chronic: Fp; Nm.
**Smooth,** Red, shining: Fp; Nm.
**Swelling,** with: Nm; Sil.
**Vesicular:** Km; Ks.
**ERYTHEMA:** Km; Np; Sil.
**ESCAPE, impulse,** to: Fp.
**ESTRANGED, family** from her: NM; Ns.
**Wife,** from his: Ns.
**EUSTACHIAN TUBES:** FP; KM; Sil.
**Catarrh:** Km; **KS;** NM; SIL.
**Inflammation:** KS; NM; SIL.
**Itching:** Km; SIL.
**Obstructed:** Km.
**Tickling,** Inducing swallowing and cough: Sil.
**EXACTING** (Critical): Sil.

EXAGGERATES, Her symptoms: Kp.

EXALTATION: See Cheerful.

EXANTHEMATA: Fp; Km; Ks; NM; Sil.

Preventive, as a: KM.

EXCITEMENT (Emotional, Excitable): CP; CS; FP; KP; KS; NM; Np; SIL.

Ailments, from: Cp; KP; NM.

Evening: Fp.

Loquacity, with: Fp.

Menses, during: Np.

Mental work, from: Kp.

Sleep, Before: Nm.

Un-Natural: Fp.

EXCORIATION: CS; Ks; NM; Np.

EXCRESCENCES: Nm; NS; SIL.

Condylomata: NS.

Fungus, Cauliflower: SIL.

Haematodes: NM; SIL.

Medullary: Sil.

Syphilitic: SIL.

Red: NS.

EXERTION, Mental Agg: Kp; NM; SIL.

Physical: CP; CS; Fp; Km; KP; Ks; NM; NP; SIL.

Vision, of: Kp; Ks; NM; NP; SIL.

EXERTION Amel: Nm; Ns; Sil.

EXHALATION Agg: NM.

Amel: Nm.

Forcible: Fp.

EXHAUSTION: See Weakness

Sense of: CP.

EXHILARATION: See Cheerful.

EXOSTOSES: CF; SIL.

EXOPHTHALMIC GOITRE: Fp; Nm.

EXPECTORATION Agg: Cp.

Amel: Sil.

Acrid: Nm; SIL.

Air, cold, open Amel: Cs.

Albuminous, clear: Cs; FP; Km; Kp; Ks; NM; Np; SIL.

Balls, of: SIL.

Bath After, Agg: Cs.

Bloody: Cs; FP; Km; Kp; Ks; NM; Np; SIL.

Acrid: SIL.

Bright red: Fp; Sil.

Brown: Sil.

Dark: Fp.

Erection, after a violent: Nm.

Fall, after, a: FP.

Menses, during: Nm.

Pale: Sil.

Purulent: Sil.

Streaked: FP; NM; Sil.

Brownish: Sil.

Copious, Profuse: Cp; CS; Fp; Sil.

Corrosive: Np; SIL.

Day time only: Fp; SIL.

Difficult: Fp; KS.

Easy, Raising: Ks; NS; Sil.

Eating, After Agg: Sil.

**Evening: KM.**
**Flies,** from mouth: Km.
**Foamy,** Frothy: Fp; Kp; Nm; Sil.
**Frequent:** Sil.
**Gelatinous:** SIL.
**Glairy: NM;** NS.
**Globular:** Cf; Sil.
**Granular:** Sil.
  Offensive: Sil.
**Grayish:** Nm.
  White: Km.
**Greenish:** Cs; FP; Kp; Ks; Nm; Np; **NS; SIL.**
**Hard:** Ns; SIL.
**Hawked** Up Mucus: NM; SIL.
**Hot,** Burning: Sil.
**House,** In Agg: Cs.
**Loose:** KS; SIL.
**Lumpy:** Cf; **CS;** Nm; SIL.
**Milky:** KM; SIL.
**Mucus:** Cf; CS; Fp; Kp; KS; NM; Np; NS; SIL.
  Bloody: CS; NM; Sil.
  Gray, greenish: Km; Ks; NS.
  Translucent: Sil.
**Offensive:** Fp; KP; Nm; NP; SIL.
  Fetid: Kp; Sil.
**Orange:** Kp.
**Painful,** As loosened: Nm.
**Profuse,** Copious: Cp; **CS;** Fp; SIL.
**Purulent:** Cp; CS; Fp; KP; KS; Nm; Np; Ns; **SIL.**

**Ropy:** NS.
**Sago-like:** Sil.
**Salty:** Kp; Nm; Np; Sil.
**Slips,** Back again: KS.
**Soap suds,** like: Kp.
**Sour:** Nm; Np.
**Starchy:** Sil.
**Sticky,** Tough, viscid: CS; Km.
**Swallow,** Must, what has been loosened: **KS.**
**Taste,** Bitter: Nm.
  Copper, like: Nm.
  Flat: NM; Np; NS.
  Greasy, oily, fatty: SIL
  Ingesta, of: Sil.
  Metallic: Nm.
  Nauseous: Nm; Sil.
  Putrid: Fp; Np; Sil.
  Repulsive: Nm.
  Salty: Kp; NM; Np; Sil.
  Sour: Nm.
  Sweetish: Kp.
**Thick:** Cs; Fp; Km; Kp; Ks; Np; Ns; **SIL.**
**Tough:** Cf; Sil.
**Transparent:** Cs; Km; **NM;** SIL.
**Tubercles:** SIL.
**Viscid:** Cs; Fp; Km; Kp; Ks; Nm; Np; Ns; SIL.
  Whitish: Km.
**Walking,** while Agg: Nm.
**Watery:** KS.
**White:** Cs; Km; Kp. NM; Sil.

**Yellow:** Cf; **CP; CS;** FP; KP; KS; Nm; NP; SIL.

Lumpy: Cf.

tiny; Cf; Kp.

**EXPLOSIONS:** See Blows, shattered.

**EXPRESS himself** cannot: Kp; Nm.

**EXPRESSION:** See under Face.

**EXTENSION:** See Stretching.

**EXTERNAL AUDITORY**

**Canal:** See Ears.

**EXTREMITIES:** See Arms, Legs.

**EXUDATION:** CP; Fp; KM; Kp; KS; NM; SIL.

**Fibrinous:** Km.

**Hard:** Km.

**EYE BROWS:** See Brows.

**Lashes,** Falling: CS; Sil.

Ingrown (Entropion): Nm; Sil.

**EYE LIDS Agglutinated:** Cs; Kp; Ks; Np; **SIL.**

**Bleeding:** Nm.

**Burning,** Margins, of: Kp; Ns.

**Chemosis:** See Swollen.

**Close,** Desire, to: SIL.

Difficult, to: SIL.

Headache, with: NM.

Must: Sil.

Spasmodic: NM; Sil.

**Cyst** On: Fp; SIL.

**Drawn** Together sensation: Mp.

**Eruptions,** on: Ks; Nm; Sil.

Pimples: Nm.

Pustules: Nm.

Scabs, crusts: Km.

Scaly, herpes at margins: **KS.**

**Everted** (Ectropion): NM; Sil.

**Excoriation:** NM.

**Falling,** Drooping of: Kp; Mp; Sil.

**Foreign,** Body, between upper and eye-ball: Fp.

**Granulations:** Km; NM; NS; SIL.

**Hair** Falling (Eyelashes): CS.

**Hardness:** Sil.

**Heat,** In: Cp.

**Heaviness:** NM; Np; NS; Sil.

Left: Kp.

Lying Agg: Nm.

Night: Fp.

**Inflammation:** CS; Ks; NM; Sil.

Margins: NM.

**Inversion:** Nm; Sil.

**Itching:** Np.

Margins: Cs; Np; NS.

**Narrowing,** Space between: Nm.

**Nodes,** Margins, in; Sil.

**Opening,** Difficult, at night: Nm.

**Pain,** Pressing: Np; Sil.

**Paralysis: KP.**

Left: Kp.

Right; Mp; Nm.

Upper: MP.

**Quivering:** NM; Np; Sil.
Reading, while: Np.
Right, Upper: Nm.
**Redness:** Fp; NM; Ns; Sil.
Margins: Ks; NM; Sil.
**Spasms:** Cp; MP; Sil.
**Stiff:** Nm.
**Styes:** Cf; Fp; Kp; SIL.
Induration, from: Sil.
Lower: Fp; Kp.
Recurrent: **SIL.**
Right: Fp; Nm.
**Suppuration,** on edges: Km; Nm.
**Swollen:** FP; Kp; Ks; NM; Np; Ns; Sil.
Meibomian glands: Sil.
Painless: Sil.
**Thickening:** NM.
**Tumours:** NM; SIL.
Cystic: Fp; SIL.
Sebaceous: CP.
Nodules: Sil.
Tarsal: Sil.
**Twitching:** MP; NM; SIL.
Menses, Before: NM.
Right: NM.
**Ulceration:** Nm; Np.
Margins: NM.
Under surface: Sil.
**EYES: NM.**
**Right:** Nm.
**Alternating** between: SIL.
**Backward** (Drawing, etc): Sil.
**Boils,** Over left: Nm.

**Burning,** Smarting: Fp; Kp; Mp.
Evening: Nm.
Sand, as from: Nm.
Steaming out, sensation: Ns.
**Cancer:** SIL.
Fungus: **SIL.**
Medullaris: Sil.
**Closing Amel:** Sil.
Difficult: Sil.
**Coition** Agg: Mm.
**Cold:** Cp.
**Contractive:** Nm; Sil.
**Crawling,** In: Ns.
**Crossed** As if: Nm.
**Crying** Hard as if: Nm.
**Distortion:** Cp; Ks; SIL.
Spasms during: Sil.
**Drawn** Backwards as if: Sil.
Together, as if: **NM.**
**Dryness:** Kp; Ks; NM; Np; NS; Sil.
Afternoon: NS.
Evening: Ns; Sil.
Morning: SIL.
Reading: Kp.
**Dull:** Kp.
**Enlarged,** Distended as if: Cp; **NM.**
**Eruptions,** About: Ks; Sil.
Boils: SIL.
Crusty: Km; Nm.
Itching: **NM.**
Spongy: Nm.

**Forced:** Out of head with cough, as if: Km.
and, brain, with: Sil.
**Foreign** body, as of a: Cp.
**Formication:** Ns.
**Heat: SIL.**
**Heaviness,** Menses, before: NM.
during: Nm.
**Inflammation:** CP; CS; Fp; Kp; Ks; **NM;** Np; Ns; **SIL.**
Acute: FP.
Chronic: **SIL.**
Cold, from: Cp.
Cold, Agg: Sil.
wet weather agg: Sil.
Dentition, during: Fp.
Foreign bodies from: **SIL.**
Gonorrhea: Cs; Ks; Ns.
Purulent: Ns.
Scrofulous: CP; **CS;** NM; NP; NS; **SIL.**
Sympathetic: Sil.
**Injected:** Nm.
**Injury** after effects: Cs: NS: **SIL.**
**Itching:** Cp; Cs; NM; Np; NS; **SIL.**
.Evening: Cp; Sil.
Morning: NM; NS.
rising, after: NM.
**Lachrymation:** See Lachrymation.
**Light** Agg: Ns.
**Looking** Down Agg: Nm.
Fire, at: Ns.
Pieces of paper at: Cs.

Sharply: NM.
Steadily: NM.
upward: Sil.
White objects at: Nm.
**Morning** Agg: Nm; Sil.
Waking on: Nm.
**Motion,** Movements, constant: Sil.
Convulsive: MP.
Involuntary: MP.
**Motion** of Eyes Agg: Kp; **NM;** Sil.
**Moving,** Something in: Cp.
**Open** half: Fp; NM.
**Opening** difficult: Sil.
Headache, during: Nm.
**Over:** NM; Sil.
**Right:** Nm.
**Pain:** Cp; Cs; Fp; KP; Ks; MP; **NM;** Np; Sil.
Aching: Cf; CP; CS; Fp; KP; NM; Np; Sil.
Afternoon, Agg: Sil.
Air, cold Agg: MP; SIL.
Air, open Amel: Nm.
Backwards, goes: Mp; Sil.
Boring: Nm.
Burning, biting: Cs; Fp; Kp; Ks; **NM;** Np; Ns; SIL.
afternoon: Ns.
12 to 3 p.m.: Nm.
evening, pressure and sand in as if: Nm.
Coition, after, Agg: Nm.
Crampy: **NM; SIL.**

Cutting: Np; Sil.

Drawing: Cp; Kp; **NM;** Sil.

backward: Sil.

stiff sensation in muscles: **NM.**

string as with, to back of head or into the brain: Sil.

Eyes, closing Agg: Sil.

Amel: Cf.

Evening reading while Agg: NS.

Fine work Agg: Nm.

Foreign body as from: **CP;** Cs; NM; SIL.

Heat, during Agg: NM.

Hiccough Agg: Sil.

Light Agg: NM; Ns; **SIL.**

artificial: CP; NM.

day: SIL.

gas: Cp.

strong: SIL.

Looking: See Looking.

Night in bed Agg: Sil.

Occiput extending to: Nm.

Paroxysmal: Sil.

Periodic: NM.

Pressing: Cs; Kp; Ks; **NM;** Np; Ns; SIL.

forward: Km.

head, extending, to: Nm.

menses, during: Np.

outwards: NS; Sil.

right: NM.

4 P.M. daily: Sil.

11 P.M.: Nm.

Right: NM; SIL.

sudden: Km.

Sand, as from: Fp; Km; Kp; **NM;** Np; SIL.

morning: **NM;** Sil.

Sore, bruised: CP; CS; Kp; Nm; Np; Sil.

evening: Np.

extending to canthi: Nm.

reading agg: Np.

Stitching, shooting: Fp; Km; Kp; NM; Np; Ns; SIL.

right: NM.

temple, to: Kp.

Sudden: Sil.

Sunlight Agg: KP; NM.

to sunset, agg: Nm.

Tearing: Kp; Ks; Ns; SIL.

Touch Agg: Mp.

Turning, sideways Agg: SIL.

Twilight Agg: Nm.

Urination, profuse Amel: Fp; SIL.

Vision, exertion on: Nm; SIL.

Vomiting Agg: Sil.

Warmth Agg: NM.

Warmth Amel: MP; SIL.

Writing Agg: Cf; **NM.**

4 P.M: Cf; NM.

**Paralysis** of muscles: NM.

Internal recti: **NM.**

**Perceptive** Power lost: Kp.

**Photophobia:** See Photophobia.

**Protrusion:** Cp; Cs; FP; Km; **NM.**
  Exophthalmus: Fp; NM.
**Pulsation:** SIL.
  Paroxysmal: Sil.
**Redness:** CP; CS; KP; **KS; NM;** Np; NS; Sil.
  Around: SIL.
  Evening: Km.
  Injuries, after: Sil.
  Reading, sewing: Nm.
  Vomiting, hiccough Agg: Sil.
**Reflex** Symptoms: Kp.
**Restless:** Kp.
**Sand** in, as if: Km; Nm.
**Scrofulous** affections of: Nm.
**Sensitive** Cold air, to: Sil.
**Smaller** left, as if: Nm.
**Smarting,** as from smoke: Nm.
**Smoke,** fire of: Kp.
**Soreness,** Tendency to: Sil.
**Staring:** Kp; Np; Sil.
**Stiffness:** Cp; Nm; Sil.
**Strabismus** Squint: Cp; Kp; MP; NP; Sil.
  Brain diseases after: Kp.
  Convergent: Mp.
  Diphtheria after: Kp.
  Divergent: **NM.**
  Sense of: NM.
  Worms, due to: Np.
**Suffused:** Fp; Nm; Sil.
**Sunk** Into head, as if: Cs.
**Sunken:** Fp; Kp.

**Swimming** In cold water: Sil.
**Swollen:** Kp; NM.
  As if: Cp; NM.
**Tension** (Glaucoma): NM; SIL.
  Coition, after: Sil.
  Decreased: Nm.
**Tired,** As if: Nm.
**Torn** out as if: **SIL.**
**Trembling** (Nystagmus): Mp.
**Turning,** Agg: Sil.
**Twitching:** Kp.
  Menses, before: NM.
**Watering,** as if: Ns.
  Full of: Sil.
**Weak:** Kp; NM; Ns; SIL.
  Coition after: Nm.
  Emission after: Nm; Np.
  Light, Agg: Np.
  Reading, writing Agg: Nm.
**Wipe** must frequently and pull at lashes: Nm.
**Writing** Agg: Cf; Nm.
**FACE: MP;** NM.
  **Abscess: SIL.**
  Antrum of: **SIL.**
  **Anemic:** Cp; Nm; Sil.
  **Angioma:** Cf.
  **Besotted,** Stupefied: NM; Sil.
  **Bloated:** Km; NM; Np.
  Fever, without: Np.
  **Bluish:** Cp; Km; Kp; Mp; NM; Np; Sil.
  Circles, around eyes: Cp; **Fp; Kp; NM; NP.**
  Cough, during: MP.
  Red: CP.

**Blushes,** Shyness from: Kp.
**Brown,** Yellowish at the edge of hair: Kp; NM.
Forehead, (Chloasmae): Kp.
**Cancer:** Sil.
Epithelioma: KS; Sil.
Lupus: Km; Sil.
Scirrhus: Sil.
**Careworn:** Kp.
**Chapped:** Sil.
**Chlorotic: CP;** Fp; Kp; KS; **NM.**
**Chloasmae:** Kp.
**Cobweb,** on as if: Nm.
**Colour,** Changing: Nm.
**Cyanotic: NM.**
**Deathlike** (Hippocratic): Fp.
**Desires** to wash with cold water: Cs.
Amel, thereby: CS.
**Dirty:** Km; Kp; Sil.
**Distorted:** Kp; Ks; SIL.
Colic and pain from: Mp.
**Down,** on Hysteria, in: Nm.
**Drawn:** Ks; Sil.
**Earthy:** CP; Fp; Kp; NM; Np; **SIL.**
**Emaciated:** Nm; Np; Sil.
**Eruptions:** CF; CP; CS; Kp; Ks; **NM;** Np; SIL.
Acne: CS; Km; NM; **SIL.**
Biting: Nm; Sil.
Burning: Nm.
scratched when: Ns.
Comedones: Nm; SIL.

Eczema: CS; **NM; SIL.**
occiput, spreading, from: Sil.
Forehead: CP; Fp; NM; Np; Sil.
Freckles: Sil.
Herpes: Cf; Cs; Ks; **NM;** NS; SIL.
circinate: NM.
Itching: CS; NM.
Papules: Sil.
Pimples: CP; CS; **NM;** NP; NS; SIL.
burning, touched, when: Ns.
forehead: CP; Nm; NP.
red: Cp; Nm.
shooting pain, touched when: Cp.
Pustules: Cp; Cs; NP.
forehead: Kp; NM.
Rash: NM.
Rough: Nm.
Scurfy: Cs; SIL.
Syphilitic: SIL.
Tubercles: Sil.
suppurating: Sil.
Urticaria: NM; Sil.
Vesicles: **NM;** Ns; SIL.
burning: Nm.
forehead: Nm.
**Erysipelas:** NS.
Gangrenous: Sil.
Phlegmonous: SIL.
**Expression,** Confused: Nm.

Haggard: Kp; NM; SIL.
Looks in mirror to see: Hm.
Old looking: **NM.**
Suffering: Km; Kp; Ks; NM; Ns.
Wretched: Nm.
**Greasy:** Cp; Kp; NM.
**Hair,** growth of on child's face: Nm.
**Hairy,** Hysteria during: Nm.
**Heat:** CP; Cs; FP; Km; NM; Np; SIL.
Afternoon to 6 p.m.: Fp.
Burning: Np.
and redness on left: Nm.
as if with coldness: Nm.
Chill, during: CP; Np.
Cold body, with: CP.
limbs, with: CP.
Eating, after: Sil.
Flashes of: Cs; Fp; Km; Kp; Ks; Sil.
menses, during: Nm.
sitting while: Fp.
washing with cold water after: Sil.
**Hectic spots:** Sil.
**Hippocratic:** Fp.
**Induration:** Sil.
**Itching:** Cs; Kp; Ks; Nm; Np; NS; SIL.
Biting: Nm; Np; Sil.
Right: Kp.
Stinging: Cs; Ks; NM; Np; SIL.

**Lead coloured:** NM.
**Nodule,** on: Cs.
**Pain** (Prosopalgia): CP; Cs; Fp; Km; KP; KS; **MP; NM;** Np; Ns; **SIL.**
Right: CP; Km; KP; MP to left: Cp; Nm.
Afternoon, 2 P.M. Agg: Mp.
Air, Cold Agg: Kp; **MP;** Ns.
open, Agg: KP; Mp; Sil.
Air, open Amel: KS; Nm; Ns.
Alternating with pain in shoulder: MP.
Attacks of repeated pain: MP; Sil.
Bed, in Agg: MP; SIL.
Below eyes (infra-orbital): Mp; Sil.
Boring: **SIL.**
Burning: Np; Sil.
rising from bed, after: Nm.
Chewing, when Agg: Km; MP; **NM;** Sil.
Cold application Agg: **MP; SIL.**
exposure, to Agg: MP; SIL.
from becoming, Agg: Cs.
Cold Application, Amel: Cs; Fp; KP.
Cramp like: MP.
Cutting: Cs.
Damp weather from: CP; NS; SIL.
Day time Agg: Mp.

Draft Agg: Cp; Kp; Mp; SIL.
Drawing: Kp; Ks; Nm; SIL.
Eating, After Amel: Kp.
Eating, sour Agg: Km.
  while Agg: Mp.
Extends cheek bones, to:
  Sil.
  chest to: Sil.
  other parts to: Cp.
Forenoon 11 A.M. TO 2
  P.M.: Mp.
Heat of stove amel: **SIL.**
Inflammatory: FP.
Infra-orbital: Mp; Sil.
Jerking: Mp.
Lancinating: **MP;** Sil.
  more frequent gradually:
  Km.
  right: Mp.
Light Agg: Mp.
Lying while Agg: Sil.
Lying Amel: Cp.
Menses, during Agg: NM;
  Sil.
Motion Agg: Cp; FP.
  jaw, lower of: Mp; Nm.
Motion Amel: Kp; Mp.
Mouth, opening, Agg: Mp.
Night Agg: Cp; MP; SIL.
  bed, driving him out of:
  .MP.
    rest, during: Mp.
Noise, Agg: Cp.
Paralysis, with: Km; Kp;
  **NM.**

Periodical: MP; **NM.**
Pressing: Fp; Nm.
Pressure, Amel: Mp.
  rubbing: Ns.
Pulsating: Fp; Sil.
Quinine, abuse of: Nm.
Rheumatic: CP; SIL.
Sleep, Amel: Mp.
Sore, bruised: NM.
  as if: Sil.
Stinging: FP.
Stitching: Fp; KM; Kp; MP;
  Nm; Np; Sil.
  left: NM.
  right: MP; Np.
Stooping, Agg: Fp.
Storm, before: SIL.
Stormy weather: Ns; **SIL.**
Sun, comes and goes with:
  NM.
Suppressed ague: **NM.**
Talking: Kp.
Tearing: KM; Kp; Ks; **MP;**
  NS; SIL,.
  right: MP.
Tooth-ache after: Nm; Sil.
Touch, Agg: Km; Mp; Nm;
  Sil.
Touch Amel: Kp.
Walking, Amel: Kp.
Warm room, Agg: **KS.**
Warmth, Amel: CP; Kp;
  **MP; SIL.**
Washing, Agg: Sil.
Wind, Agg: Mp.

dry, cold: **MP.**
south, warm, moist: KS.
**Pale: CP;** CS; **FP;** KP; KS;
**NM; NP;** Ns; **SIL.**
Menses, after: NM.
Red, alternating: Fp.
**Paralysis:** Kp; Nm.
Begins with face ache and
tenderness of affected side:
Km.
Neuralgia, after: Km.
One sided: Kp.
Right: Km; Kp; Sil.
Twitching of muscle, with:
Km.
**Perspiration:** CP; Cs; Fp; Kp;
Ks; NM; NS; **SIL.**
Cold: CP; Nm.
Eating, while: NM.
After: Ns.
Exertion, on: Sil.
Hot drinks after: Sil.
Side, not lain on: Sil.
Sleep, on falling: Sil.
**Puffy:** See bloated.
**Pulsation:** FP.
**Red:** FP; Kp; Ks; NM; Np; Ns;
SIL.
Alternating, paleness: Fp; Np.
Circumscribed: Fp; Kp; Ks;
Nm; Sil.
Cough, during: Mp; Sil.
Dark red, eating after: Sil.
Erysipelatous: Sil.
Eyes, about: Sil.
Fever, without: Np.

Glowing: Sil.
open air in but pale in
house: Nm.
Headache during: FP; Mp;
NM; Sil.
Heat of fire, from: Nm.
Menses, during: Cp; Fp.
One sided: Nm.
alternating sides: NP.
Pain, during: Fp.
**Sad:** Kp.
**Sallow:** CP; Fp; **NM;** NS.
**Shiny:** NM.
Oily: NM.
Spots, eruptions, after: Nm.
**Sickly:** Cs; Km; Ks; NM; Ns;
Sil.
**Spots: SIL.**
Bluish: Kp.
Brown: Np.
Pale: Sil.
Red: SIL.
White: Sil.
**Spotted,** blotched: Sil.
**Suffering:** Sil.
**Sunken:** Fp; KM; Kp; Ks.
Dinner, after: Nm.
**Swelled:** FP; Km; Kp; **NM.**
Bees, stings, as from: Mp.
Hard: Sil.
Intermittents, in: Nm.
Oedematous: FP; NM.
Painful: Km.
Scarlet fever, in: KS.
Tooth-ache, from: CS; **SIL.**

**Swelling:** Cs.
**Tension:** Km; Kp; NM.
**Twitching:** Km; Kp; NM.
  Coughing, when: Km.
  Eating: Km.
  Speaking, when: Km.
**Ulcers:** Km; Nm.
**White,** Nose and Mouth, about: Np.
**White** of an egg dried on as if: Nm.
**Wrinkled:** Nm.
  Forehead: Nm.
**Yellow:** Ns.
**FAG, Enervation:** Kp.
**FAILURE, feels,** himself a: Sil.
**FAINTNESS, fainting:** Cp; Fp; Kp; NM; SIL.
  **Coition,** after: NP.
  **Cold,** from taking: SIL.
  **Crowded room,** in: NM.
  **Exertion,** on: Nm.
  **Fever,** During: NM.
  **Hysterical:** NM.
  **Lying** on side while: Sil.
  **Menses** Before, from pain: Ks.
  During: Nm.
  **Night: SIL.**
  **Riding,** While: Sil.
  **Sense,** of: **NM.**
  **Sitting,** While: Ns.
  **Smoking,** On: Sil.
  **Standing,** While: Sil.
  **Stools,** After: Ns.

**Thunder-storm,** Before: Sil.
**Walking,** While: Ns.
**Warm room,** in: NM.
**FALLING apart,** as if: Cp.
  **Forward:** Nm.
  **Space** Through, as if: Sil.
  Lying on left side Agg: Sil.
**FALLOPIAN TUBES**
  (Salpingitis): Fp; Km; Sil.
  **Serum** or **pus,** Escapes, from uterus: SIL.
**FALSE Labour** Pains: Kp.
**FALTERING, Hesitates:** Kp; Sil.
**FANATICISM:** KP.
**FANCIES, Absorbed** In: Sil.
  **Evening:** Np; Sil.
  **Exaltation,** of: SIL.
  **Frightful:** SIL.
  **Vivid:** Nm.
  Falling, asleep when: Nm.
**FANNED, As** if: Ns.
**FANNING Agg:** Cp; MP; **SIL.**
**FANNING Amel:** Ks.
**FANTASY:** See Delusions.
**FAR OFF Feeling:** Cp.
**FASTIDIOUS:** Sil.
**FASTING Agg:** Cs; Kp; NP.
  **Amel:** Ks; Nm.
**FATIGUE Agg:** Fp; Kp; Mp.
  **Scientific** labour from: Kp.
**FATS:** See Under Food.
**FATTY DEGENERATION:** Ks.
  **Heart,** of: Kp; Ks.
  **Muscles,** of: Kp.
**FAULT FINDING:** Sil.

**FAVUS:** Km.
**FEAR: CP;** Cs; Fp; Kp; Ks; NM; Np; Ns; Sil.
  **Alone** of being: Kp; Ns.
  Lest he injures himself: Ns.
  **Anxious,** Restless: Nm.
  **Apoplexy,** of: Fp.
  **Bad,** News, of hearing: CP; Np.
  **Crowd,** In a: Fp; Kp; NM; Ns.
  **Dark,** of: Cp; Cs.
  **Death** of: Cs; Fp; Kp; Ks; Nm.
  **Disease** of impending; Kp; Nm; Np.
  **Evil,** of: Cs; FP; Km; Kp; NM; Ns.
  **Falling,** of: Ks; Sil.
  Walking, when: Nm.
  **Financial** loss of: Cf.
  **Future,** of: NM.
  **Getting** up from sitting: Cp.
  **Happen** something, will: Kp; NM; NP.
  **Insanity,** of: Cs; NM.
  **Lightning:** Sil.
  **Lying,** when: Sil.
  **Men,** of: Kp; Nm.
  **Menses,** during: NM.
  **Misfortune,** of: Cf; Cs; Fp; Nm; Np; Ns.
  **Motion,** of: Mp.
  Downward: Sil.
  **Night:** Np.
  **Noise,** From: NS.
  Night: Ns.

  **Palpitation,** with: Nm; Sil.
  **People,** of: Fp; Kp; Ks; NM; Sil.
  **Pins,** Pointed objects: SIL.
  **Places,** Buildings, of: Kp.
  **Pointed** Objects: SIL.
  **Poisoned,** Being: Nm.
  **Poverty** of: Cf.
  **Reason,** loss of: Nm.
  **Recurrent:** Nm.
  **Robbers,** of: NM; Sil.
  **Sleep,** to go to: Nm.
  **Space:** Kp.
  **Suicide,** of: NS.
  **Thunder-storm:** Sil.
  **Touch,** Contact: Mp.
  **Trifles,** of: NM.
  **Undertaking,** of: Sil.
  **Walking** of: Nm.
  **Work,** of: Kp; KS; Nm; Sil.
  Literary: SIL.
**FEATHER, dust:** SIL.
**FEATHER BED** Agg: SIL.
**FEEBLE:** See Weak.
**FEELS too** hot: Ks; Nm.
**FEET:** Sil.
  **Abscess:** Sil.
  **Arches:** Sil.
  **Arthritic** nodosities: Ns.
  **Bunions:** Km; **SIL.**
  **Caries,** of bones: **SIL.**
  **Chilblains,** Suppuration: Sil.
  **Cold** Agg: Sil.
  **Coldness:** Cp; Cs; FP; KM; KP; KS; NM; NP; NS; SIL.

Bed, in: SIL.

Burning, with: Sil.

Day time: SIL.

  burn at night: Np.

Evening: Km; Sil.

Fever, During: Ks.

Headache during: Fp; Nm.

Icy: Np; SIL.

Knees to: Nm.

Left, then right: Sil.

Menses during: Np; **SIL.**

  soles, to: SIL.

Mental exertion, on: Cp; NM; **SIL.**

Right: Nm.

Suppressed foot sweat from: SIL.

Tales, cold through, feet: SIL.

Walking while: Sil.

**Constriction:** Nm.

  Cramp like: NM.

**Convulsions:** NM.

**Dryness:** Sil.

**Edge,** Outer: Ns.

**Emaciation:** Nm.

**Eruptions,** Boils: Sil.

  Herpes: NM.

  Itching: Sil.

  Scabs: SIL.

  Scurfy: SIL.

  Vesicles, black: Nm.

**Fidgety:** Kp; Sil.

**Flat foot** (Broken arches): Cp; Sil.

**Formication:** NM; Np.

  Extending over body: Nm.

**Frost** bitten As if: Kp.

**Heat:** Nm; Np; NS; SIL.

  Burning: NS; Sil.

  Menses, during, at night: Np.

  Evening: Sil.

  Soles, with: Sil.

**Heaviness,** Kp; **NM;** Np; Ns; Sil.

  Menses, during: Nm.

  Standing, while: NM.

  Walking, amel: NM.

**Inflammation:** Sil.

  Dark red: Sil.

  Erysipelatous: Sil.

  Sensation of: Nm.

  Walking, while: Sil.

**Itching:** Nm; Np.

  Back of: Nm; Ns.

  Undressing amel: NS.

  Scratching amel: Ns.

**Jerking:** Ns.

**Lameness:** Sil.

  Pregnancy, during: Sil.

**Motion,** Difficult: Nm.

**Numbness:** Cp; Cs; Fp; Kp; Ks; Nm; Np; SIL.

  Left: Nm.

  Ascending, steps on: Nm.

  Riding, while: CP.

  Sitting: Cp.

**Odour,** offensive, perspiration without: SIL.

**Pain:** Cs; NM; NS; SIL.
  Alternately: Np.
  Back of: Ns; Sil.
  Blow, as of joints: Nm.
  Burning: Cs; Kp; KS; NM; Ns; SIL.
    back of: Sil.
    perspiration, with: SIL.
  Crampy: Cp; Fp; Nm; Np; SIL.
    walking, while: Sil.
  Drawing: Nm; Np; Ns; Sil.
  Extending upward: Nm; SIL.
    tibia to: Ns.
  Gouty: NS.
  Joints, of: Nm; Ns.
  Motion, amel: KS.
  Pressing: Ns.
  Rheumatic: Ns.
  Sciatica, with; Mp.
  Shooting: Fp; Sil.
  Sitting, while: Ns.
  Sore, bruised: Nm; Ns; SIL.
    arch, in: Sil.
    back, of: Sil.
  Sprained, as if: Nm; Sil.
  Standing, agg: Sil.
  Stepping on: Cp; NM.
  Stitching: CP; FP; KS; Nm; Ns; SIL.
  Tearing: Kp; NM; Np; **NS; Sil.**
  Ulcerative: NM; Ns.
  Walking agg: Nm; **SIL.**
    open air, in, amel: Nm.

**Paralysis,** Sensation of: Nm; Sil.
**Perspiration: CS;** Kp; Ks; NM; Np; **SIL.**
  Cold: CS; Km; KP; KS; SIL.
  Constant: SIL.
  Destroys shoes: Sil.
  Excoriating: SIL.
  Menses, after: SIL.
  Offensive: Cs; Nm; **SIL.**
    sour: Nm; Sil.
  Profuse: **SIL.**
  Suppressed: NM; **SIL.**
**Pulsation:** Nm.
**Redness:** SIL.
**Restlessness:** Kp; NM; Ns; Sil.
  Walking, Amel: NM.
**Sensitive:** Cs; Fp; SIL.
**Stiffness:** Cs; Fp.
**Suppuration:** SIL.
**Swelling:** Cs; Fp; Kp; Ks; NM; Np; **SIL.**
  Ascending, while: NM.
  Evening agg and amel: Sil.
  Left: Sil.
  Morning: Sil.
  Oedematous: Cs; NM; NS.
  Red: Sil.
  Right: Kp.
**Tension:** Nm.
**Tickling: SIL.**
**Tingling,** prickling: Cp; Nm; Sil.
**Trembling:** NM.

**Twitching:** Ns; Sil.
  Sleep, during: Ns.
**Ulcers:** Sil.
  Back of: **SIL.**
**Uneasy,** must move constantly: Nm.
**Weakness:** NM; Sil.
  Coition, after: Cp.
  Fever after: Cp.
  Lying, amel: NM.
  Morning: Nm.
  Riding, while, amel: NM.
  Sitting, amel: NM.
  Standing, while: NM.
  Walking, amel: Nm.
**Wetting** of Agg: Nm; **SIL.**
**FELON:** See Fingers, Felon.
**FEMALES affection** as, in General: **CP;** Fp; Kp; NM; SIL.
**After Pains:** Fp; Kp; Mp; NM.
**Coition,** Agg: Fp; Nm.
  Aversion, to: Fp; Kp; Ks; **NM.**
  Menses, after: NM.
  Enjoyment absent: NM.
  Nauseating: Sil.
  Orgasm, Painful: Nm.
  Painful: Fp; NM.
**Conception,** Difficult (Sterility): FP; NM; Np; SIL.
  Acid secretions, vagina from: Np.
  Copious menses, from: NM.
**Conception,** Easy: Nm.
**Crawling:** Cp.

**Desire,** Sexual, diminished: Fp; NM; Sil.
  Increased: CP; KP; Nm; Np; Sil.
  nursing, when: Cp.
  plethora, from: Sil.
  Insatiable: CP.
  menses, after: Kp.
  before: CP.
  Suppressed, ill effects: Kp.
**Desire** Sexual Violent (Nymphomania): CP; SIL.
  Involuntary orgasm, with: Nm.
  Spinal irritation, from: Sil.
**Sterility:** See Conception, Difficult.
  Sycotic: Ns.
  Weakness from: Sil.
**FEMALE ORGANS,** in General: Cp; NM; Sil.
**Disagreeable** Feeling: Sil.
**Dragging:** NM.
**Dryness:** Fp; Nm.
**Fullness:** Cp.
**Hair,** Falling from pubis: **NM.**
**Itching:** **NM;** Sil.
**Labour** like Pains: Cp; Kp; Nm; SIL.
**Labour pains** ceasing: NM.
  Cramps in legs, with: Mp.
  Excessive: Mp.
  False: Kp.
  Ineffectual: Kp.
  Spasmodic: Mp.
  Weak: Cf; Kp; **NM.**

**Lying** Agg: Cp; Km; NM; Ns.
**Lying** on back, Amel: Kp; Nm.
**Pressure** Amel: MP.
On back; Nm.
**Sore,** Sensitive: Cp; Mp; Nm; Sil.
**Swollen:** CP; NM; Ns.
**Thighs,** to: **CP;** Nm.
**Upward:** Cp.
**FEROCIOUS:** NM.
**FESTERING:** Nm; Sil.
**FESTINATION:** Mp.
**FETOR ORIS:** Kp; Nm; **SIL.**
**FEVER: FP:** **NM;** Ns; **SIL.**
**Abscesses,** Multiple, with: Sil.
**Adynamic:** FP; SIL.
**Afternoon** Agg: Km; Nm; Sil.
2 P.M. to 3 P.M.: Km.
**Air,** open Amel: NM.
**Alternating,** with chills: Kp; Nm; Ns; SIL.
With hot twitches: NM.
**Anger,** Brought on by: Nm.
**Autumnal:** NM.
**Before, Agg:** Nm; Sil.
**Bilious:** Mp; NM; Np; NS; Sil.
**Black water:**
**Catarrhal:** FP; Km.
**Cerebro-spinal:** NM; **NS.**
Tubercular: Sil.
**Chicken-pox:** Fp; Km; Nm; Ns; Sil.
**Chills,** Alternating, with: Kp; Nm; Ns; SIL.

Hot twitches, with: NM.
Followed by heat: **NM;** NS; Sil.
then sweat: NM; NS.
with sweat: Nm.
Then heat without thirst: Nm.
Then sweat without intervening heat: Nm.
**Chill,** With: KS; Nm; NS; **SIL.**
Without: FP; Nm.
**Cold,** from taking: NM; SIL.
**Continued,** Typhoid etc.: Fp; Km; Nm; KP; Ks; SIL.
Abdominal, icterus, with: NS.
**Coughing Agg:** Nm.
**Covers** warmth Agg: Nm.
**Day,** Evening, Agg: Sil.
Every: Nm.
**Dentition,** During: Fp; **SIL.**
**Descending:** Cp.
**Drinking,** warm Agg: Nm; Sil.
**Dry,** Burning: Cp; Fp; Kp; Ks; Ns; Sil.
**During,** Agg: Nm.
**Dysenteric:** Fp.
**Evening,** Lasting All night: Sil.
**External** Heat: **SIL.**
**Forenoon,** 11 A.m.: Nm.
Thirst and chilliness with: Sil.
**Gastric:** Fp; Km; Kp; Ks; Ns.
**Hectic:** CP; **CS;** Fp; KP; KS; **SIL.**

High, Hyperpyrexia: **NM; Ns; SIL.**
Delirium, with: **NM.**
Sleep, during: NM.
Stupefaction and unconsciousness: **NM.**
**Inflammatory:** Fp; Sil.
**Influenza:** FP; Sil.
Weakness, after: Kp.
**Intermittent** (Malaria): CP; Cs, **KS;** Mp; **NM; NS;** SIL.
Chronic inveterate: NM.
Enlarged, liver and spleen, with: Nm.
Long lasting hea' with: Sil.
Quartan: **NM.**
Quotidian: **NM.**
Spoiled: Nm.
Stage, partial irregular: Nm.
Tertian: **NM;** Sil.
**Internal heat:** FP; Kp; SIL.
Blood vessels, In: Nm.
**Irritative:** Nm.
**Long** Lasting: Cf; Nm; Sil.
**Manual Labour** Agg: Nm.
**Measles:** FP; Km; KS; Sil.
**Menses,** Before, and during Agg: Nm.
Suppressed: Sil.
**Mental** Exertion Agg: Sil.
Amel: Nm.
**Milk** (Lactation): **SIL.**
**Morning:** Nm.
9 A.M. to 12 Noon: Km.
and 5 P.M.: Km.

**Night** Agg: Ks; Sil.
**Noon:** Km; Sil.
**Pain,** in general, during: Sil.
**Paroxysms,** Increasing in severity: NM.
**Perspiration,** Absent: Kp; KS; Nm; Sil.
With: Nm; Np; NS.
**Puerperal:** Fp; Km; KP; Sil.
Vulvitis, with: NS.
**Remittent:** NS.
**Room,** in Amel: Sil.
**Rubbing,** Amel: Nm.
**Scarlet:** Fp; Km; Kp; Ks; Nm; Sil.
**Septic:** Fp; Km; **KP;** Sil.
**Shivering,** with: Mp.
**Shuddering,** with: Nm.
**Sleep,** during, Agg: Nm; Np; SIL.
**Small-pox:** Cs; Km; Kp; NM; Sil.
Black: Sil.
**Storm,** Approach, of Agg: Sil.
**Subnormal,** Persistent: Kp.
**Summer,** Hot Season, Agg: Nm.
**Thermic:** NM; **SIL.**
**Uncovering** Agg: Ns; SIL.
Amel: Nm.
**Urethral:** Sil.
**Warm room,** Agg: Nm.
**Washing** Agg: Sil.
**Worms,** From: Sil.
**Yellow:** Fp; Kp; NS.
**Zymotic:** **KP;** Ks.

---

**FIBROIDS: CF;** CP; CS; SIL.
**FIBROUS TISSUE,** Ligaments: Cf; KM; SIL.
**FICKLE** (Inconstant, Irresolute): Cf; Cp; Cs; Km; Kp; Ks; NM; SIL.
    **Ideas,** In: Nm.
**FIDGETY:** Kp; Sil.
**FIGWARTS:** NS; SIL.
**FILM:** Km; Nm.
**FILTHY, Untidy,** Dirty: Sil.
**FINANCIAL Loss Agg:** Cf.
**FINE,** Sensation as of a hair or thread: NM; Np; **SIL.**
**FINGERS:** SIL.
    **Around:** Cp.
      Ulceration: Sil.
    **Atrophy:** Sil.
    **Blue:** Nm; SIL.
    **Burning:** SIL.
      Third, middle joint: Np; Sil.
    **Chapped: NM.**
      About, the nails: **NM.**
    **Chilblains:** Fp; Km; Kp; Sil.
    **Children,** Put in mouth: Cp.
    **Clenched:** MP.
      Epilepsy, During: MP.
    **Clubbing:** Cf; SIL.
    **Coldness,** Chill during: NM.
    **Contraction:** Fp; SIL.
      Epilepsy, during: MP.
      Flexor muscles: SIL.
      Second finger: Sil.
      Spasmodic: MP.
    **Convulsions:** Nm.

**Cracks:** Nm; Sil.
    Nails, around: Nm.
**Cramps:** NM.
    First finger: Np.
    Playing piano or violin: MP.
    Writing, while: MP.
**Desquamation:** Nm.
**Discolouration,** Dark: Nm.
    Easy: Cf.
    Spots: Sil.
**Dryness:** Nm; SIL.
**Emaciated:** Sil.
**Eruptions:** KS; Sil.
    Boils; Sil.
    Eczema: Sil.
    Phagedenic blisters: sil.
    Rash: Sil.
    Vesicles: KS; NM; Ns; Sil.
      first finger: Sil.
      ulcer, becoming: Sil.
**Felon,** Panaritium: **NS;** SIL.
    Chronic tendency: Sil.
    Cold water Amel: NS.
    Deep: SIL.
    Injury, from: Ns.
    Parturition, after: Sil.
**Formication:** NM; SIL.
**Hair,** on, as if: Nm.
**Helplessness:** SIL.
**Inflammation:** Nm; SIL.
    Nails around: NM; NS.
**Itching:** Nm; Sil.
**Joints:** Cf; Nm.
    Boring, in: Ns.
    Closing Agg: Nm.

Distorted: **CP; CS;** NM; NS; SIL.

Drawing, in: NS; Sil.

Inflammation: Np.

Knuckles: Nm.

Pain: Nm; Np; Ns.

Paralysis: SIL.

Pressing: Ns.

Sore: Nm.

Sprains: Cp.

Swollen: Cs; Ns.

Tens on: NM.

**Lameness:** Km.

**Middle:** Nm.

**Nails:** See Nails.

**Nodes:** Km.

**Numbness:** Fp; Nm; Np; SIL.

First, second, third, fourth: Nm.

Night at, waking on: Nm.

**Pain:** Cp; Cs; Ns; SIL.

Ball of: Cp.

Cramps: MP.

Drawing: Ns, SIL.

elbow to: Nm.

First, finger: Np; S!L.

Fourth, finger: Cp; Np.

Paralytic: SIL.

Pressing: Ns.

Rheumatic, heart goes to: Np.

Shooting: Np.

Sore, bruised: Nm.

**Paralysis:** Cp; Sil.

Sensation of: Nm.

Pulsation: Nm; Ns.

**Sensitive:** Nm.

**Skin,** Tight: Mp.

**Stiffness:** Cs; Nm; Ns; **SIL.**

**Stitching:** NM; Np; Ns; Sil.

Ball of: SIL.

Splint, as from: Sil.

Twitching: Ns.

**Suppuration** Last finger: Ns.

**Swelling:** Cs; Np; Ns; Sil.

**Tearing:** Cp; Kp; Nm; Np; Ns; Sil.

Spinning, Agg: Ns.

Ulcerative: **SIL.**

**Tingling,** Prickling: Cs; **NM; SIL.**

**Tips:** CP.

Burn: Nm.

Cracks: Nm; Sil.

Dry, as if made of paper: SIL.

Formication: **NM;** Ns.

Itching: Nm.

Numbness: Kp; Mp; Nm.

Pain: Nm.

Pulsation: Ns.

Sensitive: Cp.

Sore: Cp.

Stiffness: Mp.

Stitching: Cp; Nm; NS.

Suppuration, as if: Sil.

Tingling: Nm; NS.

Warts on: NS.

**Trembling:** Nm.

**Twitching:** Sil.

**Ulcers:** Nm; Sil.
Nails, around: NS; **SIL.**
**Warts:** NM; NS; Sil.
**Weakness: NM.**
Drops, things: NM; SIL.
grasping, when: SIL.
**Working** with, Grasping, sewing, etc. Agg: Cp; MP; NM; SIL.
**Writing** Agg: Mp.
**FIRE LIKE:** Cp; Nm; Sil.
**FISHY:** Nm; Ns.
**FISSURE:** Cf; Sil.
**FISTULA:** Cf; Cp; Ns; **SIL.**
**Chest** Symptoms, with: Cp; Sil.
**Glands,** of: SIL.
**FITFUL, changing** Moods: Cs; Sil.
**FIXED IDEAS:** NM; SIL.
**FLABBY FEELING:** CP; Cs; Kp; Ks; Sil.
**FLACCID:** Cp; Kp.
**FLATULENCE:** Cf; CP; **CS;** Fp; Km; Kp; KS; NM; Np; **NS; SIL.**
**Abdomen,** Lower in: Nm; Sil.
Right side: NS.
Left side: Nm.
**Bath,** After: Cs.
**Breakfast** after: Np; NS.
**Confinement,** after: Ns.
**Eating,** after: Cs; Kp; Np.
**Evening:** Cf.
**Here** and **There:** Nm; Ns.
**Hysterical:** Kp.

**Lying,** Amel: Cf.
**Menses,** During: Kp.
**Milk,** After: Ns.
**Morning: NS.**
**Night,** Preventing sleep: Km.
Colicky pain, with: Mp; Ns.
**Noisy,** Rumbling: Nm; **NS; SIL.**
**Obstructed;** CP; KP; Ks; NM; Np; NS; **SIL.**
**Offensive:** Nm; Sil.
Morning: NS.
**Painful:** Mp; NS.
**Passes,** Constantly: Mp.
**Pregnancy,** in: Cf; Cp.
**Pressing,** Rectum, on: Ns.
**Pushing:** NS.
**Riding** In carriage: Cf.
**Stool,** After: Cs.
During: Nm; Ns.
**Wandering:** Nm; Sil.
**FLATUS Discharge** of: FP; KP; KS; NM; NP; **NS; SIL.**
**Afraid** To pass lest feces escape: Nm; Np; Ns.
**Copious:** NM; Mp.
**Cutting,** Pain, with: SIL.
**Diarrhea,** During: Cp; Np; **NS;** Sil.
**Difficult:** Cp; Ns; Sil.
**Drinking,** After: Cp; Nm.
**Headache,** During: Cp; Nm.
**Hot:** Fp.
**Loud:** Kp; **NS.**
Sputtering: **NS.**
Stool, during: **NS.**

**Motion,** from: Nm; **SIL.**
**Offensive:** CP; KP; Ks; **NM;**
  **NS; SIL.**
  Sour: Nm.
  Spoiled eggs: Nm.
  Sulphurous: Ks.
**Passing, Amel:** NS.
**Pinching,** with: Sil.
**Rarely:** SIL.
**Stool,** Before: Nm.
  During: **NS.**
**Stool,** Urging to but only
  flatus is passed: **NS.**
**Walking,** While Agg and Amel:
  Sil.
**FLEETING Pains:** MP.
**FLESHY:** See Excrescences.
**FLOATING, Flying,** As if: Cs;
  NM.
**FLOWING,** like water, as if: Sil.
**FLUIDITY:** See Secretions, in-
  creased.
**FLUSHES:** Cs; Ks; Nm; **NS.**
**FLUTTERING:** Cs; KP; **NM;**
  **NS.**
**FLYING to pieces:** Sil.
**FOAMY, frothy;** NM; Ns; **SIL.**
**FOETID:** See Offensive.
**FOETUS Lying crosswise:**
  **Movements,** as if:
    Cause nausea and vomit-
      ing:
    Disturb sleep:
    Lively:
    Painful: SIL.
    Violent: Sil.

**FOGS** (Cloudy Weather): CP;
  CS; MP; **NS;** SIL.
**FONTANELLES Open** (Tardy
  Closure): **CP; SIL.**
  **Across** the Eyes: Kp.
**FOOD & DRINKS Agg** & **Amel**
  **Acid:** See Sour.
  **Alcoholic Agg:** Km; NM;
  **All Disagree:** Fp; Np.
  **Artificial:** Cp.
  **Beans,** Peas **Agg:** NM; Sil.
  **Beer Agg:** Km; Sil.
    Amel: Np.
  **Bitter** Agg: Np.
  **Bread** Agg: Nm.
    Black, Agg: Nm.
    Butter and Agg: Nm.
  **Butter** Agg: Nm; Np.
  **Cabbage** Agg: Nm; Ns; Sil.
  **Cake** Agg: Fp; Km.
  **Cereals** Agg: **NM;** Ns.
  **Coffee** Agg: CP; Fp; Nm; Ns.
    Cold, Amel: NM; Sil.
    odour of Agg: NM.
  **Cold Drinks** Agg: Cf; CP;
    Km; Kp; MP; Np; SIL.
    Coffee Amel: NM; Sil.
    Food Agg: Cf; CP; Km; Nm;
      Np; NS; **SIL.**
  **Condiments:** CP; Nm; NP.
  **Dry:** Sil.
  **Farinaceous: NM; NS.**
  **Fats:** Fp; Km; NP.
  **Fish** Agg: NS.
    Herring: Fp; Nm.

**Flatulent:** Nm; Ns; Sil.
**Frozen,** Ice Agg: CP.
**Fruits:** Cp; Np; **NS.**
**Hot** Agg: Ns.
  Amel: MP.
**Ice:** CP.
**Legumes** (Beans): NM; Sil.
**Liquids** Agg: NM; SIL.
**Maple sugar:** Cs.
**Meat:** Fp; SIL.
  Smoked: SIL.
**Melons:** Ns.
**Milk** Agg: **CS;** Kp; Mp; NM;
  NP; NS; SIL.
**Onions:** K౦.
**Pastry:** Km; Ns.
**Pork:** NM.
**Potatoes:** NS.
**Raw:** Sil.
**Rich:** KM; Nm; NS.
**Salt** Agg: **NM;** SIL.
  Amel: Nm.
**Sight** or Smell Agg: Sil.
**Smoked:** SIL.
**Sour:** Fp; Mp; Nm; NP.
**Sourkraut** Agg: Nm.
**Starchy:** Ns.
**Sweets,** Sugar Agg: Np.
**Tea** Agg: Fp; Nm.
**Thought** of Agg: NM.
**Tobacco** Agg: **NM;** SIL.
**Uncooked** (Raw): Sil.
**Vegetables** Green Agg: NS.
  Raw: Sil.
**Vinegar:** Nm; Np.

**Warm** Agg: Nm; Sil.
**FOOLISH:** Cp; Sil.
**FORCED, APART:** Cp; Nm; Sil.
  **Out,** As if: Km; NM; SIL.
**FORCEPS delivery,** After: Kp;
  Sil.
**FORE ARMS Left:** Ns.
  **Compression:** Ns.
  **Contraction,** wrist, near: Sil.
  **Eruptions,** Boils: NS; Sil.
    Eczema: SIL.
    Herpes: NM.
    Pimples: Cp; Nm; NS.
      burning, itching: Sil.
    Urticaria: NM; Sil.
    Vesicles: Sil.
      burning: Sil.
  **Hanging** Down Amel: Sil.
  **Heaviness:** Nm.
  **Induration:** SIL.
  **Lameness:** Nm; Sil.
  **Motion** of Agg: Nm.
  **Numb:** Km; NM.
  **Pain:** Cs; MP; Nm; Ns; Sil.
    Aching: Cp; Sil.
    Broken as if: Cp.
    Burning: Nm; NS.
    Cramps: Cp.
    Drawing: Cp; MP; Nm; Np.
    anterior part: Ns.
    downward, extend: Nm.
    left: Sil.
    Extending to extensor: Sil.
    radius, to, hanging down
    agg: Nm.

tendons, to: Sil.
ulna, to: Cs.
Jerking: Sil.
Paralytic: Sil.
Pinching: Nm.
Pressing: Ns.
Sitting while agg: Ns.
Sore, bruised: Cp; Sil.
radius, to: SIL.
Stitching: SIL.
Tearing: Cp; Kp; Nm; **NS;** SIL.
ulna to near elbow: Sil.
Warmth Amel: Sil.
Writing, Agg: **MP.**
**Paralysis:** Cp; **SIL.**
Left: Cp.
**Sinking** Down: Nm.
**Spots:** Nm.
Purple: Kp.
**Swelling:** FP.
Nodular: Nm.
Red: SIL.
**Tension,** Extensors in, while writing: **MP.**
**Tingling:** Sil.
**Trembling,** Concomitant: CP.
**Twitching:** Nm; Sil.
**Weakness:** Nm.
Right: Sil.
**FORBODINGS:** NM; SIL.
**FOREHEAD:** CS; KP; **NM; SIL.**
**Aching:** Cp; Kp; **NM; SIL.**
**Acne: SIL.**
**Adhesion** of Skin: SIL.

**Band,** Constriction: Mp; NS.
**Brown,** Yellow: Kp.
At the edge of hair: Kp; Nm.
**Crawling:** Cs; SIL.
**Eyes,** or Temples, to: Kp.
**Formication:** Cs; Fp; Nm; SIL.
**Frowning:** Nm.
**Heat,** Burning: Nm; Sil.
**Jaw,** Lower to: Nm.
**Nose** to: Cp.
**Occiput** to: Kp; Nm.
**Pimples:** Cp; Nm; NP.
Red: Nm.
**Pustules:** Kp; Nm.
**Sweat,** Cold: Kp.
**Swelled:** Sil.
**Veins:** Cf.
**Vesicles:** Nm.
**Weight,** In, As if: NM; Sil.
**Wrinkled:** Kp; NM; Sil.
Brain symptoms, With: KP.
Chest symptoms, With: Sil.
Headache, during: Nm.
**FOREIGN BODIES:** Cf; Sil.
**FORGETFUL:** CP; Cs; FP; KP; KS; NM; NP; Sil.
**Dampness,** Exposure, from: Sil.
**Eating,** after: Nm.
**Eating,** Amel: Sil.
**Mental,** Exertion from: Nm.
**Sexual** Excess, after: NP.
**Words,** of, while speaking: Kp; NM.

**FORGETS Errand** etc.: See Memory, Weak

**FORGOTTEN Something** Constantly as if, he had: Nm.

**FORMICATION Crawling:** Cp; Cs; Fp; Ks; Nm; Np; SIL.

**Bad** News, after: Cp.

**From feet,** upwards: Nm.

**FRACTURES:** CP; **SIL.**

**FRAGILE:** CP; SIL.

**FRAIL AS** if body were: CP; KP; Nm; NP; Ns; SIL.

**FRIGHT** (See Fear): Cp; KP; Nm; Sil.

**FRIGHTENED Easily:** KP; Ks; NM; Np; SIL.

**Feeling,** As if she had been: Cp.

**Night: NM.**

**Trifles,** At: Ks.

**Waking,** On; Mp.

**FROST Air Agg:** Nm; NS; SIL.

**FROTHY, foamy:** NM; Ns; SIL.

**FULLNESS:** Km; Nm; Sil.

**FUNGUS GROWTH:** See Excrescences.

**FURIBUND** (Delirium Maniacal): Nm.

**FURRY** (Coated): Nm.

**FURY** (Rage): Nm.

**Headache,** with: Nm.

**FUSS, Aversion** for: Nm.

**FUSSY:** Cp.

**GAGGING Retching:** Cp.

**Breakfast,** After: Cp.

**Gulping,** Of white mucus with: Km.

**GAIT Anxious:** Nm.

**Falls,** Easily: Nm.

**Gallinaceous,** Ambulatory: Mp; **SIL.**

**Infirm:** MP.

**Slovenly:** Sil.

**Stooped,** Bent: Nm.

**Stumbles** Easily: Kp.

**Unsteady:** Np.

Backwards: Sil.

**GALL BLADDER:** Mp; Ns.

**Clawing:** NS.

**Crawling:** Ns.

**Stones:** Mp; **NS.**

Colic: NS.

Prevent formation: Cp.

**GANGLIA** (Bursae): Cf; Km; **NM; SIL.**

**GANGRENE:** Fp; Kp; Sil.

**Blue** Part, threatened with: Sil.

**Cold:** Sil.

**Mustard** Application, from: Cp.

**GARLICKY Odour,** Taste etc.: KP.

**GASTRIC FEVER:** Fp; Km; KP; Ks; Ns.

**GASTRIC ULCER:** Kp; NM; Np; NS; Sil.

**GASTRITIS:** Fp; Ks.

**Alcoholic:** Km.

**Chronic:** Sil.

**Enteritis,** With: Fp; Km; Kp; Ks; SIL.

Hot, Drinks, from: Km.
GATHERED, Together: See Constriction.
GAY: See Cheerful.
GENITALS (Both sexes): Cp; Fp; NM; SIL.
Burning: Cp; NM; Ns; Sil.
Cold: Nm.
Crawling: Cp.
Eruption: Nm; Np; Ns; Sil.
Fumbles: Kp; Sil.
Inflamed: Fp; Kp; Mp; NM; Sil.
Itching: KS; NM; NS; SIL.
Offensive: KP; SIL.
Sensitive: KP; NM; SIL.
Sweat, Moisture, on: CP; SIL.
Thighs Down: Nm.
Varicose: Cf.
Weakness, stool, after: Cp.
GENTLE (See Timid): Kp.
GESTICULATES Convulsively: Ns.
GESTURES, Makes (See Grasping): Cp; Kp.
Ridiculous: Kp.
GHOSTS: Ks; Nm; SIL.
GIDDY: See Vertigo
GIRDLE Pains: Km; KS; SIL.
GLABELLA Puffy: Sil.
GLANDERS: Sil.
GLANDS: Cs; Km; Kp; SIL.
Abscess: CS; SIL.
Atrophy: Kp; Sil.
Cervical: Km; SIL.

Constriction: Nm; Sil.
Fistulae: SIL.
Hard: Cf; Sil.
Inflamed: Kp; SIL.
Inguinal (Bubo): Km; SIL.
Itching: SIL.
Mesenteric Enlarged: Ns.
Hardness: NS.
Pulsation: Cp.
Tabes mesenteric: CP; CS; NS.
diarrhoea with: Cp.
Numbness: Sil.
Pain: Ks; NM; Sil.
Pulsation: SIL.
Sensitive: Sil.
Stitching: NM; Sil.
Submental: Sil.
Suppuration: CS; SIL.
Ulcerative: Sil.
GLANS: See Penis.
GLAUCOMA: NM; SIL.
Coition, After: SIL.
GLEET: CP; Cs; Fp; Km; Ks; NM; NS.
GLISTENING: Cf; Nm; Sil.
GLOBUS, Hystericus: Cs; FP; Ks; NM; Np; SIL.
GLOOMY: See Sadness.
GLOSSITIS: See Inflammation, Tongue.
GLOTTIS, Spasms of (Laryngismus Stridulus): CF; CP; Fp.
GLUEY: Km; Ks; Nm.

**GLUTTONY:** CP; CS; NM; NP; SIL.

**GNAWING:** KS; NS; Sil.

**GODLESS,** Want of Religious feeling: Kp.

**GOITRE:** CF; CS; Mp; NM; NP; NS; SIL.

**Constriction:** CS.

**Exophthalmic:** Fp; Km; NM.

**Heart:** Fp; Nm.

**Right** Sided: Ks; Sil.

**GONORRHEA:** CS; FP; KS; NM; **NS;** SIL.

**Chronic:** CP; CS; KS; **NM;** SIL.

**Ill effects** of: **KS;** NS; SIL.

**Suppressed:** NM.

**GOOSE SKIN:** NM; Ns.

**GOSSIPING:**

**GOUT:** CP; CS; Fp; Kp; NM; Np; NS; SIL.

**GRANULAR APPEARANCE:** Nm.

**GRANULATIONS Exuberant:** Cs; Km; SIL.

**Poor:** Sil.

**Warty:** Sil.

**GRASPING Agg:** MP; Nm; Ns; Sil.

**Cold** objects: NM; Sil.

**GRAY, Dirty** (Skin, Discharges, etc.): KM; Sil.

**GREESY Oily** (Skin, Discharges, etc.): Kp; NM; Sil.

**GREEDY, Avaricious:** Cf.

**GREEN, Greenish:** (Discharges, etc.): **CP;** Km; Nm; NP; **NS.**

**Turns:** Cf; NS.

**GRIEF:** NM.

**Ailments,** from: CP; Kp; **NM.**

**Boisterous:** Nm.

**Cannot,** Cry, from: NM.

**Condition,** About his future: NM.

**Financial** Loss, from: Cf.

**Prolonged:** Nm.

**Silent:** NM.

**GRIMACES:**

**GRINDING Pain:** NM; SIL.

**Teeth** of, during sleep: Kp; Np.

**GRIPING Pain:** MP.

**GRISLY:** Sil.

**GRIT want** of: Sil..

**GRITTY feeling:** Nm.

**GROANING:** Nm.

**GROPING In** The Dark:

**GROUND** or **Stair** come up to meet him: Sil.

**GROWING Pains:** CP; Sil.

**GROWLING:** Km.

**GROWTH Affected:** CP; SIL.

**GROWTHS New** (Tumours): See Excrescenses, Cysts, Tumours.

**GRUMBLING, His** Value is not understood: Cs.

**GUILT sense** of: Sil.

**Crime,** of: Fp; Nm; Sil.

**Trifles,** About: Sil.

**GULLET:** See Oesophagus.

**GUMMATA, Nodes:** Cf; Sil.

**GUMS Abscesses:** SIL.

    Recurrent: SIL.

**Aphthae: NM.**

**Bleeding:** Cs; Fp; Km; KP; Ns; **NM;** Ns; SIL.

    Cleaning when: Cs.

    Easily: KP; NM.

    Scurvy: NM.

**Blisters** On: Ns.

**Boils:** Cf; Cs; Km; NM; Np; Ns; **SIL.**

    Before pus begins: Km.

**Burn** like fire: Ns.

**Coldness,** Upper: Sil.

**Detached,** from teeth: KP; NS.

**Epulis:** NM.

**Excrescences:** Nm.

**Fistula:** NM; **SIL.**

**Grass** at: Sil.

**Inflammation:** Cp; Fp; NM; **SIL.**

**Nodosities:** Ns.

**Pain:** SIL.

    Burning: NS; **SIL.**

    eating when: Nm.

    Cold air agg: SIL.

    Pressing: SIL.

    Sore: Cs; Nm; **SIL.**

        cold and warmth agg: **NM.**

    Touched when: Sil.

    Ulcerative: SIL.

**Pustules:** Ns.

**Putrid:** Nm.

**Receding:** KP; NS.

**Red:** Fp; Kp; Ns.

**Scorbutic,** Spongy: Km; **KP;** Ns.

**Seem** Bright: Kp.

**Sensitive:** NM.

**Spongy:** Kp.

**Squeezed** Feeling: Nm.

**Suppuration:** Ns; Sil.

**Swelling:** CS; Fp; Kp; **NM;** Ns; SIL.

    Bluish red spongy between **lower** incisors, **begins on** left and extends to right, bleeds often: Nm.

    Decayed teeth, around: Cs.

    Extraction of teeth after: Sil.

    Movable: Ns.

    Painful: Sil.

    Painless: Ns.

    Shifting: Ns.

**Tumours** painless, movable: Ns.

    In place of two bicuspids: **SIL.**

**Ulcers: NM;** Np; SIL.

**Vesicles:** Ns; **SIL.**

**GURGLING** (Meteorism): Fp; NM; Np; SIL.

    **Gushing** Stools, then: Ns.

    **Motion,** Amel: Nm.

**GUSHING:** Cf; Cp; Mp; **NM; NS;** Sil.

**HABITS Intemperate Agg:** Km; Kp; NM; SIL.
**Dirty:** Sil.
**HACKING Cough:** CF; Cp; Cs; Fp; Kp; Ks; **NM;** Np; SIL.
**Stool:** Np.
**HAEMATEMESIS:** Cs; FP; Km; Kp; Np; Ns; **SIL.**
**Blood,** Clotted: Km.
Dark: Km.
**Menses,** Suppressed, during: Nm.
**HAEMATOCELE:** Cf; CS; SIL.
**HAEMATODES:** NM; **SIL.**
**HAEMATOMA:** Cf: Sil.
**HAEMATURIA:** Fp; KM; NM; Sil.
**HAEMOPHILIA:** Kp; Ns; Sil.
**HAEMOPTYSIS:** See Expectoration, Bloody.
**HAEMORRHAGE: CS;** FP; KP; **NM;** SIL.
**Acrid:** Sil.
**Blood,** Does not coagulate: KP; Nm.
**Clotted:** Cs; Sil.
Quickly: Km.
**Dark,** Thick: Km.
**Orifices,** from: Fp.
**Passive,** Oozing: Fp.
**Streaked:** Sil.
**HAEMORRHAGE** (Bleeding) **Agg:** Nm.
**Amel:** Fp.
**HAEMORRHOIDS:** See Piles.

**HAIR: NM;** SIL.
**Baldness:** SIL.
Spots, in: Sil.
Young people, in: Sil.
**Blonde:** Sil.
**Falling:** Fp; Kp; **KS; NM;** Np; **SIL.**
Bregma, from: Nm.
Bunches, in: Cp.
Children, in: Nm.
Combing, Agg: Sil.
Forehead: NM; Sil.
Headache, after: Sil.
Lactation, during: Nm.
Occiput: Sil.
Parturition after: NM; Sil.
Pubes, from: Nm.
Spots, in: NM.
Temples: Nm.
**Grey,** Early: NM; Sil.
**Letting** Down, **Amel:** Km; Kp.
**Margins,** Edge, at: Kp; Nm.
Brown stripe: Kp.
**Painful:** Cp; Nm.
Combing, when: Fp; Ns.
Touched, when: Nm; Ns.
**Sticks,** Together: NM.
**Tangled,** Tousy: Nm.
**HAIR Combing,** or Brushing **Agg:** Sil.
**Cutting Agg:** Ns.
**Touching Agg:** Nm; Ns.
**HAIR, Sensation** of: NM; Np; **SIL.**
**HALITOSIS Offensive**

Breath: Cs; **KP;** Ks; **NM;** NS; Sil.

**Morning:** Sil.

**HALLUCINATIONS:** See Delusions.

**HAMMERING:** Nm; SIL.

**HAMSTRINGS, Short:** CP; **NM;** Np.

**Menses,** After: Np.

**HANDS, Laying** on part **Amel:** Nm; Ns.

**HANDS Awkwardness:** Cs; Sil.

Drops, things: Nm.

**Back** of: Km; NM.

**Blood,** Rushes to: Ns.

**Brittle** Skin: NM.

**Brownish** Spots: Kp; Nm.

**Burning:** See Heat.

**Callosities:** Cf; Nm; Sil.

**Chapped,** Fissured: NM; SIL.

**Coldness: CP;** Cs; **FP; KM; KP;** Ks; **NM; NP;** Ns; Sil.

Chill, during: Sil.

Water, in: Mp.

**Contraction:** Sil.

**Cracked** Skin: Ks; **NM; SIL.**

**Cracking** of tendons on back of: Km.

**Cramps:** Mp; NM; Np; Sil.

Exertion on: SIL.

Grasping cold, o..: Nm.

Left: Np.

Writing: **MP;** NP; Sil.

**Desquamation: NM.**

**Dryness:** CP; NM.

**Eruptions:** KS; NM; NS.

Back of, on: KS.

pimples: Cp.

pustules: SIL.

vesicles: KS.

**Boils:** Cs.

**Brown:** Nm.

**Eczema:** SIL.

Elevated: Nm.

Herpes: Nm.

Moist: Ks.

Pustules: Nm.

Urticaria: NM; Ns.

whitish: Nm.

Vesicles: KS; NM; NS; SIL.

corroding: Sil.

denuded spots, on: Nm.

phagedenic: Sil.

**Formication,** In back of: Nm.

**Fullness:** Ns.

Knitting, while: Ns.

**Heat:** Fp; KP; Ks; Nm; NP; Ns; Sil.

Bed, in: Sil.

Cold, during: Ns.

Left: Nm.

Reading, while: Fp.

**Heaviness:** Nm; Sil.

**Inflammation:** Nm; SIL.

**Itching:** KS; Sil.

Back, of: Ns.

Rubbing, after: Nm.

**Jerking:** Nm.

**Lameness:** Nm; Ns; **SIL.**

Exertion, after: SIL.

Writing, while: SIL.

**Motion,** Convulsive, involuntary: NM.

**Numbness:** Cp; Cs; Fp; Kp; Ks; NM; SIL.

Lying on, or on hard substance: Nm.

Motion, Amel: Nm.

Putting in pockets: Nm.

Right: Kp; Nm.

**Pain:** Cp; Ns.

Aching: Cp.

Burning: Cs; KS; Nm; Np; Ns.

back of: Ns.

nettles as from: Nm.

Drawing: Np; Ns; SIL.

cramp like: SIL.

arms or fingers to: Ns.

joints, in: Np; Ns.

Extending, joints to: Ns.

Grasping anything: NS.

Morning agg: Sil.

pressing: Nm; Ns; Sil.

ulnar side: Ns.

Shooting: Cs.

Sitting, while agg: Ns.

Sore, bruised: Cp; Nm; Sil.

Sprained as if: Sil.

Stitching: Cs; Nm; NS; Sil.

ball of: Sil.

fine: Nm.

itching: Nm.

Tearing: Cp; Kp; Nm; **NS;** SIL.

ball of: Sil.

between second and third finger: Ns.

Walking, while agg: Ns.

Waters, in agg: Mp; Nm.

Writing, while: **MP;** SIL.

**Paralysis:** Cp; Nm; SIL.

Left: Cp.

Sensation of: Ns; Sil.

**Perspiration:** CS; NM; Np; **SIL.**

Cold: CS.

Copious: **SIL.**

Offensive: SIL.

**Prickling:** Kp.

**Pulsation,** Back of: Ns.

Motion, Amel: Ns.

**Purple** Spots: Kp.

**Red:** Ns.

Spots: Nm.

**Restlessness:** Cs; Nm.

**Skin,** Brittle: NM.

Cracked: Ks; NM; **SIL.**

Hard and rough: Nm.

Withered: Nm.

**Stiffness:** CS; Sil.

Nodular: Nm.

Right: Nm.

**Tension:** Prickling: Cp; Nm; Ns.

Night: Sil.

**Trembling: CP;** CS; KP; Ks; MP; **NM;** Np; Ns; SIL.

Concomitant as a: Cp.

Emotions, from: Nm.

Headache, with: Cp.

Holding objects, on: SIL.
Manual labour: Sil.
News unpleasant: Nm.
Pains, during: Cp.
Rubbing, Amel: NM.
Sitting, while: Sil.
Taking hold on: SIL.
Threading, needle when: SIL.
Using them, from: SIL.
Vomiting, with: Cp.
Waking, on: Ns.
Writhing while: NM; NP; Ns; SIL.
**Tumours:** Sil.
**Twitching:** Nm; Ns.
Sleep, during: Ns.
**Ulcers:** Sil.
**Warts:** Kp; NM; Ns; Sil.
**Weakness:** Nm; Np; NS; Sil.
Grasping objects, on: Nm; Ns.
Lying on hard substance: Nm.
Night, after fever: Ns.
Paralytic: SIL.
Writing, when: Sil.
**Wens:** Sil.
**Writing,** when, cramps: **MP;** Np; Sil.
Lameness: SIL.
Pain: **MP;** SIL.
Trembling: NM; NP; Ns; SIL.
Weakness: Sil.

**Yellow:** Ns; SIL.
**HANGING DOWN limbs**
**Agg:** MP; Nm.
**Amel:** Nm; SIL.
**HAPPY seeing others**
**Agg:** CS.
**HARD BED sensation:** FP; SIL.
Parts Feel soft: Ns.
**HARDNESS induration:** CF; KM; SIL.
Injury, after: Cf.
Pressure, Constant, from: SIL.
Stony, hard: Cf; Km.
**HARSH:** Cs; Nm.
**HASTE:** See Hurry.
**HATRED** (Cruelty, Malice): Cs; Kp; NM.
Husband and baby of: Kp.
Persons, of who had offended: Nm.
who do not agree with him: Cs.
**HAUGHTY:**
**HAUTEUR** Pride, Arrogance:
**HAWKING:** Cf; Cp; Kp; Ks; NM; Np; NS; SIL.
Agg: Sil.
Amel:
Breakfast, after: Cp.
Bitter: Nm.
Drawn From posterior nares: Nm.
Eating, Agg: Sil.
Lumps, Cheesy: KM; Kp; SIL.

Foul: Km; Kp; Ns; Sil.
yellow beads: Sil.
Greenish: Fp; Sil.
Gluey, viscid: Nm; Ns.
**Salty:** Nm.
**Singing,** Before: Cp.
**Sleep,** during: Cp.
**Sweetish:** Mp.
**Talking** While: Cp.
**Vomiting,** with: Cp.
**HAY FEVER:** Kp; Ns; Sil.
**HEAD Affections** in General:
CS; MP; NM; SIL.
**One sided: KP;** NM; SIL.
Alternating: Nm; Sil.
Begins on one goes to other
and Agg: Nm.
Left: Cp; Nm; Ns; Sil.
Right: Nm; Sil.
**Absent** As if:
**Abdominal** Irritation from: Sil.
**Aching:** See Pain
**Air Cold Amel:** Fp; Ks.
Open Amel: KP; KS; NM;
Np.
**Air wind** Through: **NM.**
Blowing on or Flowing, night:
Sil.
**Alive as if** in: Sil.
While walking: Sil.
**Alternating, Arms** Pain in
with: Sil.
Teeth, pain in with: Kp.
**Anger Agg: NM.**
**Animal fluids,** Loss of, from:
Cp; NM; SIL.

**Appearance** of Lump, on
scalp with: Sil.
**Ascending Agg:** Nm; Np;
**SIL.**
Into: Nm; **SIL.**
Left: Sil.
Right: Nm.
**Asleep,** As if: Nm.
**Backward** Extending: Kp; Nm.
**Bald** (See Hair): Sil.
Premature: Sil.
**Ball, lump,** knot: Sil.
**Band,** Hoop: Ks; NM.
**Bandaging:** See Binding.
**Base** of: Nm; Ns; Sil.
**Bathing** from: Sil.
**Bathing,** Washing, Agg: CP;
CS.
**Bending** Backwards.
Agg: Ks.
Amel: NM; SIL.
Down Agg: Fp; Nm.
One side on, Agg: Ks.
**Big** (Enlarged): Sil.
Body wasted, with: Sil.
**Bilious** Diarrhea, with: Ns.
**Binding** Up the Hair Agg:
Km; Kp; Np; **SIL.**
**Binding** Head tightly Amel:
**SIL.**
**Blow,** Shock thrust, as of:
NM.
**Boiling,** Bubbling, as if: Ks;
Sil.
**Boring,** Digging: Kp; KS; Nm;
NS; Sil.

**Breakfast** After Agg: Nm.
**Breathing** Deep Agg:
**Brittle** As if: Nm.
**Bubbling,** As if: Ks; Sil.
**Burning:** CP; Kp; Ks; Nm; Ns; SIL.
**Cap,** Hat, as if on: CS; Mp.
**Catarrhal:** Fp; Km; Nm.
**Cheerful** Excitement Amel: Kp.
**Chill** after Agg: **NM.**
Before: NM.
During: Fp; KS; NM.
**Chilliness,** With: Sil.
**Chronic:** Cp; Nm; Sil.
Old person: Cp.
**Coition Agg:** Nm; **SIL.**
After: Sil.
**Cold Applications** Amel: CP; Fp; NM; Ns.
Foot bath Amel: Ns.
Taking Agg: KS; SIL.
**Coldness:** Ns; Sil.
**Colicky** Pain, with: NS.
**Combing** Hair Agg: Sil.
**Concussion** From: Cs; Fp; NS.
**Confusion:** Sil.
**Constant,** Continuous: Nm.
**Constipation,** From: CP; Km; **NM;** NS.
**Constrictive:** Cs; Fp; KS; NM; Ns; SIL.
**Contents,** of, As if liquid: Mp.
**Contradiction,** From: Nm.

**Cool** Feeling in with: Cp; Sil.
**Coryza,** with: Fp; Kp; Ks; Sil.
Suppressed, from: Sil.
**Cough** Agg: **NM.**
**Creeping** In scalp, to vertex: Ns.
**Crushed** As if, shattered to pieces: Nm; Ns; SIL.
**Damp Day** Agg: Ns.
**Darkness** Amel: Mp; Sil.
**Delirium,** with: Sil.
**Dentition** Agg: Cp; Sil.
**Displaced,** As if: Nm.
**Distensive,** full: CP; Cs; Fp; Kp; Ks; Nm; Ns; Sil.
**Disturbances** of Vision, with: Nm; Sil.
**Diuresis,** With: Sil.
**Dizziness,** with: Ns.
**Downwards,** Nose, eye: Sil.
**Draft Agg: SIL.**
**Dragging** in: Nm.
**Drawing:** CP; Kp; Ks; Nm; Np; SIL.
Eyes together: NM.
**Drinking** hot tea Amel: Fp.
**Drinking** Quickly, from: Nm.
**Drowsiness,** with: Nm.
**Dull:** Nm; Ns; Sil.
**Earache** with: Fp.
**Eating** before Agg: **SIL.**
During Agg: Nm; Ns.
**Eating** Amel: Nm; Sil.
After Amel: Cp; Kp.
**Electric shocks** spasms before: Mp.

**Emotions excited** from: FP; Kp; **NM;** Sil.

**Empty Hollow:** Nm; Np.

Menses during: Fp.

**Empty** Feeling in stomach: Kp.

**Enlarged** expanded as if: NM; SIL.

**Eructations,** with: Sil.

**Evening** Agg: Sil.

Amel: Cf; Nm.

**Exertion,** Mental, Agg: CP; Mp; NM; **SIL.**

Physical, Agg: Cp.

**Exhaustion,** with: Sil.

**Eyes,** Closing Agg: Fp; Sil.

Amel: NM; SIL.

Extending into: SIL.

Pressure on Amel: Nm.

**Eye strain** from: Kp; Ks; NM; NP; **SIL.**

**Eyes,** Forced out as if: Sil.

**Face Flushed** and hot with: Sil.

Pale: Nm; Sil.

**Falling** Forward on stooping: Ns.

Left Temple, to: Ns.

**Fasting,** From: Ks; SIL.

**Fatty** Food from: Km; Nm; Np.

**Fever** with: Fp.

**Flatulence** with: Cp; Ns.

**Followed** by Blindness: Sil.

**Foot ball** during Agg: Ns.

**Foot steps** by, Agg: Sil.

**Forenoon** Agg: Cs; Ks; Nm.

**Forward** Extending, right: SIL.

**Frowning** Agg: NM.

**Gastric** Disturbances Agg: Cp; Cs; Kp; Ks; Ns; **SIL.**

**Getting** Cold, on: Nm; Sil.

**Gnawing:** Nm; Ns.

Spots, in: Ns.

**Grasping,** Vise, in: Ns.

**Grief,** From: Nm.

**Gums** Painful, with: Nm.

**Haemorrhage** From: Sil.

**Hair,** Bristling, of: Sil.

Pins sticking, under: Kp.

**Hair** Down, Amel: Km; Kp.

**Hair** Falling, with: Sil.

**Hanging** As if by a piece of string, at the nape: SIL.

**Hat,** Pressure of, from: CP; SIL.

As if, on (sensation): Cs; Mp.

**Hawking** Up white mucus: Km.

watery mucus: Nm.

**Heat,** From: Fp.

After Agg: NM.

During Agg: **NM; SIL.**

**Heat** Amel: **MP;** SIL.

**Heat:** CP; CS; Fp; Kp; Ks; NM; Np; SIL.

Burning: Sil.

Chill after: **SIL.**

during: Ns.

Cold bath Amel: Nm.

Forehead: Cs; Kp; Ks; Nm.

Hands cold, with: Nm.

Menses, during: FP Nm; Ns.

Mental exertion, from: SIL.

Night: SIL.

Occiput: NM; Ns.

Reading while: Ns.

Rising up: Ns.

from abdomen: Ns.

Smarting of hair roots: Cp.

Toes, descending to: CP.

Vertex: Fp; Nm; Np; NS.

menses, during: NS.

thinking, while: NS.

Warm room, in: CS; KS.

**Heaviness:** CS; Fp; Km; KP; Ks; **NM;** Ns; SIL.

Loss of sleep, as from: Nm.

**Hold** Up, unable to: CP; Nm; SIL.

**Hollow:** See Empty.

**Hot** Application, Amel: MP.

**Humour,** Bad with: Sil.

**Hungry,** When: Kp; Sil.

**Hydrocephalus:** CP; Kp; NM; Sil.

Impending: Fp.

**Increases** and **Decreases** with the sun: NM.

And decreasing gradually; Nm.

Suddenly and decreases suddenly: Mp.

**Injuries,** After: NM; **NS;** Sil.

Mental symptoms: NS.

**Injuries** Mechanical: CS; NM; **NS.**

**Jaw,** into: Sil.

**Jerking:** Kp; Ks; NM; Sil.

Fright, from: Nm.

From one side to another: Ns.

Right, to: NS.

**Lancinating,** Vertigo, with: Nm.

**Laughing** Agg: Nm.

**Leaning** Against, while: Nm.

**Lifted** By hair, she had: Sil.

**Lifting:** Sil.

**Light** Agg: Nm; Ns; Sil.

Day Agg: Sil.

**Limbs** Heavy, with: Sil.

**Looking,** Bright objects at Agg: SIL.

Downward Agg: Nm.

Fixedly, at anything: NM.

Sideways Agg: Nm.

Upward Agg: Cs; SIL.

**Looseness,** Feeling of: NM; Ns.

Forehead, in: Nm.

Shaking the head, on: Nm.

Stooping, on: Ns.

feel as if brain fell forward: Ns.

**Lying** while Agg: Np; NS.

Occiput, on Agg: Kp; Nm.

**Lying** Amel: Nm; Ns; Sil.

Back, on: Kp.

Dark room, in: Ns; SIL.

Head high with: NM.
side on: NM.
Occiput on: Kp.
**Menses** Appearing Amel: Kp.
Before, during Agg: Fp; Kp; Nm.
Commencement, at Agg: NM.
**Mental** Exertion Agg: Np; Sil.
Amel: Cp; Nm.
**Mental** Weakness, with: Cp; Sil.
**Midnight,** After to 10 A.M.: Nm.
2 A.M. to 3 A.M. Agg: Km.
**Morning** Amel: Nm.
Rising on Amel: Nm.
**Motion** Agg: Fp; **NM;** SIL.
Arms of: Nm; Sil.
Eyes of: NM; SIL.
Quick from: Nm.
**Motion** Gentle Amel: Kp.
Head of: Kp.
**Motions** in: Km; Kp; Ks; Nm; Ns; SIL.
Ascending stairs, while: Nm.
Moving the head by: Ks; Nm.
Sitting while: Sil.
Step-making or stumbling: SIL.
Stooping, on: NS.
Walking, while: SIL.
**Motions** of: CP.
Forward: Nm.
Involuntary: Nm.

Nodding: NM.
Rolling: Fp; SIL.
moaning with: Fp; SIL.
Sideways: Ns.
**Nausea** with: Cs; **NM;** Np; **SIL.**
Chilliness, and: Mp.
Vomiting, and: Mp.
**Nail,** As from: Mp; Nm.
**Nervous:** KP; Mp; **NM;** SIL.
Exhaustion: Kp; Sil.
**Night** Agg: **SIL.**
**Noise,** Clanging, As if: Sil.
Creaking, preventing sleep: Cf.
**Noises** in head with: Kp.
**Noon** Agg: Cp; Nm.
Until evening: Sil.
**Nose-Bleed** Amel: Fp; Sil.
**Numbness,** Tingling of lips, tongue and nose with: Nm.
**Numbness** as if: Cp; NM; Sil.
Forehead: Sil.
Occiput: Cp.
**Nursing** infant after, Agg: Sil.
**Odours,** strong Agg: Sil.
**Open,** As if: Sil.
Vertex, would: Np.
**Optical** Defects with: Mp.
**Outward,** extending: Sil.
**Oversensitiveness:** SIL.
**Pain** Aching dull heavy: CP; CS; Fp; Kp; **KS; NM;** Np; Ns; **SIL.**
Blow, shock, as of a: NM.

Boring, Digging: Kp; Ks; Nm; NS; Sil.

Bruised sore: CP; Fp; KM; Kp; Nm.

   spots, in: Sil.

Bursting: Km; Kp; Ks; NM; Np; Ns; SIL.

Constrictive, crampy: Cs; Fp; KS; NM; Ns; SIL.

   net, as if in, a: Kp; Nm.

   string, as if by: NM.

Cutting, stabbing: KM; Nm; Sil.

Hammering: Nm.

Maddening: Nm.

Nails, as from: Mp; Nm.

Paroxysmal: Fp; Kp; Mp; Np; SIL.

Periodical: Cs; **NM;** NP; Ns; SIL.

   every day: NM; SIL.

   every other day: Nm.

   every seventh day: Sil.

Pinching: Np; Sil.

Pressing: See heaviness.

   asunder: Cp; Sil.

   cap like: Mp; Ns.

   stone, as from: NM.

   vise, as if, in: **NM.**

   weight, as from: Km; Sil.

Shattered, as if: Nm; Ns; SIL.

Shooting: Mp; NM; Sil.

Stitching: Fp; KM; **KP; KS;** NM; NP; Ns; SIL.

   to chest and neck: NM.

Stunning, stupefying: Kp; Ks; NM; Np; SIL.

Sutures, along: CP.

Tearing, rending: Cp; CS; Fp; KS; **NM;** Np; Ns; SIL.

   head around: Cp; Cs.

   teeth, to: Km.

Throbbing, pulsating: Nm.

Ulcerative: Nm.

Violent: Kp; Ks; NM; SIL.

Wakes up from sleep: Sil.

   frequently: Kp.

Wandering: Mp; Ns.

Wound, as from: Mp.

**Paralysis** Of one side, after coition: Sil.

**Perspiration**, With: NS.

**Perspiration**, Amel: NM; NS.

**Perspiration**: CP; CS; **KM;** KP; Ks; **SIL.**

   Coughing, on: Sil.

   Forehead: Kp; Nm; Np; Sil.

   chill during: NS.

   cold: Kp.

   eating after: Ns.

   offensive: Sil.

Mental exertion, on: KP.

Musty: **NM.**

Occiput: SIL.

Reading, while: Ns.

Sleep, during: CP; SIL.

   on falling asleep: SIL.

Sour: **SIL.**

**Pressure** Amel: Mp; NM.

Eyes on, Amel: Nm.

Hard, Amel: Mp.

**Pricking**: Nm.
 Needles, like: Nm.
**Pulled,** as if hair were: Sil.
 Occiput, from: Kp.
**Pulsation,** Throbbing: Cp; Cs;
 Fp; Kp; KS; Nm; Np; **SIL.**
 Chest and neck, to: Nm.
 Hammers, as from little: NM.
 Nausea, vomiting, with: Nm.
 before 10 a.m.: Nm.
**Pushed** Forward, as if: Fp.
**Pushing**: Nm.
**Reading Agg**: Cs; **NM**; Ns;
 Sil.
**Rest** Agg: Ns.
 Amel: Ns; Sil.
**Resting** Head, quietly on arm
 while: Nm.
**Restlessness**: Sil.
**Rheumatic**: Ks; NM; SIL.
**Rising** After, Amel: Kp.
**Rising,** Lying from, Agg: Cs;
 NP; **SIL.**
 Sitting, from: Sil.
**Rocket,** Had passed through:
 Kp.
**Rope,** Tight round: Nm.
**Running** From: Nm.
**Saliva** Profuse, with: Nm.
**Scalp,** Adherent to cranium as
 if: Mp; Sil.
**School** Girls, in: **CP**; Nm.
 Diarrhoea with: Cp.
**Screw,** Driven through, as if:
 NS.

**Separated,** From body, as if:
 Nm.
**Sexual** Desire, suppression:
 Kp.
**Shaking** As if: Kp; Mp; Sil.
 Scalp of: Sil.
 stepping heavily and walk-
 ing when: SIL.
**Shaking** Head, from: Cs; Fp;
 Ks; Nm; Sil.
**Shattered,** As if: Sil.
**Shocks,** Electric sparks from
 as if: Mp.
**Sitting** Agg: Fp; Sil.
 Amel: Nm.
**Skull** Cap, sensation: Ks; Mp.
 4 p.m.: Cs.
**Sleep,** Falling to Agg: Sil.
 During, Agg: Ns.
**Sleep,** Amel: Nm.
**Sneezing,** After, during Agg:
 Nm.
**Sneezing,** Amel: Cp.
**Spirituous** liquors, from: Cs;
 Nm; SIL.
**Step** Every, were felt in: Cp;
 Nm.
**Stepping** Hard, mis-steps agg:
 Cp; NM; SIL.
**Stiffness**: Nm; Ns.
 Evening, in bed: Sil.
 Motion, on: Ns.
 Occiput: Sil.
**Stool,** Pressing, at, from: Cp;
 Nm; SIL.
 After: Sil.

**Stooping**, Agg: Fp; Km; Nm; Sil.

**Students**: Kp; Mp.

**Summer**: NM; NS.

**Sun**, Exposure to: Cs; Fp; Nm.

**Supporting** Head Agg: Nm.

**Swashing**, As of water, in: Mp.

**Sweat**, On: Km; **SIL.**

**Swollen**, Distended, feeling: Nm.

**Talking** Agg: Cs; **NM**; SIL.
Amel: Sil.

**Tea** Amel: Fp.

**Thick**, As if: Nm.

**Throbbing**, In: See Pulsating.

**Tingling**, Vibration: Sil.

**Tired** Feeling: Fp; Kp; Nm.

**Tobacco** Smoking Amel: Cp.
Sucking, craving for: Cp.

**Toothache** With: Nm.

**Trembling**: Mp.

**Turning** Body Agg: Nm; Sil.
Eyes, sideways: Sil.
Head: NM.
Suddenly: Sil.

**Turning** and Twisting, as if: Sil.

**Twisting**: NM.

**Unconsciousness**, With: NM; SIL.

**Uncovering** Agg: Kp; Mp; NM; Np; **SIL.**

**Urination**, Profuse Amel: Fp; SIL.

**Urination**, Profuse, with: Sil.

**Vertigo**, With: Fp; Ns; Sil.
Lancinating pains with: Nm.

**Vexation**, Irritation, with: Kp; Nm; Sil.

**Vibration**, Tingling: Sil.

**Visual** or Eye symptoms with: Sil.

**Vomiting** Agg: Fp.
After, Agg: Ns.
Amel: Ns; Sil.

**Vomiting** With: Km; NM; Sil.
Bile: NS.
Slime: Np.
Sour: Np.
Transparent mucous: Cp; Nm.
Undigested food: Fp; NP.

**Walking**, While Amel: Nm.

**Walking**, Air, open Agg: MP; Sil.

**Warmth**, External Amel: MP; Sil.

**Washing** Agg: CP; CS; Sil.
Feet, cold water, Amel: Ns.

**Waving**: Mp; Nm; Sil.
Occiput: Sil.

**Weakness**, As if: Nm.
**Walking** in Sun: Nm.

**Weakness**, With: Sil.

**Whirling**: Sil.

**Wine** Agg: Km.

**Wrapping** Agg: Fp.
Amel: Km; Kp; Mp; Nm; SIL.

**Wrinkling** Forehead, Agg: Nm.

**Yawning**, Stretching with: Kp.
  After Amel: Nm.
**HEAD EXTERNAL**: CP; SIL.
  **Right**: Sil.
  **Occiput**: SIL.
  **Abscess** of scalp: SIL.
  **Bald**: SIL.
    Spots in: Ks.
    Young people, in: Sil.
  **Caries** of bones: Cp; Cs; NM;
    SIL.
  **Coldness**, Chilliness: CP; Cs;
    Fp; Ks; NM; Sil.
    Air, as from cold: Nm.
    Covering, Amel: Nm.
    left: Nm.
    Icy: Cp.
    Occiput: **CP**; Sil.
    Vertex: **CP**; Cs; Fp; Ks; NM;
    SIL.
  **Drawing** Back and forth of
    scalp: Nm
  **Drawn**, away: Sil.
    Backward: NM; NS; Sil.
    Sideways: Sil.
  **Eruptions**: Cs; Kp; KS; NM;
    Np; SIL.
    Bleeding, scratching on: Cs.
    Boils: SIL.
    Carbuncles: SIL.
    Crusta lactea: Cs; Km; Sil.
    Crusts, scabs, white: KM;
    **NM**.
      yellow: Cs; **KS**.
      favus (scald head): Cs;
      Km; Sil.

Hard: Nm.
Impetigo: Cp; Sil.
Margins, at the hair: NM.
Moist: Ks; NM; SIL.
  glutinous: NM.
  yellow: **KS**.
Nodes: **SIL**.
Occiput: NM; SIL.
Pimples, hair, under: Cs.
Ringworm: Ks; Sil.
Scurfy: Nm.
  black: CP.
  white: Nm.
Suppurating: Cs; Sil.
Tubercles, on scalp: Nm;
  Sil.
**Falling**, Forward, of head:
  NM; SIL.
**Formication**: CP; Cs; Ns;
  SIL.
  Vertex: Cp; NS.
**Fungus**: CP.
**Hard** Scalp: Fp.
**Heat**: CP; CS; Fp; Kp; NM;
  Np; SIL.
  Burning: Sil.
  Chill after: **SIL**.
    during: Ns.
  Cold bath, Amel: Nm.
  Forehead: Cs; Kp; KS; Nm.
  Hands, cold with: Nm..
  Menses, during: Fp; Nm;
    Ns.
  Mental exertion, from: Kp;
    SIL.
  Night: **SIL**.

Occiput: NM; NS.
Reading, while: Ns.
Rising, up: NS.
abdomen, from: Ns.
Smarting, hair roots, of: Cp.
Toes, descending, to: CP.
Vertex: FP; Nm; Np; NS.
menses, during: NS.
thinking, while: NS.
Warm room, in: CS; KS.
**Hold** Up, unable, to: CP; Nm; SIL.
**Itching**: CS; Fp; Kp; KS; NM; SIL.
Burning: Sil.
Crawling: Sil.
Forehead: Nm; Sil.
Occiput: **SIL.**
Rubbing Amel: Nm.
Scratching Agg: SIL.
Amel: Nm.
Spots, in: SIL.
Warmth of bed, Agg: SIL.
**Large**: CP; SIL.
Emaciation of body, with: Sil.
**Motions**, of: CP.
**Sensitive**: Sil.
Cold air, to: Fp; Km; NM; **SIL.**
Combing, hair: Ns.
Draft to: CP; Ks; **SIL.**
Touch to: Cp; Fp; NM; Ns; SIL.

**Shocks**, Blows, jerks: Fp; Km; Kp; KS; NM; Np; Ns; SIL.
Coughing, when: NM.
Electric, like: Mp; Ns.
Forehead, in: Nm.
finger, as if, with: Nm.
Sides: Ks; Ns.
Talking, while: Nm.
Vertex: Fp.
**Swollen**, Glands of: **SIL.**
Scalp; puffy beneath: SIL.
**Symptoms**, Alternate with, abdomen: Cp.
**Thin**, Cranium: CP; Cs.
**Twitching** Muscles: Np; Ns; Sil.
Evening and night: Sil.
Forehead of: Sil.
Vertex: Sil.
**Ulcers**: CP; SIL.
Occiput: **SIL.**
**Wens**: Sil.
**Wobbing**: CP; SIL.
**HEADSTRONG**: See Obstinate.
**HEALING** Difficult: Cp; Ns; SIL.
**HEARING**: Kp; NM; SIL.
**Acute**: KP; Ks; NM; NP; **SIL.**
Noises, to: Fp; KP; NP; NS; SIL.
Rumpling of paper, to: NS.
Voices and talking to: Kp.
**Bad**, Deafness, impaired: CP; Fp; Km; Kp; Ks; Mp; **NM;** NP; SIL.
Right: KS.

Adenoids from: Cp.
Alternate with sensitivity: Sil.
Blowing nose, Amel: SIL.
Change of clothing: SIL.
Cold, after: Sil.
  exposure: Km.
  from: Fp; Km.
  menses, during: Fp.
  wet weather: SIL.
Coughing Amel: Sil.
Eating Agg: Sil.
Eustachian catarrh from: KM; **KS**; Nm; SIL.
Glands swollen about the ear, from: Km.
Intermittent: Sil.
Loud report, Amel: SIL.
Measles, after: SIL.
Menses, at: Fp.
Nervous: Nm; SIL.
Noises in ear with: Kp.
Old age: Km.
Paralysis, auditory nerve: Kp; NM; SIL.
Rheumatic, gouty diathesis: Sil.
Scarlet fever, after: SIL.
Scrofulous, diathesis: Sil.
Snap report, Amel: Sil.
Spinal fever, After: Sil.
Sudden: Sil.
Swelling of external ear: Ks.
Thickening of drum: Km.
Throat affections, from: Km.
Vaccination: Sil.

Voice to human: Kp; Sil.
Warm room, Agg: Ks.
Washing Agg: Sil.
Yawning Amel: Sil.
**Difficult**: Fp; Km; NM; SIL.
Human voice, for: Sil.
**Footsteps**, Next room in: Np.
**Illusory** Sounds, Noises: Cp; Cs; Fp; Km; KP; KS; NM; NP; NS; Sil.
Air cold, from: Sil.
Blowing nose: KM; Sil.
Bubbling: Nm; Sil.
Buzzing: Cs; FP; Kp; Ks.
Chewing, when: KM; KS; NM; Sil.
Chiming: Nm.
Chirping: Km; Ks; Sil.
  intermittent fever in: NS.
Clashing: Sil.
Clucking: Sil.
Coughing, on: Sil.
Cracking: Km; Ks; NM; Sil.
  jaws moving, on: Nm.
Crackling: Ks.
Crashing: Sil.
Feet becoming cool from: Sil.
Fluttering: KP; KS; NM; Np; Sil.
  butterfly as if: Nm.
  rhythmical: Sil.
  right: Ns.
Headache, during: SIL.
Head. turning: Fp; NM; Sil.

Hissing: NS; Sil.

Humming: Fp; Kp; Ks; NM; Np; Sil.

Lying while: Fp; Nm; Sil.
   amel: Ns.

Night: Sil.

Noise: Sil.

Puffing: SIL.

Reverberating (echoes and re-echoes): KP; Ns; Sil.
   own voice: Ns.

Ringing: CS; Fp; Kp; KS; NM; Np; NS; SIL.
   bells as of: Cf; Ns; Sil.
   distant, in: Ns.
   forcing him to rise and walk about (night): Sil.

Roaring: CS; Fp; Kp; KS; NM; NP; NS; **SIL.**
   left: Nm.
   right: Ns; Sil.

Running water, like: Fp.

Rushing: KP; KS; **NM;** Sil.
   steam, escaping like: Sil.
   water-fall, like a: Np.

Rustling: Sil.

Singing: Cp; Cs; Fp; Nm; Nm; Np.
   right: Cp.

Sitting while: Nm.

Snapping: KM; SIL.
   as hearing returns: Sil.

Sneezing, Agg: Km; Sil.

Stool, after: CP.

Swallowing, when: KM; Nm; Sil.

Synchronous with pulse: Sil.

Ticking: Nm; Sil.

Tickling: Nm; Ns.

Vertigo, with: Kp; Nm; Np; Ns; SIL.

Walking, while: Nm; Sil.

Washing neck and face, cold water, from: Np.

Whistling: Sil.

Whizzing: Kp; Ks; Np; Sil.

**Lost**: Kp; Nm; Np; Ns; SIL.

**HEARING**, Talk AGG: Sil.

**HEART**: Cf; FP; NM.

**Air**, Open Amel: Nm.
   Warm Amel: Sil.

**Alternating** with: Nm; Np.
   Pain in great toe: Np.

**Angina**: Fp; Kp; MP.
   Organic heart trouble from: Cf.

**Anxiety**, In the region: Fp; Ns; Sil.

**Ascending** Agg: Nm.

**Beating,** In the region of: CP; Kp; SIL.

**Beats**, Felt all over the body: Nm.
   Shakes the body: Nm.

**Bubble** Starts from and passes into arteries: Np.

**Chest**, Holding amel: Ns.

**Coldness**, Of heart: Km; Nm.
   Icy, chill during: NM.
   In region of: NM.
   Mental exertion, Agg: NM.

**Constriction**, Contraction: Fp; Kp; Mp; **NM.**
Vise in, as if: MP.

**Coughing** Agg: **NM; SIL.**

**Crushed**, or Bruised: Mp; Nm.

**Cutting** In the region of: CP; KM.
Interrupting breathing: CP.

**Dilatation**: Cf; Fp; NM.

**Drawing**: Nm.

**Drinking**, after Agg: Nm.

**Eating**, After: Nm; Ns.

**Expiration**, Agg: Mp.

**Extending**, to spine, left: Fp.
Thighs, to: Cs.

**Fatty** Degeneration: KP; Ks.

**Fluttering**: See Trembling.

**Foramen** ovale, non-closure of: Cp.

**Gnawing**: Nm.

**Goitre** Heart: Fp; Nm.

**Go** Upward: Mp.

**Hands**, Over: Nm.

**Heat**, Flushes of, in the region: Sil.

**Heaviness**: Sil.

**Hypertrophy**: Nm.

**Inflammation** (Myocarditis): Fp.
Endocardium, of: Fp; Nm.
Menses scanty, with: Nm.
Pericardium of: Cs; Fp; Km; Nm.
chronic: Cf.

**Inspiration** Deep: CP; Ks.

**Jerks**, Thrusts: Nm.

**Joints**, Alternating with: Np.

**Lying**, Amel: Cp.

**Lying** In bed Agg: Sil.
Left side, on: Mp; NM; SIL.

**Lump**, Ball, load as of: Np.

**Mental** Exertion Agg: NM.

**Motion** Agg: Nm; Sil.

**Movement**, In, as of: Nm.

**Muscle** Exhaustion: Cp; KP.

**Old** people, in: **SIL.**

**Oppression**, As if: Kp; NS.
Morning: Ns.
Sitting: NS.

**Pain**: Fp; Kp; NM; Np.
Aching: Fp; NM; NP.
in the region of: Cp; Ks; NM.
Jerking: Nm.
Pressing: Km; NM; Ns; Sil.
Pulsating: Sil.
Sharp, shooting: Cp.
Sore, bruised: NM.
Stitching: CP; Km; Kp; Ks; Nm.
apex: NM.

**Palpitation**: CP; Cs; FP; Km; KP; KS; **NM; NP;** SIL.
Alternating with beats in head: Nm.
Anemia, vital drains: Cp; Nm.
Ascending Agg: Cs; KP; **NM.**
Audible: FP; Nm; NP.

Chest, constriction with: Cp; NM.

Dinner, after: Sil.

Dropsy, with: Km.

Eating, after: NM; Np; Sil.

Excessive flow of blood to heart, from: Km.

Excitement Agg: KP; Nm.

Exertion Agg: Fp; **NM;** Np; Sil.

Fainting, with: Nm.

Feeling of pulsation in different parts of body with: Np.

Flatulence: Kp.

Fright, after: NM.

as from: Np.

Hysteria in: NM.

Lying, side, on Agg: Nm.

left, on Agg: NM; Np.

Amel: Mp.

right on Amel.: Nm.

Menses, after, before: NM.

during: NM; Np; Sil.

suppression: Nm.

Morning: **NM.**

awakening on: Nm.

bed in: Nm.

hungry, when: Km.

Motion Agg: Fp; Kp; NM; SIL.

violent or quick: Sil.

Nervous irritation: Kp; Mp.

Night: Fp; Nm.

Noise from every strange: NM.

Paroxysmal: MP.

Pregnancy, during: NM.

Shaking the body, from: Nm.

Sleep, on going to: NM; Sil.

Standing, while: NM; Sil.

Suppressed foot-sweat from: SIL.

Throat, extending to: NM.

Tumultous, violent, vehement: KP; Ks; **NM.**

Unrequitted affection from: **NM.**

Visible:. Nm; Ns.

apex beat through:

clothing: Mp.

Waking, on: NM; SIL.

the patient agg: Nm.

startled, dream from: Sil.

Walking, rapidly on: Fp; NM.

Writing: Fp.

**Pressure** External Agg: Fp.

**Pressure** Of hand Amel: NM; Ns.

**Reading,** Aloud Agg: Nm.

**Rest,** During Agg: Nm.

**Rising,** From sitting Agg: Cp; Sil.

**Running,** Agg: **SIL.**

**Sleep,** Starting up, from Agg: SIL.

**Sneezing,** Agg: Sil.

**Standing,** Agg: Sil.

**Stone cutters,** in Agg: SIL.

**Stools,** After Agg: SIL.

**Stooping,** On Agg: Fp; Nm; SIL.

**Stopped** As it, sleep, during: Sil.

**Straightening** Up, when Agg: Nm.

**Stretching** the body, Amel: Fp.

**Suckling** Agg: SIL.

**Talking**, Aloud, agg: Nm.

**Tension**, Tightness: Nm.

**Touch** Agg: Nm.

**Trembling**, Fluttering of: NM; NP.

About the heart: Np.

Ascending Agg: NP.

Eating, after agg: Np.

Lying agg: Nm.

Menses, after: Np.

**Twitching**: Nm.

**Urinating** After, Amel: NM.

**Valvular** Diseases of: Cf.

**Walking** Amel.: Mp.

**Walking** and in open air Agg.: Nm.

**Weak**: Nm.

**HEARTBURN**: Cp; CS; **FP;** Kp; Ks; NM; Np; NS; SIL.

**Coffee**, After: Cp; Fp.

**Eating**, After: CP; NM; Sil.

**Meat**, After: FP.

**Night**: MP; Nm; NP.

**Pregnancy**, During: Nm.

**Sour** Things, after: Fp; Np.

**HEAT OF FIRE**, Sun,

becoming heated or over-heated **Agg**: Cs; FP; Km; Kp; KS; NM; NS; **SIL.**

**Body**, Of: Km.

**Room**, Of: Cs.

**HEAT** (Warmth of bed, External heat) Amel: MP; **SIL.**

**HEAT Flushes**, of: CS; Fp; KS. Nm; Np; **NS;** SIL.

**Afternoon**: Np.

**Dinner**, During: Cs.

**Evening**: NS.

Eating while: Cs.

**Menses**, During: Nm; Np.

**Sleep**, During: Nm; Sil.

**Upwards**: Ns.

**Warm** Water, dashed over as if: Nm.

**HEAT Sensation** of: **CS; KM; NM; NS.**

**Blood vessels**, in: Nm.

**Vital** lack of: CF; CP; CS; KP; Mp; NM; NP; **SIL.**

Exercise, during: Sil.

**HEAVINESS, Externally**: Km; Ks; NM; SIL.

**Internally:** Km; NM; **SIL.**

**Lightness**, Alternating with: Nm.

**Paralytic**: KP; NM.

**HECTIC Fever**: CP; **CS;** Fp; KP; KS; **SIL.**

**HEELS Aching**: Cp.

**Caries**: CP; SIL.

**Cracked**: Kp.

**Cutting**: Ns.

**Eruptions**, Blisters: Nm; SIL.

**Gnawing**, Right: Nm.

**Pain**: Cp; Nm; NS.

**Piercing**: Ns.
**Rubbing**, Amel: Ns.
**Sitting**, While Agg: Sil.
**Sore**, Bruised: Cp.
**Spinning** While, evening in Agg: Ns.
**Standing**, While Agg: Ns; Sil.
**Stitching**: Nm; Np; NS; SIL.
Itching: Nm.
**Tearing**: Ns; SIL.
**Throbbing**: Ns.
**Ulcerative** Pain: NS.
**Ulcers**: SIL.
**Walking** While Agg: Ns.
**HELD Being Amel**: Ns; Sil.
**Wants** to be: Kp.
**HEMICRANIA**: Cp; Fp; **KP**; Ks; NM; Np; Ns; SIL.
**Right**: Nm; SIL.
**Left**: Cp; NM; Ns; Sil.
**Extending** To eyes: Nm.
To forehead: Sil.
**HEMIOPIA** (Half vision): Cs; NM.
**Vertical**: Fp; NM.
**HEMIPLEGIA**: Km; Kp; Nm.
**Right**: Nm; Sil.
**HERE and THERE** (wandering): MP.
**HEPATALGIA**: See Pain, **Liver.**
**HEPATITIS**: Kp; NM; **NS**; Sil.
**HERNIA**: Cp; Ks; NM; Ns; Sil.
**Children**, in: Sil.
**Painful**, Sensitive: SIL.
**Strangulated**: Sil.

**HERPES**: See Eruptions, herpetic.
**HESITATES**: Kp.
**HICCOUGH**: Cf; Fp; Ks; MP; NM; NS; SIL.
**Bread** and **butter**, after: NS.
**Convulsive**: MP.
**Day** and **night**: Mp.
**Eating**, After: Nm; NS; Sil.
**Evening**: NS; Sil.
**Fever**, During: MP.
**Forenoon**, Eating after: Ns.
**Hawking**, Agg: Cf.
**Hot** Applications, Amel: Cp; Fp; Mp.
Drinks, Amel: Mp.
**Meteorism**, With: Mp.
**Night**: Mp; Sil.
**Noon**: Sil.
**Quinine**, After: NM.
**Retching**: Mp.
**Spasmodic**: Mp.
**Violent**, obstinate: Cf; MP; NM.
**HIDE**, Desire, to:
**Children**, Behind furniture:
**Run**, away, and:
**HIGH PLACES** (See ascending) **Agg**: CP; Kp; NM; Np; Sil.
**HIP JOINT DISEASE** (Tuberculous): **CP**; **CS**; **KP**; **KS**; NM; Ns; **SIL.**
**Pregnancy**, In: Cp.
**HIPS** (Region) **Coldness**: Sil.
**Cramps**: Nm.

**Fistulous** Opening: SIL.
**Forced** Apart, as if: Cp.
**Injuries**: Ns; Sil.
**Joint**: See Hip joint.
**Pain**: CP; Cs; KP; KS; Nm; NS; **SIL.**
  After pains: SIL.
  Ascending steps, Agg: Ns.
  Bed, motion in Agg: Ns.
    turning in: NS.
  Breathing deep, Agg: Nm.
  Cutting: Ns.
  Dislocated, as if right: Nm.
  Drawing: Cp; NM; Np.
    extends downwards: Nm.
    feet to: Mp.
    knees to: NS.
  Gouty: SIL.
  Jerking: Sil.
  Knees, to: NS.
  Left: NS.
  Lying on it, Agg: Nm.
  Piercing, left: NS.
  Pinching, only during rest: Ns.
  Pressing: Ns.
  Rheumatic: Nm.
  Rubbing, Amel: Ns.
  Shooting: Cp.
    left: Ns.
  Sitting, in the act of: Ns.
  Sprained, as if: NM.
  Stitching: Cp; Fp; NM; Np; NS; SIL.

  downward, extends: Cp; SIL.
  Stooping Agg: NS; SIL.
  Tearing: Cp; Fp; Kp; NP; SIL.
    knees, extends to: Sil.
  Walking Agg: NS; SIL.
    Amel: CF; Cp; **KS.**
  Wet weather agg: Sil.
**Paralysis**, Sensation of: Nm.
**Pregnancy**, In: Cp.
**Pulsation**: Sil.
**Rising**, Agg: Ns.
**Shocks**: Nm.
**Sitting** Down, Agg: Ns.
**Stiffness**: Nm; **SIL.**
**Suppuration**: CP; Cs; **SIL.**
**Tension**: NM.
**Tingling**, Prickling, in gluteal muscles: Cp.
**Twitching**: Sil.
**Ulcers**: Nm.
**Weakness**: Cp.
**HIVES**: See Urticaria.
**HOARSENESS**: See Under Voice.
**HODGKIN'S DISEASE**: Cf; Km; Nm.
**HOLDING** or **Being held Amel**: Ns; Sil.
**HOLLOW**: See Empty.
  **Knee**, of: NM.
    Eruptions: NM.
      red: NM.
    Pain: Cp; Nm.
      left: Np.
    Tearing: Nm.

**HOME-SICKNESS**: Cp; KP; NM; SIL.

**HOOK WORM** Disease: Sil.

**HOPEFUL**:

**HOPELESS** (See Despair): Cs; NM; Ns; Sil.

**HORNY**: Sil.

**HORRIPILATION** (Goose Skin): NM; Ns.

**HOT APPLICATIONS Amel**: Cf; MP; **SIL.**

**HOUSE in Agg**: Ks.

**HUMID, Warm**, Damp weather Agg: Cf; CP; CS; MP; **NS**; SIL.

**HUMMING, Buzzing**, whizzing: Fp; Km; Kp; Ks; NM; Np; Sil.

**HUNGER**: See Appetite.

**Agg**: **SIL.**

**HURRY Impatience**: Cs; Kp; Ks; **NM**; Np.

**HURT, Fears,** being: NS.

**HYDRARTHROSIS**: Km; Ks; Np.

**HYDROCELE**: Cf; CP; NM; **SIL.**

**Boys, of**: CS; Km; **SIL.**

**Scrofulous**: **SIL.**

**HYDROCEPHALUS**: CP; Kp; NM; **SIL.**

**Impending**: Fp.

**HYDROGENOID**: NM; **NS.**

**HYDROPHOBIA**: Mp; Nm.

**HYGROMA** (See Ganglion): Cf; Km; SIL.

**HYPERCHLORHYDRIA**: Cp; Np.

**HYPERMETROPIA**: NM; **SIL.**

**HYPERPYREXIA**: See Fever, High.

**HYPERTROPHY:** Km; Nm; SIL.

**Heart,** of: NM.

**HYPOCHONDRIAL Distension**: Nm.

**Flatulence**: Sil.

**Fullness**, Right: Nm.

**Hard**, Right: CP.

**Pain**, Aching, right: Cf; NM; **NS**; Sil.

left: Nm.

Air, open Agg: NS.

Burning: Nm.

right: Km.

Clawing: Nm.

right: NS.

Coughing, Agg: Ns.

Cramping, gripping: CS; Nm; Sil.

Cutting: Cf; Nm; Np.

Dragging, bearing down, right, when lying on left side: NS.

Drawing: Nm; Sil.

right: Nm.

Extending, back, to: Nm; Ns.

Lancinating, right: Cf.

night: NS.

Pressing: Cp; Nm; SIL.

left: Nm.

right: CP; Km; NM; SIL.

Sore, bruised: CP; Nm; NS.
right: CP; **NS;** SIL.
Stitching, shooting: Cp; NM;
Ns; **SIL.**
left: Ns.
right: CP; Nm; NS.
Twisting: Nm.
**Pulsation:** Cp; Sil.
Right: Cp; Ns; Sil.
**Sensitive:** Ns.
**Tension:** Km; NM; NS.
Right: Nm; Ns.
**HYPOCHONDRIASIS:** Kp; Nm.
**HYPOCRISY:**
**HYPOGASTRIUM Band,**
Tight around: Nm.
**Distension:** Nm; NS; Sil.
**Empty:** Ks.
Flatus passing, amel: Ks.
**Flatulence:** Sil.
**Heaviness,** Across: Nm.
Pressing in pelvis, down-
wards and backwards: Kp.
**Itching:** Nm.
**Pain,** Aching: CP; Kp; NM;
NP; SIL.
Burning, menses during: Nm.
Cramping, gripping: Km; Sil.
menses, before and dur-
ing: MP.
Cutting, menses during: Nm.
Pressing: Cp; Ks; NM; Np.
Sore, bruised: NM.
Stitching, sticking: KP; Nm.
across: KP.

**Pulsation,** Female, in: Cp.
**Shocks,** Coughing, when: Nm.
**Tension:** NM.
**Trembling:** Cp.
**HYPOPYON:** Cs; Km; SIL.
**HYPOSTASIS:** FP; Kp; NM.
**HYSTERIA:** Cs; Fp; **KP;** Ks;
NM; Np; **SIL.**
**Fainting,** Hysterical: NM.
**Twitching,** Menses, before
and during: Nm.
**ICHTHYOSIS:** Ks; Nm; Sil.
**ICE COLD:** NM; SIL.
**IDEAS Abundant,** Clearness of
mind: Cp; Fp; Ks; Np; Sil.
**Deficiency,** Of: CP; NM; Np;
Sil.
**Evening:** Np; Sil.
**Fixed:** NM; SIL.
**IDIOCY:** CP.
**IDLENESS** AGG: Nm; Sil.
**ILEO-CECAL Region:** See
Appendicitis.
**ILEUS** (Paralysis of Intestines):
KP.
**ILIAC REGION** Pain, cutting:
Np.
Stitching: Sil.
**ILIUM pain,** above crest of: Ks.
Cutting, to scapula: Nm.
Stitching: Sil.
**ILL** or **Sick feeling:** Nm.
**ILLUSIONS:** See Delusions.
**IMAGINATIONS:** See Delusions.
**IMBECILITY:** Cp; Cs; Km; KP;
NM; NP; **SIL.**

**IMMOBILE**: Fp; Kp; Nm.
**IMPATIENCE, Hurry**: Cs; Kp; Ks; **NM;** Np.
　**No one works** fast enough: Np.
　**Trifles,** about: Kp; Nm.
**IMPERTINENCE** (Rudeness, insolence) **Ailments.**
　From: Nm.
**IMPETIGO**: Nm; Sil.
**IMPETUOUS**: Fp; Kp; NM.
　**Evening**: Fp.
　**Perspiration**, with: Nm.
**IMPOTENCY**: **CS;** Kp; Ks; NM; NP; Sil.
　**Evening** and Night: Kp.
**IMPUDENCE**: Nm.
**IMPULSES** Fears, his own: NS.
**IMPULSIVE**: KS.
**INACTIVE**, Lethargic, aparthetic: Kp; Sil.
　**Coition**, after: Kp; Np.
　**Conversation**, from: Np; Sil.
**INCOHERENCE**: See Confusion.
**INCONTINENCE, Stool,** Urine, etc.: Fp; Km; KP; MP; **NM;** NP; **SIL.**
**INCONSOLABLE**: NM.
**INCOORDINATION**: Kp; SIL.
**INCREASES and Decreases**: Mp; Nm.
**INDIFFERENCE** (Apathy): CP; Cs; Fp; KP; Ks; **NM; NP; SIL.**
　**Alternating** With anxiety and restlessness: NM.

**Chill,** During: Sil.
**Loved ones,** To: Np.
**Pleasure,** To: Fp; Km; NM.
**Society,** When, in: Nm.
**To Everything**: Np.
**INDIGESTION**: See, Stomach, Disordered.
**INDIGNATION**: CP.
　**Dreams,** Unpleasant, at: Cp.
　**Pregnant,** While: Nm.
**INDOLENT** (Aversion to physical work): CP; Fp; Km; KP; Ks; NM; Np.
　**Breakfast,** After: Ns.
　**Conversation,** From: Sil.
　**Lightest** Labour seems heavy work: Kp.
　**Morning**: NM; Ns.
**INDURATION**: **CF;** KM; SIL.
　**Cellular** Tissue: Sil.
　**Glands**: CF; **SIL.**
　**Injuries,** After: Cf.
　**Knotty,** Like rope: SIL.
　**Muscles**: CF; Sil.
　**Stony**: Cf; Km.
**INDUSTRIOUS**: Cp; Ns.
　**Coition,** after: Cp.
**INFANTS**: See children.
**INFERIORITY**: Sil.
**INFLAMMATION**: FP; Km; Ks; Nm; **SIL.**
　**Blood vessels** of: Sil.
　**Bones: SIL.**
　　Chronic (osteitis deformans): CP.

**Cartilages**: NM.
**Cellular** Tissue: Sil.
**Favour**, Absorption: Km.
**Gangrenous**: KP; SIL.
**Internally**: Nm; Sil.
**Nerves**: NM; Sil.
**Periosteum**: CF; SIL.
**Serous** Membranes: Cp; NM; SIL.
**Surgical**: Sil.
**INFLUENZA**: Fp; Ks; NS.
**Weakness**, After: Kp.
**INGUINAL GLANDS**: See Inguinal region.
**INGUINAL REGION** (Groins)
**Abscess**, Bubo: Km; **SIL**.
  Suppurating: SIL.
**Clicking** Sound as if two bones slipped over each other: Nm.
**Distension**: Ns.
**Fullness**: Ns.
**Glands**, bubo. Km; SIL.
  Fistula: Sil.
  Pain: SIL.
  Sore: SIL.
  Swelling: CP; Nm; SIL.
**Heat**: CP.
**Hernia**: Cf; Cp; Nm; SIL.
  Children, in: Sil.
  Painful, sensitive: SIL.
  Strangulated: Fp; Sil.
**Internal** Ring:
  Coughing Agg: Nm.
**Pain**, Aching: Ks; NM; Ns; Sil.

  axillae, to: Ns.
  right: Ns; Sil.
  then left: Cp.
Burning: Ns.
  menses, during: Nm.
Cramping: Ns.
Cutting: Nm.
  menses, during: NM.
Drawing: Cp; Nm; Sil.
  right: Sil.
Emission, after: Np.
Menses, during: Kp; Nm.
Piercing, urging, to urinate with: Ns.
Pinching: Nm.
Pressing, right: Ns.
Sore, right: Cp.
Squeezing: Nm.
Stitching, sticking: Cs; Ks; Nm; NS.
  left: Cs; Ns.
  right: Nm.
Tearing: Sil.
**Swelling**: Sil.
  Left: Sil.
  Sensation of: Sil.
**Tension**: Nm; Ns.
  left: Nm.
**Ulcers**: Nm.
**INHALATION**: See Inspiration
**INJURIES**, cuts, blows, etc: Fp; Km; Kp; Nm; NS; SIL.
**Bites**: Mp.
**Bones**: Cp.
**Constitutional** Effects: NS.

**Glands**: SIL.
**Mental** Effects: Ns.
**Old**, Pains in: Sil.
**Pain**, Returning: Nm; NS.
**Reopening** Of old: Nm; SIL.
**Slow** To heal: SIL.
**INQUISITIVE**:
**INSANITY** (Madness): Cs; Km; KP; NM; Ns; Sil.
**Appetite**, Loss of habitual with: Km.
**Injuries** To head, from: NS.
**Mental** Labour, from: KP.
**Moaning**, With: Km.
**Neuralgia**, Disappearance of with: NM.
**Paralytic** Debility, with: Kp; Nm.
**Paroxysmal**: Ns.
**Periodical**: NS.
**Pregnancy**, In: Km; Kp.
**Puerperal**: Kp.
**INSECT bites**: NM; Sil.
**Bitten** By fleas, as if: Mp.
**Crawling**, Formication: Km; Nm; Np; Sil.
**INSECURITY** Sense of: Nm; Ns.
**INSENSIBLE**: See Unconsciousness and numbness.
**INSOLENT**: Nm.
**INSOMNIA**: See Sleeplessness.
**INSPIRATION** Agg: NM; Sil.
**Amel**: Nm.

**INSUSCEPTIBILITY**: See Numbness.
**INTELLECT**: KP; NM.
**INTEMPERANCE** Agg: Km; KP; NM; Np; Sil.
**INTERCOSTAL** Region: Mp; Nm.
**Neuralgia**: See pleurodynia:
**INTERMITTENCY**: CP; KS; NM; NS; SIL
**INTERMITTENT fever**: See under fever.
**INTERTRIGO**: CS; Ks; NM; SIL.
**INTESTINES**:
**Marble** dropped down at stool, as if: Np.
**Ulceration** of: Cp; NP.
**INTOXICATION**: Km; NM; SIL.
**INTROSPECTION**
**Introverted**: Cs; Kp.
**INTUSSUSCEPTION**:
**IRIS Discolouration**: NM.
**Inflammation**: Fp; Km; NM; SIL.
Adhesions, with: Sil.
Choroid of, with: Sil.
Hypopyon, with: **SIL.**
**Jagged**: Sil.
**IRREGULAR, Inco-ordinate**: KP; Nm; **SIL.**
**IRRELIGIOUS**: KP.
**IRRESOLUTE**: See Fickle.
**IRRITABILITY**: CP; **CS;** Fp; KP; **KS; NM;** Np; NS; **SIL.**

5 F.A.

**Alternating** with Cheerfulness: Nm.

**Breakfast**, Before: Np.

**Business**, About: Nm.

**Children**, In: CP; Kp; Sil.

**Chill**, During: Nm.

**Coffee**, After: Cp.

**Coition**, After: Kp; Nm.

**Eating**, After: Nm.

**Evening**, Amel: Nm.

**Headache**, During: Cp; Kp; Mp; Nm; Sil.

**Menses**, Before and after: Nm.

During: Kp; Ks; Nm; Np.

**Own's** Mental sluggishness: Fp.

**Perspiration**, During: Cp; Nm.

**Questioned**, When: Nm.

**Sitting**, While: Nm.

**Spoken** To, when: Nm; Ns; Sil.

**Trifles**: Km; Np.

**Waking**, on: Kp; Nm; Ns.

**ISOLATED EFFECTS**:

**ITCH, Barber's**: Mp.

**ITCHING**: CP; Cs; Kp; KS; NM; Np; NS; **SIL.**

**Air** Agg: Sil.

Cold: Ns.

**Bed,** In: Sil.

**Biting**: Cp; Nm; Np; SIL.

**Burning**: CP; CS; KS; Nm; Np; **SIL.**

**Crawling**: Cs; Kp; Ks; Nm; Np; Sil.

**Internal**: Nm; Sil.

**Jaundice**, In: NP; NS.

**Jerking**: Nm.

**Painful**: Sil.

Menses, during: Sil.

**Scratch**, Must, till it is raw: Sil.

**Smarting**: Sil.

**Spots**: NM; **SIL.**

**Tearing**: Sil.

**Tickling**: SIL.

**Uncovering**: NS.

**Voluptuous**: SIL.

**Wandering**: Sil.

**Warm**, on becoming in bed: NM; NP; **CS.**

**JADED RAKES**: NP.

**JARRING, Shaking,** stepping Agg: Cs; FP; KP; KS; NM; Np; **SIL.**

**Spine**: Sil.

**JAUNDICE**: CP; Cs; Kp; NM; Np; **NS;** SIL.

**Anger**, After: NS.

**Intermittent** Fever: Nm.

**New-born** Children: NS.

**JAWS Caries** of: Sil.

**Chewing**, Motion of: Nm.

Chill, during: Nm.

**Clenched**: SIL.

**Convulsions**, Joints, of: Sil.

**Dislocated**, As if: Fp.

**Lock-jaw**: Mp; Sil.

**Necrosis** of lower: Cp; SIL.

**Pain**, Aching, lower: Kp; SIL.

upper: CP; CS.

Boring, right: Ns.
Drawing in: Nm; **SIL.**
 lower: Nm; Ns.
Crampy, maxillary articulation: Sil.
Gnawing: Nm.
Head, to: Ns.
 other parts, to: Km.
Pressing, lower jaw: Sil.
Sore, bruised: NM; Np; SIL.
 maxillary articulation on chewing: Sil.
Stinging: Sil.
Stitching, Lower jaw: Np; **SIL.**
 joints: Nm.
**Pricking:** Nm.
**Stiffness** Lower: Ns.
**Suppuration**: Sil.
**Swelling**, Lower: CF; Cs; SIL.
**Tension**, Jaw, articulation of: Nm.
**Thickening**: Sil.
**Throbbing**, Lower: Nm.
**Twitching**, Lower, night: SIL.
**Upper**, Affections of maxillary sinus: SIL.
**JEALOUSY**: Cp; CS.
**JELLY** Body were made of: Ns.
**JERKING**, Pain: See Pain, Jerking.
**JERKING Internally:** Nm; SIL.
 **Bones**, In: Sil.
 **Convulsions**, As in: **NM;** Sil.
 **Muscles**: **CP;** Ks; Nm; Sil.
 **Sleep**, in: NM; Ns; Sil.

**JESTING**: Nm.
 **Averse**, to: Nm; Sil.
**JOINTS**: CP; FP; Kp; Nm; NS; SIL.
 **Colds**, Agg: Cp.
 **Constriction**, In: Nm.
 **Cracking**, In: KS; NM; Np; NS.
 **Cramps**: CP.
 **Dislocation**, Easy: Cf; Nm; Sil.
 **Deformed**: **CF;** CP; CS; Nm; NS; SIL.
 **Dryness**: Cs; Kp; NM; SIL.
 **Eruptions**: CS; Cp; NM; Np.
 **Gouty**: CP; CS; Fp; Kp; NM; Np; NS; SIL.
 **Gritty** feeling: Nm.
 **Night**, Amel: Mp.
 **Nodes**, Hard, around: **CF;** CP; Cs; Ks; Nm; SIL.
 **Rheumatic**: **CP;** CS; **FP;** Km; Ks; NM; Np; NS.
 **Rice Bodies**, In: Cf.
 **Small**: Np.
 **Sprained**, Easily: Nm; Sil.
 **Suppuration**: CS; SIL.
 **Swelling**, Pale (white): Km; SIL.
  Fatigue, slight, Agg: Cp; Mp.
  Oedematous, fractures, After: CF; Cp.
 **Synovitis**: Cf; Cp.
 **Tearing** Severe pain: Nm; Sil.
 **Tension**, In: Nm; Sil.
 **Tuberculosis**, of: Cp; Sil.

**Ulcerated**: Sil.
**Water**, in (Hydrarthrosis): Km; Ks; Np.
**Weak**: Cp; Kp.
**JOYOUS**: Cp; Fp; Nm; Np; Ns.
**JUMP**, Tendency, to:
**Bed**, out of:
**Bridge** crossing, when:
**Dream**, in: Cf.
**Height**, from:
**Window**, from: Nm.
**KELOID**: Cf; Sil.
**Itches**, when warm: Sil.
**KERATITIS**: See Cornea, inflammation.
**KIDNEYS** Abscess (perinephritic): Sil.
**Burning**: See Heat.
**Catarrh**: Sil.
**Heat**, in region of: NM.
Sitting, while: Nm.
**Inflammation** (Nephritis): Cs; Km; Kp; Ks; NS.
Acute, parenchymatous: Ks; Ns.
Bronchitis, with: Ks.
Chronic: Fp; Km.
Frequency, of: Kp.
Pelvis of (pyelitis): Cs; Ks.
calculus: **SIL.**
chronic: Sil.
Suppurative: Cs; SIL.
**Jar**, from: Cp.
**Lifting**, Agg: Cp.
**Pain**: Cp; Fp; Km; Kp; NM; Ns.

Blowing nose Agg: Cp.
Burning: Nm.
Burrowing: Nm; **SIL.**
Cramping: Nm.
Cutting, in ureters: Ns; Sil.
Digging, when, Agg: Cp.
Drawing, in ureters: NM.
Extending, to ureters: NM.
Griping: Nm; **SIL.**
Piercing, in both ureters with urge to urinate: Ns.
Pressing: Nm.
outward: NP.
Sore, bruised: Ns.
Stitching: Cf; Kp; Ks; NM; Np.
**Pecking** (Right): Nm.
**Pulsation**: Nm.
**Tension**: Nm.
**KILL, desire** to: Sil.
**Impulse**, sudden to, herself: NS.
**KINDNESS** agg: Sil.
**KISSES** everyone
**KLEPTOMANIA**:
**KNEADING** Bread or making similar motion Agg:
Amel: NS.
**KNEELING** and Praying: Ns.
**KNEES**: Cf; CP; NM; NS; SIL.
**Abscess**: **SIL.**
Gonarthracae: **SIL.**
**Bandaged**, as if: NM; **SIL.**
**Bed**, in Agg: Ns.
**Bending**, Knees Agg: Cp.

**Boring**: Cp; Np; NS.
**Bubbling**: Nm.
**Burning**: Ns.
 Below: Ns.
**Bursitis**: Fp.
**Caries**: Sil.
**Catch**, In: Nm.
**Coition** Agg: Nm.
**Coldness**: NM; **SIL.**
 Chill during: Sil.
 Walking in open air: Sil.
**Cold**, On becoming Agg: SIL.
 Exposed to, when: CP.
**Compression**: Nm; Ns.
**Costriction**: Nm; Ns.
**Contraction**, hamstrings: Cp;
 **NM.**
 Hollow of: **NM;** Ns.
 Lying back on, while: Ns.
**Cracking**: Nm.
 Walking while: Nm.
**Crampy**, (pain) of hollow left:
 Mp.
**Cutting**: Cp; Np.
**Cysts**, Patella: Sil.
**Drawing** Pain: Kp; Ks; NM;
 Np; NS.
 Extending, downwards: Ns.
 Hollow, of: Cp; NM; Ns.
**Eruptions**: NM; Np.
 Boils: NM.
 Crusty: Sil.
 Gritty: Nm.
 Herpes: **NM.**
 Hollow of: NM.

 red: Nm.
 Itching: Nm.
 Vesicles: Np.
**Extending**, Downwards: Kp.
**Heaviness**: Nm.
 Walking, after: Cs.
**Hollow,** of: Cp; Nm.
 left: Np.
**House** Maid's: Nm.
**Inflammation**: Sil.
 Suppressed, gonorrhoea: Sil.
**Itching**: Km; Kp; Nm; Np.
 Bend of: Nm.
 Like insect bites: Np.
**Lameness**: Cs.
**Left then Right**: CP.
**Lying**, After Agg: Np.
 Painful side, on Agg: Nm.
**Moving** Agg: Fp.
 Amel: Ns; SIL.
**Nail** Driven as if in: Nm.
**Numb**: Np.
**Pain**: CP; CS; Kp; Ks; NM;
 Np; NS; Sil.
 Aching: Nm.
 Paralytic: Nm.
 Pinching: Sil.
 Pressing: Ns; **SIL.**
  constrictive: **SIL.**
  sudden: **Ns.**
 Rheumatic: CP; Fp; Nm.
**Shuddering**: Nm.
 Walking, Amel: Nm.
**Shooting**: FP.
 Sitting, while: NM; Ns; SIL.
 Sitting, Amel: Sil.

**Sore**, bruised: Cp; Kp; Nm; Np; Ns.

Patella: Sil.

**Sprained**, As if: CP; Nm.

**Standing** Amel: Sil.

**Stiffness**: CS; Km; Nm; NS; **SIL.**

Rising, from seat: Nm.

Standing, while: Sil.

Walking, while: Sil.

**Stitching**: CS; Fp; KS; NM; Np; Ns; SIL.

Leg down: Fp.

Hollow of: Nm.

inner side as from nail: Nm.

**Stretching** Agg: Cp; Sil.

**Swelling**: CP; Cs; Ks; NM; **SIL.**

Dropsical: SIL.

Hot: FP.

Rheumatic: Cs.

Scrofulous: SIL.

Spongy: SIL.

White (Tuberculous): Cf; Cp; SIL.

**Tearing**: KM; Kp; Nm; Np; NS; SIL.

Downwards, extending: Ns.

Hollow of: Nm.

Stitch, like: Sil.

**Tension**: **NM;** Sil.

Hollow, of: NM.

Menses, during and after: Np.

Rising from seat: Cp; Nm.

Walking, while: Sil.

continued Amel.:

**Trembling**: Nm; Sil.

Ascending: Nm.

Emissions after: Np.

**Tumours of Hollow**: Cf; Sil.

**Twitching**: Np.

**Walking** On Agg: CP; Nm; Ns.

Amel: KS; Ns.

**Weakness**: Cs; FP; Ks; **NM; NS;** SIL.

Morning: Nm.

Walking, while: Nm.

**KNIFE** Sight of Agg: Sil.

**KNOT**: See Ball.

**KNUCKLES**: Nm.

**KYPHOSIS**: CS; SIL.

**LABIAE**: See Vulvae.

**LABOUR LIKE pains**: Cp; Kp; Nm; SIL.

**LABOUR PAINS Ceasing**: Kp; NM.

**Cramps**: Cp; MP.

**Cramps** In legs, with: MP.

**Excessive**: Mp.

**False**: Kp.

**Ineffectual**: Kp.

**Spasmodic**: Mp.

**Weak**: Kp; **NM.**

**LACERATIONS**: Km; SIL.

**LACHRYMAL CANAL,**

Gland and sac: Sil.

**Discharge** from sac: **SIL.**

Pus, on pressure: SIL.

**Epiphora**: NM; SIL.
**Fistula**: NM; **SIL.**
**Inflammation**, Canal: NM; SIL.
　Gland, of: **SIL.**
　Sac, of: **SIL.**
**Stricture** of Canal: NM; **SIL.**
**Swollen** Canal: NM; SIL.
　Gland, sac: **SIL.**
**LACHRYMATION**: Cp; Fp; Kp; Ks; NM; Np; NS; **SIL.**
**Affected** Side Agg: Nm.
**Air**, Cold, in: Sil.
　Open: NM; SIL.
**Cold**, Head in, with: Km.
**Cough**, With: NM; Sil.
**Headache**, During: Nm.
**Laughing**, When: Nm.
**Morning**: Nm.
**Pain**, During: Nm.
**Sneezing**, With: Nm.
**Tears**, Acrid: NM.
　Biting, smarting: NM.
　Burning: NS; SIL.
　Leave varnish mark: Nm.
**Whooping** Cough, with: NM.
**Wind**, In: Nm; SIL.
**Yawning**, When: Cp.
**LACK of POWER**: Kp; SIL.
**LACK of VITAL HEAT**: CF; **CP**; CS; **KP**; **MP**; NM; NP; **SIL.**
**Exercise**, During: SIL.
**LACTATION**: Sil.
**Milk**, Absent, scant: Cp.
　Bad, spoiled: Cf; Cp; **SIL.**

Child refuses, mother's: **CP**; Sil.
Flowing: SIL.
Salty: Nm.
Sour, acid: Cp; Np.
Suppressed: SIL.
Thin: CP; Nm; SIL.
**LA GRIPPE** (Influenza): Fp; Ks; NS.
**LAIN ON PARTS Agg**: Nm; (See Pressure Agg and Directions.)
**LAMENTING**: Kp; Nm; Mp; Sil.
**Appreciated**, Because he is not: Cs.
**LANCINATING** Pain: Km; Mp.
**LARYNX Burning**: CP; Fp.
**Catarrh**: **CP**; **CS**; KS; NM; Sil.
**Closed**, Nearly as if: Cf.
**Cold** Air, Agg: Cp; Sil.
**Constriction**: NM; SIL.
　Auditory canal scratching from: SIL.
　Sleep, during: SIL.
**Crawling**: NM.
　Dust, as from: Cs; NM.
　Foreign substance: CF; NM; SIL.
　desire to swallow with: Cf.
**Lump**: NM.
Scratching: Nm.
Tickling: CF; CP; KP; **NM**; Np; NS; SIL.
　3 to 4 p.m.: Cf.
　day and night: Nm.
　ulcerative: Nm.

**Croup**: **CS**; Kp; NM.
Recurrent: **CS.**
Spasmodic: CF; CP; Fp.
**Dryness**: Cf; Fp; Km; KS;
NM.
**Ear,** To: Nm.
**Food,** Drops into: Nm.
**Hair,** In: Sil.
**Inflammation** (Laryngitis): Cs;
FP; Km; NM.
Chronic, catarrhal: Nm.
Membranous: Fp; KM.
Singer's: Fp.
Tuberculous: Cp; Fp; Km;
SIL.
**Inspiration** Agg: Nm; Sil.
**Irritation**: CP; KM: KP; KS;
**NM**; Np; SIL.
Swallowing empty agg: NM.
**Itching**: Cf; Sil.
**Lifting** Agg: Sil.
**Mucus,** In: CP.
Copious: Nm.
Cough, each paroxysm af-
ter: NM.
Ejected with difficulty: NM;
SIL.
**Pain:** Nm.
Air, cold Agg: Sil.
Bending head backwards:
Sil.
Burning: CP; Fp.
Coughing: Nm.
Rending, tearing: Nm; Sil.
Stitching: KS.
Talking Agg: Nm.

**Paralysis** of Vocal cords: Kp.
**Rattling,** In: Fp; KS; Nm; Sil.
**Rough,** Raw: NS; SIL.
**Scraping,** Clearing: CF; CP;
CS; Kp; KS; NM; Ns; SIL.
**Singers** Of: FP.
**Soreness**: CS; KS; MP; NM;
SIL.
**Swelling,** Fibrous, painless:
Sil.
**Tickling,** In: Nm; Sil.
**LARYNGISMUS STRIDULUS**:
CF; Fp.
**LASCIVIOUS** (Amorous): Cs;
Nm; SIL.
**LASSITUDE** (inactive): Fp; Km;
KP; NM; Np; **SIL.**
**Conversation,** From: Sil.
**Heat** of Summer, from: Sil.
**Sleep,** After: Sil.
**Warm** Weather: Np.
**LATENT DISEASE:** KS; SIL..
**LAUGHING** AGG: Nm.
**LAUGHS**: Kp; NM; SIL.
**Asthma** With: Ns; Sil.
**Averse** To: Kp; Nm.
**Cause** Without: Nm; Sil.
**Evening**: Nm.
**Immoderately**: NM.
**Involuntarily**: Nm.
**Night**: Sil.
**Serious matters,** Over: NM.
**Sleep,** During: **SIL.**
Whining, and: Sil.
**Spasmodic,** Convulsive, hys-
terical: Nm; Sil.

**Weeping**, Alternately: Kp.
**LAUNDRY WORK** agg: Mp.
**LAX**: Kp; Nm; Np.
**LAZINESS**: KP; NM.
**LEAD** AGG: NS.
**LEAF**, Valve, skin, as of a: Ns.
**LEANING AGAINST** Anything,
    **Agg**: Nm; Sil.
    Amel: KP; NM.
**LEAN people: CP; SIL.**
**LEARNS easily:**
**Poorly**: CP; Nm.
**LECHEROUS, lewd**: Cs; Nm;
    SIL.
**LECTOPHOBIA** (Fear of Bed):
**LEGS** (Lower Limbs): CP; **SIL.**
    **Abscess** (Psoas): SIL.
    Joints, of: Cp; SIL.
    **Air,** Open Agg: MP.
    **Alive** Sensation: Sil.
    **Alternating**, Between: Cp; Mp;
    NM; Ns; Sil.
    Upper with: Km; **SIL.**
    **Ascending** Steps Agg: Nm.
    **Ataxia** (Inco-ordination): SIL.
    **Awakening** Agg: Ns.
    **Awkwardness**: Mp; NM; Sil.
    **Band** Around bones, as if:
    Nm.
    **Below**, Knees: Sil.
    burning: NS.
    **Bones**: Cf; CP; SIL.
    **Brown** Spots: Ns.
    **Bubbling**: Sil.
    **Burning**: Ns.

**Bursae**, Joints in: Cp; Km;
    **NM; SIL.**
    Cysts: SIL.
**Chill,** During Agg: Nm.
**Chilliness**: NM.
**Cold** Agg: MP; Sil.
    Applications, Agg: MP.
**Coldness**: CP; Cs; FP; Km;
    KP; Ks; NM; Np; SIL.
    Icy: SIL.
    Joints, of: NM.
    Menses, during: SIL.
    Painful parts: Sil.
    Standing while: Nm.
    Warm room, in: SIL.
**Compression**: Ns.
**Constriction**, Joint: NM; Sil.
**Contraction**: NM; SIL.
    Hamstrings: CP; Np.
    Joints: NM.
    Menses, after: Np.
    Spasmodic: Mp; Sil.
**Convulsion**: Sil.
**Cracked**, Skin: Nm.
**Cracking**, Joints in: KS; NM;
    Np; NS.
**Cramps**: KM; Kp; KS; NM;
    SIL.
    Chill, during: SIL.
    Exertion, after: Mp.
    Thighs, in: Fp.
**Curving** and bowing: CP;
    **SIL.**
**Dislocation**, Joints of, easy:
    Cf; **NM.**

**Distortion**, Joints of: **SIL.**
**Drawn** Apart: Sil.
  Up, flexing knees Amel: Sil.
  Upwards on abdomen, in necrosis of femur: SIL.
**Elephantiasis**: Sil.
**Emaciation**: Nm.
  Diseased limbs, of: Nm; Sil.
  Paralysed, limbs: KP.
**Emotions** Agg: **NM.**
**Eruptions**: CP; KS; Nm; Np; **SIL.**
  Bends of joints: NM.
  Boils: Nm; **SIL.**
  Desquamation: Cp.
  Dry: Cp.
  Eczema: Nm.
  Gritty: Nm.
  Groups, in: Nm.
  Herpes: **NM;** Sil.
  Joints, on: Cp; NM; Np.
  Miliary: Sil.
  Moist: Nm.
  Pimples: Cp; KS; Nm; Np;Sil.
  Rash: Nm.
  Red: Nm.
  Scabies: Cp; KS.
  Scabs: Ks; SIL.
  Vesicles: NM; SIL.
    between thighs: Nm; Ns.
    bloody serum: NM.
    corroding: Sil.
    thighs inside: Sil.
**Exertion** Amel: Nm.
**Fatigue**, Sense of: Nm.

**Formication**: CP.
  Riding: CP.
  Sitting, after: CP.
**Gait**: See Gait.
**Headache**, During Agg: Sil.
**Heat**: Nm.
**Heaviness** (Tired limbs): Cp; Cs; KP; Ks; NM; Np; Ns; SIL.
  Ascending, steps: NM.
  Fatigue, as from: Ns.
  Menses, during: Cp.
    suppressed: Nm.
  Motion, Amel: Nm.
  Pregnancy, during: Cp.
  Thighs, of: Ns.
  Walking, while: Sil.
**Inco-ordination**: SIL.
**Inflammation**, Bones: **SIL.**
  Erysipelatous: SIL.
  Joints: FP; NM; NS; **SIL.**
  Periosteum of: Cf; Sil.
  Synovitis: Fp; Sil.
  Tibia: **SIL.**
**Itching:** Kp; NM; Np; NS; **SIL.**
  Scratching Amel: Ns.
  Thighs, between: Nm.
  Touch, Agg: Nm.
  Undressing: **NS.**
**Jerking**: Ks; NM; Sil.
  Falling asleep on: Sil.
  Lying on back: Cp; Ns.
  Sleep, during: NM.
    on going, to: NM.

**Lameness**: Cp; **NM;** Sil.
Flexor muscles: Cp.
Joints: SIL.
**Lightness**, Sensation of: Nm.
**Living**, In Cold damp house
Agg: NS.
**Loose**, Sensation, bones: Nm.
**Lying** Agg: NM; **SIL.**
Affected parts, on: Sil.
Bed, in: Sil.
**Menses**, After Agg: Cp.
During Agg: SIL.
**Milk** leg (phlegmasia alba
dolens): CF; NS; SIL.
**Motion**, Convulsive: Cp.
Difficult: Sil.
Involuntary: Nm.
Lying on back, when: Cp.
on side Amel.: Cp.
Loss of power, in morning
on waking: Sil.
**Motion Agg**: Cp; Kp; Mp; Ns;
Sil.
**Motion, amel**: Cp; KP; **KS;**
Nm; NS; SIL.
slow· Kp.
**Mouse**, Running up, sensa-
tion, of: SIL.
**Night** Agg: MP; NM.
**Nodes**: Nm; Sil.
Tibia: Cf.
**Numbness**: CP; Cs; Kp; KS;
NM; Np; Ns; **SIL.**
Extending to wrist-line: CP.
to leg: Fp.

Lying on, then: SIL.
One of, pain in other: Sil.
Riding, while: CP.
Siesta, during: Nm.
Sitting: CP; Sil.
Thighs: Sil.
**Over-exertion** Agg: **SIL.**
**Pain:** CP; CS; Kp; MP; NM;
Np; SIL.
Above the knee: Sil.
Aching: CP; NM; Np.
bones in: CP; Nm; SIL.
chill during: Nm.
extensor muscles: Cp.
Alternating, with convulsive
pain in arms: Sil.
Anterior part: Ns.
Bones, in: Nm; Ns; SIL.
Boring: Np.
Breaking, brittle: Ns.
Burning: Kp; SIL.
below knee: NS.
Crampy: Fp; **KM;** MP; NM.
labour, during: Mp.
Cutting: SIL.
Downward: Kp; Mp; Nm.
Drawing: Cp; NM; SIL.
feet, to: SIL.
thighs, to: Kp; Ns.
Ending in jerking: SIL.
Inner side (thighs): Cp; Np;
Sil.
above the knee: Cp; Nm.
Jerking: Sil.
Lower part (thighs): CP.

Paralytic: NM; SIL.

Paroxysmal: MP; Nm.

Pinching: Sil.

Posterior part (thighs): NM; Sil.

Pressing: Kp; Sil.

Rheumatic: Cs; Nm.

Sciatica: CP; Fp; KP; **MP;** NM; NS; SIL.

    coldness of painful limbs with: Ns; Sil.

    hips to feet: Sil.

    suddenly comes and goes: MP.

    tonic contraction, chronic: NM.

    vertebral origin: NM; Sil.

Shooting: CP.

    downwards: Cp.

Sitting when, Agg: KS; Nm; Sil.

Sitting Amel: Sil.

Sore, bruised: Fp; Kp; NM; Np; Ns; SIL.

**Pulsation:** SIL.

**Sprained** as if: Nm.

**Standing** Agg: Ns; Sil.

**Stepping** On Agg: Sil.

**Stiffness**: Cs; NM.

**Stitching**: Cs; Fp; Kp; **KS;** NP; NS; SIL.

    Bones in: Sil.

    Downwards: SIL.

**Stooping** Agg: Nm; Ns; Sil.

**Stormy** Weather Agg: **SIL**

**Stretching** Out, Extending limbs Agg: Nm.

    Amel: Nm.

**Tearing**: Ks; NM; **NS;** SIL.

    Back and foot: Sil.

**Tension**: NM.

    Alternating with upper: Km.

    Ascending steps: Nm.

    Downwards: NM.

    Hamstrings: CP; **NM;** Np.

    Menses during: Nm.

    Tendons in, as if short: Nm.

    Walking, while: Nm.

**Thrusting**: Nm.

**Tingling**, prickling: Sil.

    Sitting while: Sil.

**Trembling**: See Trembling.

**Twitching**: Fp; Kp; Ks; NM; Np; Ns; **SIL.**

    Electric shock, as from: Nm.

    Sleep, during: Nm; Sil.

    falling to: NM.

    Wandering: NS.

**Uncovering Agg:** Sil.

**Weak:** Nm; Ns.

    Descending Agg: Sil.

**LENS**: SIL.

**Cataract**: **CF;** CP; Km; Ks; Nm; **SIL.**

    Foot sweat suppressed from: **SIL.**

    Office worker's: Sil.

    Right eye: Sil.

**LENTIGO, Freckles:** Sil.

**LEPROSY:** SIL.

**LETHARGY**: See lassitude.
**LEUCODERMA**: Cf; Nm; SIL.
**LEUCORRHOEA**: CP; **CS;** Fp; Kp; KS; **NM;** Np; Ns; **SIL.**
   **Agg:** Nm.
   **Amel:**
   **Abdominal** Pain, after: Cp; **NM; SIL.**
   **Acrid**, Corroding: CS; Fp; Km; KP; Ks; NM; NP; Ns; **SIL.**
   blisters, causing: Kp; Ns.
   **Afternoon:** Cp.
   **Backache and Weak** feeling preceding and attending: NM.
   **Biting:** Sil.
   **Bland:** Cp; Fp; Km; Nm; Sil.
   **Bloody: CS;** SIL.
   **Brown:** SIL.
   **Burning**: CS; KP; Ks; Nm.
   Abdominal pain, after: Cp.
   **Children**, In: Cp.
   **Colic**, After: Cp; SIL.
   **Copious**: Cp; Cs; Kp; NM; NP; **SIL.**
   **Cream** Like: CP; NP.
   **Day** and Night: Cp.
   **Debilitating**, Replacing menses: Nm.
   **Diarrhoea**, with: Nm.
   **Gonorrhoea**, following: NS.
   **Greenish**: KP; KS; **NM; NS.**
   **Gushing: SIL.**
   **Headache**, With: Nm.
   **Hoarseness**, With: Ns.

**Honey Coloured**: Np.
**Hypogastrium**, Cutting pain, with: **SIL.**
**Itching**, Causing: Sil.
**Lumpy**: Sil.
**Menses**, After: CP; CS; Kp; Nm; NP; Ns; SIL
   Before: CP; CS; Fp; NM; SIL.
   Instead of: Cp; Nm; SIL.
   scanty, with: Cp.
   two weeks after: CP.
**Milky:** CP; Fp; **KM;** Nm; **SIL.**
   Flowing at intervals: Sil.
**Night**: Nm.
**Offensive:** Cp; **KP;** Ks; **SIL.**
   Putrid: **KP.**
   Sour: NP.
   Sweetish: Cp.
**Orange coloured:** Kp.
**Painful:** Sil.
**Parturition,** after: Ns.
**Purulent:** Cs; Kp; KS; Ns; Sil.
**Rawness** and Itching pain with: Np.
**Smell,** Sour: NP.
   Sweetish: Cp.
**Starch** Like boiled: Nm.
**Stools** Foul with: Cp.
**Thick**: Cs; KM; Ks; NM.
**Thin**, Watery: Fp; KS; NM; NP; SIL.
**Transparent**: CP; NM.
**Unconsciousness** of: Cp.

**Urinating**, After: Sil.
During: SIL.
**Walking**, While: **NM.**
**White**: CP; CS; Fp; Km; NP.
Green, turns: Nm.
**Yellow**: Cs; Kp; KS; Nm; NP; Sil.
**Yellowish** Green: Kp.
**LEUKEMIA**: CP; KP; NM; NP; **NS**.
**Splenic**: Ns.
**LEVITATION** (floating as if): Cs; NM.
**LEWD**: See Lascivious.
**LICE** (Lousiness):
**Itching**, with:
**LICHEN**: Nm.
**LICKING**, Lips Agg: NM.
**LIE DOWN** inclination to: Fp; Km; Ks; NM; Np; NS; **SIL**.
**Eating**, after: NM.
**LIDS**: See Eye lids.
**LIENTERIC Diarrhoea**: Cs; Fp; KP; Np; NS.
**LIFE Satiety** of: NS; Sil.
**Unworthy** of: Cp; Nm; NS.
**Weary** of: KP; NM; SIL.
**LIFTED Up** Sensation: Cs; Nm.
**LIFTING Agg**: Cf; CP; CS; Fp; Km; Nm; Ns; SIL.
**Amel**:
**LIGAMENTS** (fibrous tissue): Cf; KM; SIL.
**LIGHT Agg**: FP; Kp; Mp; NM; Np; NS; SIL.
**Artificial**: NM; SIL.

**Candle**: **NP**; NS.
**Day**: Nm; **SIL**.
**Gas**: Ns.
**Stained** glass: Ns.
**Subdued**: Ns.
**LIGHT Desire** for: Nm; Sil.
**Sun**: Km.
**LIGHTNING Pains**: Km; Mp.
**LIMBS Upper**: See arms.
**Lower**: See legs.
**Alternatig** Upper and Lower: Km; **SIL**.
**Cold**: CP.
Digestion, affected, with: Cp.
**Crawling**: Cp.
**Drawn** Up: Nm.
**Drawing** Up Agg:
Amel: MP.
**Elevating** Amel: NM; SIL.
**Numb**: Cp.
**LINEA Nasalis**: See Face pale.
**LINEAR Pains**: Km; KP; Sil.
**LIPS**: NM; Sil.
**Bleeding**: Nm.
**Bluish**: Fp; Nm.
**Burning**: CS; Fp; NM.
Smokers in: Nm.
Touched when: Fp; NM; SIL.
**Cancer**: Ks; SIL.
Epithelioma: Km; Sil.
lower: Sil.
**Chapped**: **NM.**
**Cold Sores**: Cf.
**Corners**, Cracked: MP; NM; **SIL**.

Eczema: Sil.
Eruptions: Cf; NM; SIL.
  scabs: SIL.
Excoriated: Km; Nm.
Indented: Sil.
Indurated: SIL.
Inflamed: Sil.
Nodosities: Sil.
Pain, burning: Ns.
  sore: Sil.
Swelling: NM; Sil.
Twitching: Mp.
Ulcers: NM; SIL.
**Cracked**: Cp; CS; Kp; Ks; **NM;** SIL.
Middle of: NM.
**Crawling**: NM.
**Crusty,** Scaly: Nm; SIL.
**Discolouration**, Bluish: Fp; NM.
  Chill, during: NM.
  Pale: FP; Np.
  Red, upper: Nm.
**Drawn** up: Nm.
**Drooping**: Kp.
**Dryness**: Fp; Km; Kp; NM; Ns; SIL.
  Burning and desquamation with: Ns.
**Egg** Albumin, on: Nm.
**Eruptions**: Cf; Cs; Km; Ks; **NM;** Np; Ns; SIL.
  Crusts, scabs: Kp; Nm; **SIL.**
  Eczema: NM.
  Herpes: CF; NM; Sil.

Lower: NM.
Mouth, around: Cf; Km; **NM;** Np; Ns; SIL.
Pimples: Kp.
  mouth, around: SIL.
Scabs, around: SIL.
Tubercles, about, mouth: Sil.
Upper: NM; SIL.
Vesicles: Cs; Kp. Ks; **NM;** Ns: Sil.
  lower: Cs; Ns.
  mouth, around: **NM;** NS.
  upper: Kp; Mp.
  blood blisters: NM.
**Excoriated**: KP; Nm.
**Indented**: Sil.
**Induration**: Cp; Sil.
  Upper: Cp.
**Itching**, Lower: Sil.
  Mouth, around: Np.
  Swelling, with: Kp.
**Jerking**, Twitching: Mp.
  Convulsions, during: Sil.
**Licks**: Nm.
**Nodosities**: Sil.
**Numbness**: NM.
**Pain**, Burning: Ns.
  Lips, inside: Cs.
  Lower: Nm.
  Sore: Nm.
    inside: Cs.
  Stinging: Sil.
  Upper: CP.
**Peeling**: Km; Kp; Ks; NM; Ns; Sil.

**Pouting**, Thick: Nm.
**Rough**, Upper: Nm.
**Salty**: Nm.
**Sensitive**: Nm.
**Slimy**: Km.
**Sordes,** On: Kp; Nm.
**Swelling**: Km; Kp; Ks; **NM; SIL.**
  As if: Kp.
  Lower: Ks; Sil.
  Red: Fp.
  Upper: Cp; Kp; **NM.**
**Tingling**: NM.
**Twitching**, Around, mouth: Mp.
**Ulcers**: Km; Kp; NM; **SIL.**
  Lower: Sil.
**LITHEMIA**: Ns.
**LIVELY**: See Cheerful.
**LIVER**: CF; CP; Ks; NM; NS; Sil.
**Abscess: SIL.**
**Air,** Open **Agg:** NS.
**Atony,** of: Km.
**Atrophy:** KM; NM; NS.
**Backward**, to scapulae: Ns.
  right, to: NM.
**Ball**, Lump, in: NS.
  Below: Ns.
**Bending**, Forward Amel: CF; Nm.
**Bile** Ducts: Np.
**Breathing**, Deep Agg: NS.
**Bursting**: Ns.
**Cancer**: Sil.
  Jaundice, with: Kp; Ns.

**Cirrhosis**: Km; Sil.
  boils, with: Np; Sil.
**Coughing** Agg: Ns.
**Cutting**: Cf.
**Enlarged**: Fp; Ks; NM; **NS;** Sil.
**Fullness**: KM; Nm; Ns.
  Chronic: Ns.
**Hard,** indurated: Sil.
**Heaviness**: Ns.
**Inflammation**: Kp; NM; **NS;** Sil.
  Chronic: NM; **NS.**
**Jarring**, Agg: Ns.
**Lying Back**, on Amel: Np.
  Left side: Ns.
**Pain** (hepatalgia): CF; CP; CS; FP; Kp; Ks; NM; **NS; SIL.**
  Mental labour, after: **NS.**
  Sitting, Agg: Cf.
  Touched, when, Agg: NS; Sil.
  Vexation, after: NS.
  Waking, while: NS; Sil.
**Pressing**: CP; CS; NM: SIL.
**Sclerosis** of: Np.
  Diabetes and succession of boils with: Np.
**Stiffness**, Sense of: Nm.
**Stitching**, Sticking: CF; CP; Cs; Kp; Ks; NM; NP; NS; SIL.
**Swelling**: Nm; **NS;** Sil.
  Mental exertion, after: Ns.

**Throbbing**, Beating: Ns; Sil.
**Twisting**: NM; NS; SIL.
**Waxy:**
**LIVER SPOTS**: KP.
**LIVID**: See Blue.
**LOAD**: See Heaviness.
**LOATHING**: See Aversion.
**LOCATION LOST**: See Confused.
**LOCHIA Acrid**: Sil.
  **Bloody**: Sil.
    Grows light and again becomes: Sil.
    Child nurses, when: SIL.
  **Hot**: Sil.
    Ceases when lying: Sil.
  **Offensive**: KP; Sil.
  **Protracted**: NM.
  **Red**: SIL.
  **White**: NM.
**LOCK-JAW**: Mp; Sil.
**LOCOMOTOR** Ataxia: MP; NM; Sil.
**LOINS:**
**LONELY:**
**LONGING**: See Craving.
**LOOKED at Agg**: NM; Sil.
**LOOKING About Agg**: Sil.
  **Downward**: Fp.  .
  **Long**, Anything at: Nm.
  **Moving** Objects, at: NM.
  **Steadily**: NM; SIL.
  **Upward**: Sil.
  **White** Objects, at: NM.
  **Window**, Out of: NM.

**LOOSE As if**: Km; Nm; Ns; Sil.
  **Flesh,** From bones: Nm.
**LOOSE, Lax**: Cp; Kp; NM.
**LOQUACITY** (Talkative): Fp; Nm.
**LOSS OF MEMORY**: Cp; Cs.
**LOSS OF VITAL FLUIDS AGG**: CP; KP; Nm; NP; SIL.
**LOVE Ailments** from disappointed: CP; KP; **NM.**
  **Sick** With one of her own sex: Cp; Nm.
  **Silent** Grief from disappointed: **NM.**
**LOWER LIMBS**: See Legs.
**LUMBAGO**: See Lumbar Back.
**LUMBAR BACK**: CP; Cs; KP; Np; SIL.
  **Abscess**: CP.
    Psoas: Sil.
  **Aching**: Cf; Cp; KP; Np; Ns; SIL.
    Erect on becoming: Nm.
    Waist line: Nm.
  **Affected** By everything: KP.
  **Breaking**: Nm.
  **Broken**, as if: NM.
  **Burning**: Kp; Np; Sil.
    Up the spine:
    Between scapulae: Sil.
  **Caries** of Vertebrae: SIL.
  **Chill** Starts, in: NM.
  **Coldness**: Nm.
  **Cramp** Like pain: Sil.

**Cutting**: Cp; NM.
**Drawing**: Cs; Km; Kp; NM; SIL.
**Everything** Agg: Cp.
**Feet**, To: Km.
**Heat**: NM.
Flushes of: Cp.
**Heaviness**: Kp.
**Hip**, To: SIL.
**Itching**: NM.
Burning, to abdomen and thighs: Nm.
**Lameness**: NM; Sil.
**Lancinating**, Injury, after: Ns.
Motion, Amel: Ns.
**Morning**, Rising, bed from: Km; **NM.**
**Night: NS; SIL.**
**Numbness**: SIL.
Loss of sensation in morning or on rising: NM.
**Pain**: Cf; CP; Cs; FP; Km; KP; KS; MP; NM; NP; NS; SIL.
Penetrating: Nm.
Pressing: Cp; Cs; Nm; Sil.
menses, during: Fp.
Sore, bruised: CP; NM; NS; SIL.
morning, rising till evening: Ns.
Stitching, shooting: CP; Cs; Kp; MP; NM; Np; **SIL.**
Tearing: CP; Kp; NS; **SIL.**
Ulcerative: Ns.
(Agg and Amel see Back)

**Paralysis**: NM.
Sensation of: NM.
**Perspiration:** SIL.
**Pressure** Amel: Nm.
**Radiating**, from: Sil.
Down the legs: SIL.
Scapulae to right: Nm.
Thighs to: Nm.
**Restlessness**: CF.
**Separating**, As if: CP.
**Stiffness**: Nm.
**Swelling**: Sil.
**Tension**: NM; Sil.
**Weakness** of Spine: CF; **CS;** Ks; **NM;** Np; SIL.
Emissions, after: Np.
Morning: Sil.
Sitting: FP.
**LUMBO-SACRAL** Region:
**Pain**: Sil.
**Stiffness:** Nm.
**LUMP**: See Ball.
**LUMPS, Lumpy effects:** Cs; Sil.
**LYING Agg:** Cp; Fp; Km; Nm; **NS.**
**After:** Sil.
**Back**, On: KP; MP; Nm; NS; **SIL.**
**Bed**, in: Km; Kp; Ks; NM; NP; **SIL**.
**Moist** Floor, on: Cp; **SIL.**
**Side**, On: Nm; NS; **SIL.**
Left: **NM;** Np; Ns; SIL.
Painful: Cf; Km; Kp; Nm; **SIL.**
Right: Km; MP.

**LYING Amel:** CP; Fp; kP; MP; **NM: SIL**

**Abdomen,** On: CP.

**Back,** On: NM; NS; Sil.

**Bed,** In: NM; SIL

**Doubled,** or Bent: MP.

**Hard** Surface, on: Nm.

**Side,** on: Cp; Nm; SIL.

    Left: Nm.

    Painful: Mp; Sil.

    Painless: Cf; Km; SIL.

    Right: **NM;** SIL.

**LYING-IN women** (Puerperal state): NM; Sil.

**Uncomfortable,** As if: Sil.

**LYMPHANGITIS:** Km; Kp; Sil.

    **Acute** glandular infiltration, and hard swelling: Km.

**LYMPHATIC VESSELS:** Km; Kp.

**LYPOTHEMIA** (Mental exhaustion from grief): CP; Kp; **NM.**

**MADDENING** pain: NM.

**MADNESS:** See Insanity.

**MAGNETISED, Desires,** to be: SIL.

**MAGNETISM Amel:** Sil.

**MALAR BONES Caries:** Ks.

    **Inflammation:** SIL.

    **Pain,** Zygoma: Cp; Ns.

    Burning: Nm.

    **Swelling:** Nm.

**MALARIA:** See Fever Intermittent.

**MALE** (Genitals): NM; NS; SIL.

**Condylomata: NS.**

**Cowperitis:** Sil.

**Crawling:** Cp.

**Disagreeable** Feeling in: Sil.

**Erections:** See Erections.

**Eruptions:** Nm; Sil.

    Eczema: Nm.

    Herpetic: Nm; Sil.

    Itching: Nm.

      moist spots: SIL.

    Miliary: SIL.

    Moist: Nm; Sil.

    Pimples: Nm; Sil.

    Vesicles: Np.

**Flaccidity** (Relaxation): Mp; Sil.

**Hair,** falling from pubis: **NM.**

**Irritability** Excited: **NM; SIL.**

**Itching:** Ks; Nm; NS; Sil.

    Burning: Nm.

    Night: **NM.**

    Urination, during: Sil.

**Masturbation,** Disposition for: Nm,

    Ill effects, of: CP; Nm.

**Odour,** Stinking: NM.

**Pain,** Cutting, compressing: Sil.

**Perspiration:** Sil.

    Offensive: Nm.

**Throbbing,** In: Cp.

**Voluptuous** Feeling in: Cp.

**Weakness,** Sensation of: Cp; NM.

    Stool, after: CP.

**MALICE**: See Hatred.

**MALIGNANCY**: See Cancerous affections.

Suspected: Kp.

**MALINGERING**:

**MAL-NUTRITION**: CP; Nm; SIL.

**MAMMAE**: CP; NM; SIL.

**Right**: SIL.

**Left**: Nm.

**Alternating**, Sides:

**Abscess**: SIL.

Gangrenous, offensive pus: Kp.

Nipples, of: SIL.

**Atrophy**: NM; SIL.

**Bleeding,** Nipples: Sil.

**Cancer**: SIL.

Epithelioma: Cp; SIL.

Itching, with: SIL.

Scirrhus: SIL.

**Cicatrices**, Old: Cf.

Suppurating: Sil.

**Cracks**, Of Nipples: Sil.

**Distension**, Sensation: Sil.

**Drawn** in like a funnel, nipple: Sil.

**Dwindled**, Emaciated: Nm; Sil.

**Enlarged**, As if: Cp.

**Eruptions**, On: Nm.

**Excoriation**, Nipple: Cp; SIL.

**Fistula**: SIL.

**Fullness**: CP.

**Indurated**, Hard: Cp; **SIL.**

Left: **SIL.**

**Inflammation**: Cf; Cs; Fp; Km; SIL.

Nipples: SIL.

Pus formation, before: Km.

**Inverted,** Nipples: Ns.

**Itching:** Nm; Sil.

**Milk**, Bad spoiled: Cf; Cp; **SIL.**

Flowing: SIL.

Mother's child refuses: CP; Sil.

Salty: Nm.

Sour, acrid: Cp.

Suppressed: SIL.

Thin: CP; Nm; SIL.

**Nodules**, Sensitive, in: Cf; Cp; Nm; **SIL.**

Left: CP.

Right: SIL.

Hard: CF; Sil.

Soft: Km.

Walnut like, in male: Cp.

**Pain**: CP; Km; SIL.

Left: Sil.

Nipples: CP.

Region of: Ns.

Burning: CP.

nipples: SIL.

Cutting: Cp.

right, under: Kp.

Drawing, from nipple all over the body: Sil.

**Menses**, Before agg: KM.

**Nursing**, while the child: SIL.

**Pregnancy**, during: CP.

**Pressing**, in region of: NM.

**Sitting**, while: Ns.
**Sore**, bruised: CP; Km; Nm; **SIL.**
nipples: CP; SIL.
sensitive: Ks.
**Stitching**: KP; NM; SIL.
left: SIL.
nipple: SIL.
under: Nm.
stitching region, of: Sil.
uterus, pain with: Sil.
**Perspiration**, Night: Sil.
**Retraction**, Nipples, of: Ns; **SIL.**
**Small**, Undeveloped: See. Atrophy.
**Swelling**: Nm; **SIL.**
Cicatrices, of: **SIL.**
Menses, before: KM; Ks.
**Tumours**: SIL.
Left: CP.
Like a walnut in male: Cp.
**Ulceration**: SIL.
Nipples: SIL
**Warts,** little around, after. Nursing: Sil.
**MANIA**: KP; Nm.
**Periodical**: Ns.
**Mono**: Sil.
**MANIA-A-POTU:** Cs; Fp; Kp; **NM;** Sil.
**MARASMUS** (Emaciation): NM.
**Infants,** bottle fed: Np.
**MARRIAGE** the Idea seemed unendurable: Kp; Nm.

**MASSETERS contracted**: Nm.
**Cramp:** CP; MP.
**Stiff**, Hard: Sil.
**MASTITIS**: See Mammae, Inflammation.
**MASTODYNIA**: See Mammae, Pain.
**MASTOID**: See Ear, Behind.
**Caries**: SIL.
**Inflammation**: Cp; Fp; Km; Mp; Sil.
**Periosteitis**: Cf.
**MASTURBATION, Disposition,** (Males): Nm.
**Females**: Kp; Nm.
**Ill effects** of: CP; Kp; NM; **NP;** Sil.
**MEAN** (Avaricious): Cf.
**MEASLES**: FP, Km; Ks; Sil.
**Bronchial** and **pulmonary** symptoms with: Fp; Km; KS.
**Complications** or sequelae of: FP; Ks.
**Haemorrhagic**: Fp.
**MEAT WATER** Like: Fp; Ns; SIL.
**MEATUS Agglutination**, of: Cp; NM.
**Burning**: Cf; Ks; NM
**Cutting**: Ns.
**Induration** (Hard): Cp.
**Inflammation**: Nm.
**Itching**: Km; Kp; NM; Sil.
**Pain**: NM.
**Pouting**: Nm.

**Stitching**: Nm.
**MEDICINES Abuse** of: See Drug, Abuse of.
**Refuses** to take: KP; SIL.
**Sensitive**: KP.
**MELANCHOLY**: See Sadness.
**Brooding**: Cs; Nm; Kp.
**Death**, fear of, with: Kp.
**Financial**: Cf.
**Puberty**, During: Cp; Nm.
**Religious**: Kp.
**MEMBRANE**: See Mucous and serous membranes.
**MEMORIES**, Disagreeable, recur: Kp; Nm.
**MEMORY, Affection**, in general: KP, **NM.**
**MEMORY Active**: Cp; Kp; Np; Sil.
**Involuntary** recollection: Nm.
**Loss** of and Power of thought suddenly after lunch: Cs.
**MEMORY, Weakness** of: Cp; Cs; Fp; **KP;** Ks; NM; NP; SIL.
**Do,** for what was about to: Cp; Cs.
**Done,** for what has just: CP.
**Expressing**, oneself, in: NM.
**Happened,** for what has: NM.
**Labour,** for mental: **NM;** SIL.
Fatigue, from: Nm; SIL.
**Occurrence** Of the day: Nm.
**Periodical**: Nm.
**Read,** For what has: NM.
**Say,** for what is about to: NM.

**Sudden** and Periodical: Cs.
**Thought**, for what has just: Nm.
**Words**, for: KP; NM; Sil.
**Write,** for what is about to: NM.
**MEN Dread** of: Nm.
**MENIER'S Disease**: Fp; Km; Sil.
**MENINGITIS Acute** and **Chronic**: Cp; NM; Ns; Sil.
**Spinal**: NM; NS.
**Tubercular**: CP; Nm; SIL.
**MENSES after Agg**: NM; Np; Sil.
**At the start** of: **CP;** Nm; SIL.
**Before: CP;** Km; **NM;** Np; Sil.
And after: Km; NM.
**During**: Cp; Km; KP; NM; Np; SIL.
**Suppression**: Sil.
**MENSES After Amel**: Cf; Kp; Mp.
**At the start** of: Mp.
**MENSES Disturbances** in general: NM.
**Amenorrhoea** (Menses absent): Cp; Cs; FP; Km; KP; Ks; NM; Np; Ns; **SIL.**
Anemia, from: Cp; Nm.
Change of climate, from: Cp; SIL.
Colic, with: Ns.
Constipation, with:
Mental shock, from: Kp.
Months, for: Sil.

**Abdomen,** Weight in: KS.

**Acrid**: NS; **SIL.**

**Anger,** Brings on the flow: Nm.

**Appear,** As if would: CP; Nm.

**Before,** the Proper age: CP; Nm.

**Between** Periods: **SIL.**

**Black**: Cp; KM; Kp; Ns.

Red: Ks.

**Bloody,** Mucus: NS.

**Bright Red:** CP; Fp; Km; Ks; Sil.

**Burning,** Hot: Sil.

**Choleric** Symptoms, with: Sil.

**Clotted**: CP; KM; NM; Ns.

**Coagulating,** Not: KP.

**Copious**: **CP;** Cs; FP; KM; KP; KS; **NM;** Np; Ns; SIL.

Emotions, excitement: Nm; SIL.

Exertion agg: CP.

Fibroid, from: Cp. Sil.

Icy coldnes of body with: Sil.

Night: **NM.**

Nursing the child, when: SIL.

Plethora, in: Sil.

Pregnancy, during: Kp.

Puerperal (Post-partum): Cf; Fp.

Short duration, of: Nm; SIL.

Standing in water, from: Sil.

Walking Agg: Nm.

**Dark**: CP; Cs; Fp; KM; Mp; Nm.

First, then bright red: Sil.

**Delayed,** Puberty at: CP; Cs; KP; **NM;** SIL.

**Early:** Fp; Mp; Nm.

Scanty, and: Nm.

**Face,** flushed, with: Cp; FP.

**Fearsome**: Nm.

**Fluid** blood, Containing clots: Ns.

**Foul**: See Offensive.

**Frequent,** Too early, Too soon: CP; CS; FP; KM; KS; **NM;** Np; SIL.

Every two weeks: Cp; Kp; Nm.

three weeks: Fp; Ks; Nm.

Scanty: Cp; Nm.

**Headache,** Congestive

symptoms concomitant: Fp; Kp; NM.

**Indelible**: Mp.

**Intermittent**: Fp; Ns; Sil.

**Interrupted** And reappearing: Mp.

**Irregular**: Cp; Cs; Fp; Kp; SIL.

Every two or three months:

**Knee cords,** Shortening with: Np.

**Lactation,** During: CP; Sil.

Nursing the child while: Sil.

**Late,** Delayed: CP; Cs; FP; Km; KP; KS; **NM;** NP; NS; **SIL.**

Profuse, and: SIL.

Prolonged, and: Cs.

Too, and too scanty: Kp.

**Lying,** Ceases on: Sil.

**Membranous**: Nm.

**Mental excitement**, concomitant; Np.

**Night**, Only: Nm.

More: Nm.

**Offensive**: Cp; **KP**; Ks; SIL.

Strong: Kp; SIL.

**Painful** (Dysmenorrhoea): CP; Fp; Km; KP; KS; MP; Nm; Np; Ns; Sil.

Convulsions, with: Nm.

Fainting, with: Ks.

Flow, amel: Mp.

Forenoon, only: Nm.

Irregular: NM.

every two weeks, or so: Cp; Fp.

Membranous: CP; MP; Nm.

Premature: MP; Nm.

Spasmodic, neuralgic: MP.

Urination, frequent urge, with: Fp.

Wet feet, from getting: Nm.

**Pale**: Cs; FP; Kp; **NM**; Np; Sil.

**Plethora**, in: Sil.

**Pregnancy**, During: Kp.

**Protracted**, Too long: NM; Sil.

**Return** After menopause: Nm.

**Scanty**: Cs; FP; KM; KP; KS; NM; Ns; SIL.

Day or two then profuse: Nm.

**Short** Duration of: Kp; NM; Ns; Sil.

**Spasms**, Twitching with: Cs; Nm.

**Stains**, Leaving: SIL.

**Stringy**: Mp.

**Suppressed**: Cp; Cs; FP; KM; Kp; KS; NM; **SIL**.

Agg: Sil.

Anemia from: Kp; Nm.

Feet getting wet, from: NM.

Love, disappointed, from: NM.

Vicarious, bleeding with: Ns; Sil.

**Tarry:** Km; Mp.

**Urinary** Symptoms, with: Cp; Mp.

**Viscid**, Thick: KM; KP; Mp.

**Walking**, Only while: Ns.

**Water**, Standing, in from: Sil.

**Watery**, Thin: FP; Kp; NM; Np.

**Weeks**, Every three: Fp.

**MENTAGRA**: Cp.

**MENTAL Depression**: See Sadness.

Exertion Agg: Cp; KP; NM; SIL.

Exhaustion, Prostration: Cp; Cs; **KP**; NM; **NP; SIL**.

Reading from: SIL.

Talking, from: CP.

Writing, after: SIL.

**MERCURY Abuse** of: Nm; NS; SIL.

**MESENTERIC GLANDS**

Enlarged: Ns.

**Induration**, hard: NS.

**Pulsation**: Cp.

**Tabes mesenterica**: CP; CS; NS.

Diarrhoea, with: Cp.

**METASTASIS**: Cs; Ks; MP; Sil.

**METEORISM, Gurgling**: Fp; NM; Np; Sil.

**Gushing**, Stools, then: NS.

**Motion**, Amel: Nm.

**METRITIS** (Endometritis) Acute: Sil.

**Chronic**: Kp; Ks; Nm; SIL.

**Peri and Para** metritis: Sil.

**MICTURITION**: See Urination.

**MIDDLE EAR Acute catarrh**: FP; KM; Sil.

**Chronic**: KM; Sil.

**Suppurative**, Acute: Cs; FP; Km; Sil.

Chronic: Cf; **CS;** Km; Kp; KS; Nm; Sil.

**MIGRAINE**. (Hemicrania): Nm; Ns; Sil.

**MILDNESS Gentleness**, tenderness: Kp; **NM; SIL.**

**MILIARY Eruptions**: Nm

**MILK**: See Lactation.

**Agg and Amel**: See under food.

**Crust** (Head external): Cs; Km; Sil.

**Leg** (phlegmasia, alba dolens): CF; NS; SIL.

contractions with: SIL.

**MIND Affections** in General: **CP;** Cs; **KP; NM;** Np; Ns; **SIL.**

**Acute**, Physical weakness with: Sil

**Anger**, Suppression, Agg: Cp; Fp; Kp; NM; Sil.

**Anticipations**, Agg: Nm.

**Blank**: Fp.

**Childish** (Foolish): Cp; Sil..

**Diarrhoea** Amel: Cp; Ns.

**Digestive** Affections with: Np.

**Eating** Amel: CS; KS; NP.

**Exertion**, Physical Agg: CP; KP; Nm; Sil.

**Eyes**, Closing; Agg: Sil.

**Filthy**: Sil.

**Heart**, Alternating with: Nm; Np.

**Laughing**, Agg: Nm.

**Menses**, Before and During Agg: Nm.

**Stools**, Amel: Ns.

**Syphilis** Agg: Cf; SIL.

**Uterus**, Alternating with: NM; SIL.

**Walking** on Agg: CP; KS; NM; Sil.

**Walking**, Open air, in Agg: Cp; Kp; Nm; SIL.

**Yawning** Amel: Cp; Kpl Sil.

**MINER'S DISEASE**: Sil.

**MIRTH** (Hilarity, Liveliness): Cs; Fp; Kp; Nm; Np.

**Alternating**, with Irritability: Nm.

Sadness, and nose-bleed amel: Km.

**Changing** suddenly to melancholy: Cs.

**Evening**: Cs; Nm.

**MISANTHROPY**: Nm.

**MISCARRIAGE**: See abortion.

**MISERABLE Makes himself** by brooding over imaginary wrongs: Cs; Kp.

**MISERLY** (Avaricious): Cf.

**MISFORTUNE**: See under fear.

**MISTAKES Localities** : Nm; Sil.

**Reading**, in: Sil.

**Speaking** in: Cp; Cs; Kp; NM; Sil.

Intend, what he does not: Nm.

**Words**, Misplacing: Kp; Ks; NM; Sil.

**Writing**, in: CP; KP; Ks; NM; Sil.

Repeating, words: CP.

**Wrong** answers, gives: Cp.

Words, using: Cp.

**MOANING**: Km.

**Children**: Cp.

**Pain**, with: Sil.

**Sleep**, in: Cp.

Loudly: Nm.

**MOISTNESS**, Increased: See Secretions.

**Skin**, of: Nm; Sil.

Spots, in: **Sil.**

**MOLES**: SIL.

**MOLLITIS** Ossium (softening of bones): Cf; CP; **SIL.**

**MONOMANIA**: Sil.

**MONS VENERIS**: Nm; Sil.

**Eruptions**: Sil.

**MOOD alternating**: Fp; Nm.

**Changeable**, Variable: Cs; Kp; Ks; Nm; Sil.

**Repulsive**: Sil.

**MOON PHASES Agg: SIL.**

**New Agg**: Sil.

**First** quarter AGG.: Nm.

**Full**: Nm; SIL.

**MORNING Agg** (4 to 9 a.m.): **CP; FP; KP; NM; NP; NS; SIL.**

**MORNING Sickness**: FP; Kp; NM; Np; **NS**; Sil.

**MORPHINISM**: Np.

**MORTIFICATION** (Chagrin)

**Ailments**, after: **NM.**

**MORVAN'S DISEASE**: Sil.

**MOTION absent**: Kp.

**Agile**: Cp.

**Automatic**: Sil.

**Averse** To: **CS;** Kp; NM; **SIL.**

**Difficult:** Sil.

**Disorderly**: Mp; NM; Sil.

**Erratic**: KS; Mp; NM; SIL.

**Oscillatory**: Mp.

**Tumultous**: Nm.

**MOTION Walking Agg**: CP; CS; FP; Km; Kp; MP; NM; NP; NS; **SIL.**

**Affected** parts of: Nm; SIL.

**At** the beginning: KP; **SIL.**
**Continued**: Kp.
**Rapid,** Violent: Sil.
**MOTION Amel**: Cp; Fp; KP; **KS;** Ns.
**Continued**: CF; Sil.
**Slow,** Gentle: KP.
**MOTION, Air open,** AGG: Mp.
**Amel**: KS.
**Beginning**: KP; **SIL.**
**MOTTLED, Patchy**: Km; NM.
**MOULD As** if forming over whole body: Sil.
**MOUTH** (See throat): Km; Kp; KS; NM; Sil.
**About**: NM.
Eruptions: Km.
**Angles,** droop: Kp; Nm.
**Aphthae**: KM; Ks; NM; Sil.
Borax, abuse of, from: Ns.
Children, in: KM.
Glands swelling, with: Km.
Thrush: Km.
**Bitter**: Sil.
**Bleeding**: Fp.
**Breath**: See Breath.
**Cold** Sores: Cf; NM.
**Dry**: Cp; Cs; KP; Ks; **NM;** Np; **NS; SIL.**
Morning: Ns.
Night: Nm.
Saliva, increased with: Nm.
Thirst, with: **NM;** Ns.
without: SIL.
Walking open air, in: Sil.

**Froth,** Foam, from: Nm; Sil.
Absent in spasms: Sil.
Sleep, during: Sil.
**Gangrenous**: Kp; Sil.
**Grasps**: Sil.
**Heat**: Ks; Nm; Ns; Sil.
**Inflammation**: Cs; Fp; Kp.
**Mucous Membranes** pale: NM.
Red: Fp; Km.
**Mucous,** Slime, in: Cs; Kp; Ks; **NM; SIL.**
Balls, of: Mp.
Morning: Cs; Sil.
Viscid: Nm; NS.
While: Km; Ns.
**Numbness**: Np; NS.
One sided: Nm.
Prickling with: Np.
**Pain:** Kp; Nm.
Burning: Kp; NM; Ns.
lips, inside: Cs.
pepper, as from: Ns.
Sore: Kp; **NM.**
spot: Sil.
inside right cheek: Cp.
**Prickling**: Np.
**Ranula**: Cf; NM.
**Roughness**: NS.
**Scalded,** As if: Mp.
**Sensitive,** To touch: NS.
**Spitting,** Constant: Nm.
**Sticky,** Viscid: NM.
**Stomacae**: NM; SIL.
**Swelling**: Cs; Kp; Sil.

Erysipelatous, after extraction of teeth: Sil.

**Twitching**: Mp.

**Ulcers** (See Apthae): Km; Nm.

Ashen grey: Kp.

Biting: Nm.

Burning: Nm.

Flat: Nm.

Nursing mothers, in: KM.

Painful: Nm.

touch, to: NM.

Syphilitic: KM.

White: Km.

**Vesicles**: Cs; Km; NM; Np; Ns.

Biting: Nm.

Blood: Nm.

Burning: NM; Ns.

Cold things, Amel: NS.

**MOUTH** Open, hangs, jaws drop: Cp; KP; Nm.

**MOUTH Opening Agg**: Sil.

**MOVEMENTS**: See Motion.

**MUCOUS COLITIS**: Kp.

**MUCOUS MEMBRANES**: Km; Fp; NM; Ns; Sil.

**Dark**: Fp; Nm.

**Dry**: NM; SIL.

**Pale**: Fp; NM.

**Patches**: Km; NM.

**Raw**: Km; Nm.

**Secretions**, Altered: Cs; NM; Sil.

Increased: NM; SIL.

**Ulcerated**: Fp; Km; NM; Sil.

**Vesicles**: NM.

**MUDDLED**: See Confusion.

**MUMPS**: FP; Km; Kp; Mp; NM; SIL.

**Fever**, Without: Km.

**Metastasis**, Testes to: Km; Nm.

**Persistent**: Sil.

**Suppuration**, With: NM; **SIL.**

**MUSCAE VOLITANTES**: Kp; **NM; SIL.**

**MUSCLES**: CP; Kp; MP; NM; Ns; SIL.

**Atrophy**: CP; **KP.**

Progressive: KP.

**Cramps**: Cp; MP; NM; Ns.

**Indurated**: Cf; Sil.

**Jumping**: Mp; NM; Ns; Sil.

**Knots**: KP; MP; Ns.

**Lax,** Flabby: Cp; Km; Kp; Sil.

**Obey** Feebly: Kp.

**Short** (Contractions): Km; Nm.

Congenital: Nm.

**Sore**, From dancing etc.: Cp; Cs; KP; NM; Np; Sil.

**Stitches**: NM; SIL.

**Tense**: Km; NM; SIL.

**Undeveloped**: NM.

**Weak,** Feeble: CP; Cs; **KP;** Mp; **NM;** NP; NS; Sil.

**MUSIC Agg:** Nm; Np; NS.

**MUSTY, Mouldy**: Sil.

**MUTINISM: CP;** Nm; SIL

**MUTTERING**: Nm.

**MYXEDEMA**: CP; Sil.

**NAEVI**: Cf; Nm.
**NAIL**, Plug: Nm.
**NAILS**: Cp; NM; SIL.
  **Blue**: Fp; NM; SIL.
    Chill during: NM.
  **Brittle**: SIL.
  **Corrugated**: SIL.
  **Cracks** on: NM; SIL.
    Around: Nm.
  **Crippled**: SIL.
  **Crumbling**: SIL.
  **Distorted**: SIL.
  **Dryness**: Sil.
  **Edge** Of: Cp.
  **Exfoliation**: SIL.
  **Falling**: Sil.
  **Felon**, (Onychia, Paronychia):
    FP; NM; NS; SIL.
    Beginning in nail: SIL.
    Chronic tendency: Sil.
    Cold application amel: Nm.
    Deep: Sil.
    Hang-nails from: NM.
    Maltreatment from: SIL.
    Periosteitis: Cp; SIL.
    Splinters from: Sil.
      under: Sil.
    Suppurative, stage: SIL.
    Tendons affected: Ns; SIL.
    Thumb: SIL.
  **Gray**: SIL.
  **Growth** Interrupted: Ks; Sil.
  **Hang-nails**: NM; NS; Sil.
  **Hypertrophied**: Cf.

**Ingrowing** (Toes): Km; MP;
  NM; SIL.
  Ulceration with: SIL.
**Injury** from Splinter of glass:
  SIL.
**Pain**: CP; Nm; SIL.
  Burning: Nm.
  Drawing, under: Nm.
  Edges, along: Cp.
  Root, of: CP.
  Stitchig: NM; Sil.
  Tearing: SIL.
    under: Cp.
  Ulcerative: CP; NM; Ns;
    SIL.
    splinter, as from: SIL.
**Redness** (Toes): Nm.
**Roughness**: SIL.
**Sensation** of Splinter under:
  SIL.
**Sensitive**: NM; SIL.
**Split**: SIL.
**Spotted**: SIL.
**Thick**: SIL.
**Tingling**, Under: Ns.
**Ulcers: NM; Ns; SIL.**
**White** Spots: SIL.
**Yellow**: SIL.
**NAPE**: See Neck.
**NARROW Opening**: Cp; Sil.
**NASO-PHARYNX** (Posterior
  Nares): NM.
  **Closure** Of: Cs.
  **Discharge**, from: **NM**; Np.
    Thick: Km; NP; NS.

Tough, viscid: Km; Np.
Yellowish, green: CS; Km;
   **NM**; NP; NS.
**Dryness**: Cp; NM; SIL.
**Food**, Sensation of, in: SIL.
on swallowing: SIL.
**Itching**: Kp.
**Lump**, in: Nm.
**Rawness**, inspiration Agg: Fp.
**Scraping**: KP; NM; Ns.
**NATES**: See buttocks.
**NAUSEA**: CP; CS; FP; Kp; KS;
   MP; NM; Np; SIL.
**Afternoon**: Sil.
4 p.m.: Cp.
**Anxious**, Deathly: Fp.
**Breakfast**, After: Cp.
During: NM.
**Chill**, Before: Nm.
During: Nm.
With: Km.
**Coffee**, After: CP; NM.
**Coition**, During: Sil.
**Concomitant**, As a: NS.
**Confusion**, With: Cp.
**Continuous**: Nm; NS; **SIL.**
**Cough**, During: Kp; Ks; Nm;
   Np.
**Descending**: NS.
**Drinking**, After: NM; Sil.
Cold drinks, after: Ks; NM.
**Eating**, After: FP; Kp; Ks; NM;
   NS; Sil.
Before: NS.
While: Sil.

**Epigastrium**, in the: NM; Sil.
**Eructations**, Amel: Kp.
**Evening**: NM.
Bed in, drinking water after:
   **NM.**
**Exertion**, After: Sil.
**Faint** Like: NM; Sil.
**Fever**, During: Nm.
**Fish**, After: Nm.
**Food**, On looking at: Sil.
**Headache**, During: CP; Cs;
   Kp; KS; NM; Np; Ns; Sil.
**Lying**, Down, on: Nm.
Amel: Sil.
Right side, abdomen on
   amel: Nm.
Side, on amel: Nm.
**Menses**, Before: NM.
During: Kp; Nm.
Suppressed, with: Nm.
**Morning**: Nm; Sil.
Rising, on: Fp.
**Nursing**, After: SIL.
**Pain**, During: Nm.
**Periodic**: Nm.
**Pregnancy**, During: Fp; Kp;
   NM; SIL.
**Pressure** On painful spot,
   from: Nm.
**Riding** In carriage: CP.
**Rising**, On: NS.
**Salt**, On thinking of: NM.
**Sea-sickness**: Nm.
**Shivering**, With: Km.
**Shuddering**, When: Nm.

**Sleep**, Before: Ns.
  During: Fp.
**Smoking**, After: CF.
  While: Nm; Sil.
**Stools**, After: NM; Sil.
  During: Sil.
**Stooping**, On: Cp.
**Sudden** Attack of: Fp.
**Throat**, In: Fp; Sil.
**Urinating**, Amel: Np.
**Vaccination**, After: **SIL.**
**Vexation**, After: Nm.
**Wakes** Him at night: Fp.
**Walking**, After: NM; SIL.
  Air, open in: Ns.
  While: Fp; NS; Sil.
**Warm room**, on entering after being in open air: Cs.
**Yawning**, when: Nm.
**NAVEL and REGION**
**Constriction**: Sil.
  Region of: Nm.
**Contraction**: Nm.
**Discharge**: CP; NM.
  Bloody fluid (in new born): CP.
**Distension**, Inflation: Nm.
**Empty feeling**, about: Co.
**Festers**: Cp.
**Moisture**, at: Cp.
**Pain**, Aching: CP; NM; **NS**; Sil.
  Bruised, beaten as if: Cp; Nm.
  Burning: Cp.

Crampy: Nm; Ns.
Cutting: Km; NM; SIL.
Dragging: Cp.
Extending to rectum: Nm.
Flatus passing, Amel: Cp.
Pinching: Sil.
Pregnancy, during: Cp.
Sore, bruised: CP; Nm; Sil.
Stitching: Sil.
**Protrusion** On, as if hernia would, form: Nm.
**Retraction**: Cp.
**Tension**: Nm.
**Ulcers**: Sil.
**NEAR SIGHT** (Myopia): NM; Np.
**NECK and NAPE abscess**: Sil.
  Old cicatrices, of: SIL.
**Across** the Back: Cs.
**Air**, Draft, unbearable: CP; **SIL.**
**Alternating** Sides: Cp.
**Arms**, To: Nm.
**Boils**: Sil.
**Bruised**, As if: Nm; Ns.
**Burning**: NS.
**Clavicles**, To: NS.
**Coldness**: NS; **SIL.**
  Creeping: Sil.
**Cramp** like Pain: CP.
  Right to left: CP.
  Vertex to: Cs.
**Crick**: Fp.

**Drawing**, Pain: CP; NM; NS; Sil.

Spasmodic: NM; NS.

**Ear**, to: Cp.

**Emaciation**, of: CP; NM.

**Eruptions**: Nm; **Sil.**

Blood boils: Ns; **SIL.**

Carbuncle: **SIL.**

Eczema: SIL.

Herpes: Nm.

moist: Nm.

Pimples: Nm; **SIL.**

flattened, itching: SIL.

suppurating: Cp.

Scabs white: SIL.

Vesicles: Np.

**Eye**, to: SIL.

**Fatigue**, As if: Nm.

**Gnawing**: NS.

**Head**, To: SIL.

All over: Ns.

**Heaviness**: CP.

**Itching**: **NM;** Np; Sil.

Scratching after agg: Nm.

**Peculiar feeling**, In: Km.

**Perspiration**: SIL.

**Pressing**: NM; NS; Sil.

**Pulsating** Pain: CP; Fp; Nm; NS.

**Pulsation**: Cp.

**Short**, As if: NM; NS; Sil.

**Sore**, Bruised: Cs; Kp; Ks; **NM;** Np; NS; **SIL.**

Seventh vertebra and around: Sil.

**Sprained**, Dislocated as if: Nm.

**Stiffness**: CP; Cs; Fp; Km; Kp; KS; NM; Np; NS; **SIL.**

Air, draught of Agg: **CP.**

sitting on in, while over-heated: Km.

Dancing, after: Km.

Enlarged glands, from: Kp.

Headache, during: Nm; Sil.

Head inclined to right, shoulder raised: Ks.

Left side: Nm.

Morning, awakening on: Km.

Painful: Nm.

Yawning: Nm.

**Stitching**, Shooting, pain: Fp; NM; NP; Ns; Sil.

**Swallowing**, Agg: Cp.

**Tearing**: NS; Sil.

**Tension** (Short as if): NM; NS; Sil.

**Thin**: Cp.

**Tumours**, Malignant, on: Cp.

**Twitching**: Nm.

**Ulcers**: Sil.

**Weak**: Cp; Nm.

**Wry neck,** torticollis: Sil.

**Yawning**, Agg: Ns.

**NECROSIS** Bones of: CF; Cp; SIL.

Jaws of, lower: SIL.

**NEEDLES**: See Pain, Stitching.

**NEPHRALGIA**: See Kidney, Pain in.

**NEPHRITIS**: See Kidney, In-
flammation.
**NEPHROLITHIASIS**: Mp; **NS**;
**SIL.**
**NERVOUS Patients, Nerves**:
Kp; **MP**; Nm; **SIL.**
  **Activity**: Kp; sil.
  **Paralysis**: Kp; Nm; Np.
  **Prostration**, Neurasthenia:
  Cp; **KP**; **NM**; **NP**; **SIL.**
  Grief from: Nm.
  Sexual: Kp; Np.
**NETTED** (Birth mark): Cf; Nm.
**NETTLE RASH**: Mp; NM; Sil.
**NEURALGIA**: See Pain.
  **Brachial**: Cs; MP; Nm; Ns;
  Sil.
  **Caries**, From: Cf; Sil.
  **Ciliary**: Nm; Sil.
  **Coition**, After (male): Kp; NP.
  **Crural**: See Sciatica.
  **Injury**, From: NS.
  **Intercostal**: Mp; Nm.
  **Menses**, During: Cp; Nm.
  Suppressed from: Nm.
  **Operations**, After: Cp: Fp;
  NS.
  **Orbital**: Nm; Sil.
  **Palpitation**, with: Kp; Mp.
  **Paralytic** Weakness and trem-
  bling with: CP; Mp; **NM;**
  NP; NS; SIL.
  **Peripheral**: Cp; Kp; MP; NM.
  **Prodrome**, As a: Sil.
  **Shingles**, after: Nm.
  **Stump**, of: NS; Sil.

**NEURASTHENIA**: CP; KP; Nm;
Sil.
**NEURITIS Injury** after: NS; Sil.
  **Multiple**: Nm; SIL.
  **Optic**: Kp; Sil.
  **Retro-bulbar**: Kp; Nm; Sil.
**NEVER Well since**: Cp; Ns; Sil.
**NEVUS**: See Naevus.
**NEW cannot** do anything: Sil.
  **Growth**: See Growth, new.
**NEWS bad**: See Bad news.
  **Glad**: See Joy.
**NIBBLING Appetite**: Np.
**NICTALOPIA**: Sil.
**NIGHT SWEATS** of phthisis:
  Cp; Fp; Sil.
  **Weak** and Anemic persons:
  Fp.
**NIGHT Terrors**: Fp; Kp; NM; Np;
  SIL.
**NIPPING** (Twinges): Np; Sil.
**NIPPLES**: Cp; SIL.
  **Abscess**: Sil.
  **Bleeding**: Sil.
  **Cracks** Of: Sil.
  **Drawn** In like a funnel: Sil.
  **Excoriation**: Cp; SIL.
  **Glandular** Swelling, about: Sil.
  **Inflammation**: SIL.
  **Inverted**: Ns.
  **Left**: Ns.
  **Pain**: CP.
    Burning: SIL.
    Drawing from, all over body:
    Sil.

Sore: CP; SIL.

Stitching: Nm; SIL.

**Retraction**, of: Ns; **SIL.**

**Ulcer:** Cp; SIL.

**NIPS** (Twinges): Np; Sil.

**NODES**: Cf; Ks; Sil.

**NOISE Agg:** Fp; KP; **NM**; NP; NS; **SIL.**

**Menses**, During: Kp.

**Slightest**: Sil.

**Sudden**: Nm.

**NOMA**: KP; Sil.

**NOSE**: Cp; Km; NM; **SIL.**

**Left:** Nm.

**One side**: Sil.

**Abscess**: **SIL.**

**Acne**: Cp.

**A r**, Open, Amel: Sil.

**Alae**: See Nostrils.

**Bleeding**: See Epistaxis.

**Blow**, Constant inclination to: Nm.

**Blood**, Blowing from: Cp; NM; SIL.

**Bones**, Caries: Cs; **SIL.**

syphilitic: SIL.

Diseased: Cf.

Growth: Cf.

Pain: Nm.

burning: Nm.

sore, bruised: NM; SIL.

Periostitis: Cf.

**Boring**, Into with fingers, itching: NM; NP; **SIL.**

Until it bleeds: Sil.

**Cancer** (Epithelioma): KS; Sil.

**Coldness**: Cf; Cp; SIL.

**Constriction**: Nm.

**Crawling**, Formication: Nm.

**Crusts**: Cs; Fp; Km; Kp; NM; Np; Ns; **SIL.**

Left: Np.

Right: Sil.

Greenish, seems to come from ulcer: NS.

High up: SIL.

Painful: SIL.

**Deadness**: Nm.

**Desquamation**: NM.

**Discharges**, Albuminous: Mp; **NM**; NS.

bland: Ks; SIL.

Bloody: CS; Fp; Kp; Ks; NM; **SIL.**

infants, in: Cs.

Brownish: KS.

Burning, hot: Ks; Nm.

Clear: NM.

Copious: Km; **NM**; Ns.

Crusts, scabs: See Crusts.

Dripping: Nm; Sil.

sensation, of: Nm.

Excoriating: CS; Fp; KM; Kp; Ks; Nm; SIL.

air, in open: Ks.

Flocculent: Sil.

Flows, obstruction with: Sil.

Fluent: Cf; CP; Cs; Km; KP; Ks; **NM**; NP; NS; SIL.

day time: Sil.

indoors: Cp.

Foamy, frothy: Sil.
Greenish: Cf; Kp; Ks; SIL.
Hard, dry: Ns; SIL.
Lumpy, plugs: Mp; **SIL.**
Night: Ns.
Offensive: See Ozaena.
Purulent: CS; FP; KM; KP; **KS;** NM; NP; NS; SIL.
Salty: KS; Nm.
Slimy, mucus of: Cp; SIL.
Starch, like boiled: NM.
Sudden, gushing: Nm.
Suppressed: NM; SIL.
Thick: Cf; CS; Km; **KP;** KS; NM;. NP; **NS; SIL.**
Thin: Ks.
Viscid, tough: Km; **KS;** SIL.
Watery: Cp; Cs; KP; NM; Ns; SIL.
  left, at night: Ns.
  night: Ns.
  right, during day: Cs.
White: KM; Kp; NM.
  like white of an egg: NM.
Yellow: **CS; KP; KS;** NM; NP; NS; SIL.
  orange: Kp.
Yellowish green: CF; CS; NS; SIL.
**Discolouration**, Red: Mp; Nm; Sil.
Left side: Nm.
Spots, in: Sil.
  red, burning: Sil.
**Dryness**: Cs; Km; Kp; KS; NM; NS; SIL.

Air, in warm: Cp.
Chronic: SIL.
Painful: SIL.
Sensation of: **SIL.**
Suppressed, foot sweat after: **SIL.**
**Eruptions**: Ks; Nm; **NP; SIL.**
Acne: Cp.
Around: Sil.
Blood boils: Sil.
Burning: Nm.
Crusty, scaly: NM; Sil.
Eczema: NM; Sil.
Itching: Sil.
Nodular: Nm.
Pimples: NM; SIL.
  red, burning: Cp.
Scurfy: Nm.
Vesicles: NM; SIL.
**External**
Inflammation: NM; Sil.
  left: NM.
Itching, formication: CP; CS; Kp; Ks; Sil.
Lupus, of: Nm; SIL.
Perspiration, on: Nm.
Picking: Np.
  till it bleeds: Sil.
Pressing: Sil.
Sensitive: Sil.
  touch to: Sil.
Sore: NM; **SIL.**
  blowing on: NM; SIL.
  compressing wings: Nm.
Sunken: Sil.

Swelling: CP; CS; KP; Ks; NM; SIL.

left: NM.

Tingling: Np.

Twitching, left: Nm.

Ulcers, burning: SIL.

painful: **SIL.**

**Foreign** Body, as if in: CP; Nm; Sil.

**Hardness**: Cf.

**Heat** In left: Nm.

**Heaviness**: Sil.

**Inflammation**, Acute, catarrhal, from pollen, hay fever, rose cold, summer catarrh e c.: KP; Ks; NM; SIL.

**Inflammation**, Catarrhal, ordinary cold in head: Fp; NM; Sil.

Coryza: See Coryza.

**Itching** (Boring): Cp; Km; KS; NM; SIL.

Right: Nm.

Rubs, constantly: Sil.

**Liquids**, food returns through, swallowing when: NM; SIL.

**Numbness**: Nm.

**Obstructed**: CS; Km; KP; Ks; **NM**; Np; NS; SIL.

Adenoids, removal after Ks.

Air, open in: Cp.

Alternate with discharge: Nm; SIL.

Breathes, through, mouth: Ks.

Chronic: SIL.

Cold, after evening: SIL.

Diphtheria, in: KM.

Flow, relieved by: Sil.

Foot sweat suppressed from: Sil.

High in: Nm.

Morning: SIL.

Mucous discharge, with Km.

Night: KP; Ns; Sil.

uncovering head, day during from: NM.

Pus, with: **SIL.**

Sensation of: Ns.

Smell, loss of with: Sil.

Talking while: Sil.

Warm room: Cp.

**Odours**, From or in:

Blood of: Sil.

Offensive: CS; Np.

foetid: Sil.

morning: Np.

Sickly: Sil.

**Operations** After: Fp.

**Ozaena**: CF; KP; KS; NM; Np; NS; Sil.

Syphilitic: SIL.

**Pain**, in: Cp; Fp; Ks; Nm; Ns; **SIL.**

Biting: Cp; Sil.

Blowing; nose Agg: NM; SIL.

Burning, smarting: Kp; Ks; NM; NS; **SIL.**

Coughing Agg: Nm.

Drawing: Ns; Sil.
Dryness, from: SIL.
Eating, Agg: Sil.
Extending to brain like rays: SIL.
  forehead to: Ns; Sil.
Foreign body, as from: Cp.
Gnawing: Sil.
Inspiration Agg: FP.
Menses, during Agg: Ns.
Night: Sil.
Sore, bruised: CP; Kp; NM; Np; Ns; **SIL.**
  left: Np.
  right: Kp; SIL.
Splinter like, on touch: Sil.
Stitching: Cp.
Stooping, Agg: NM; Sil.
Tearing: Ns; Sil.
Ulcerative: SIL.
Wrapping head Amel: Nr
**Polypus**: CP; SIL.
Bleeds easily: Cp.
**Pulsation**: Sil.
**Root of**
Eruptions, vesicles: Nm.
Fullness, sense of: Np.
Pain: Fp; NM; NS; SIL.
  boring: Nm.
  drawing: Nm; Sil.
  pressing: Kp; NM.
  smarting, inside: Nm.
  stitching: Nm; Sil.
  tearing to forehead: NM.
Quivering, cheek to: Cs.

Tension: Np.
Twitching: Nm.
  visible: Nm.
**Septum**, Crusts, scabs on: SIL.
Eruptions, pimples: Nm.
Pain: Sil.
  burning: Sil.
  sore; bruised: Ks; Nm; SIL.
  stitching: Sil.
Perforation: Sil.
Ulcers, round: Cp; **SIL.**
**Sinuses** (Antrum, Frontal): Km; SIL.
  Abscess: **SIL.**
  Catarrh: Nm.
**Smell**: See Smell.
**Sneezing**: See Sneezing.
**Swelling**: Cp; Nm; SIL.
  Touch, painful to: Nm.
**Tickling**: Cp; Sil.
**Tingling**: Nm; Np.
**Tip**, Burning: Sil.
  Burrowing: Sil.
  Cold: CP; Sil.
  icy: Cp.
  Eruptions: SIL.
  Heat: NM.
  Itching: Cp; Np; SIL.
  Pale, pointed: Cp.
  Red: Nm; Sil.
  shiny: SIL.
  Sore: SIL.
  Stitching: Sil.
  extends to forehead: Sil.

**Ulcers**: Cp; Kp; Nm; SIL.
  Burning: SIL.
  High up: SIL.
  Painful: **SIL.**
  Right: SIL.
**NOSTALGIA** (Home-sickness):
  Cp; KP; NM; SIL.
**NOSTRILS Alae,** wings:
  **Cracks**: Sil.
  **Eruptions**, Vesicles: **NM**; Sil.
  **Itching**: Nm; NP; NS; Sil.
  **Rawness**: CP.
  **Redness**, Left: Nm.
  **Scurfy**: NM; NS; SIL.
  **Sore**: CP; Cs; Nm.
  **Squirming**, In as from small
    worm: Nm.
  **Swelling**: NM.
    Left: Nm.
  **Tearing**: Sil.
    Left: Sil.
**NOTHING Ails** him, says:
**NUMBNESS Externally**: CP;
  Km; Kp; SIL.
  **Gland**, In sensation of: Sil.
  **Internally**: Nm; Sil.
  **News**, Unpleasant from: Cp.
  **One** Sided: Nm.
  **Pain**, From: Nm.
  **Part**, Lain on: NM; Sil.
  **Partial**, Single parts: CP; Fp;
    Kp; NM; NS; **SIL.**
  **Suffering** Parts, of: NM; Sil.
**NURSING children**: CP; Nm;
  NP; Sil.

**Mothers**: **CP**; KP; Nm; NP;
  SIL.
  Sexual excitement in: Cp.
**NUTRITION affected**: CP; NM;
  SIL.
**NYCTALOPIA**: Sil.
**NYMPHOMANIA**: CP; Nm; Sil.
  **Involuntary** Orgasms with:
    Nm.
  **Menses**, Suppressed from: Sil.
  **Spinal** Irritation, from: Sil.
**NYSTAGMUS**: Mp.
**OBESITY**: Sil.
**OBSCENE**: Cs; Nm; SIL.
**OBSTINATE**: Cs; Fp; Km; KP;
  Ks; SIL.
  **Children**, Yet cry when kindly
    spoken to: Sil.
**OCCIPUT**: CP; Cs; KM; NM;
  NP; NS; **SIL.**
  **Left**: Nm.
  **Ascending**, Through: SIL.
  **Band**, Constriction: Nm.
  **Bathing**, Cold Amel: Cp.
  **Blow**, On as if: Km.
  **Burning**, Heat: Nm; SIL.
  **Bursting**: Sil.
  **Cold**: Cp.
  **Depression**, at: Cp.
  **Downward**: Cp.
  **Eruption**: Sil.
  **Extending**, Eyes or head to
    or in waves: SIL.
    Forehead, to: NM; NS; SIL.
    Forward, upward or vertex
      to: **SIL.**
  Neck down back: Ns.

**Lying** On AGG: Kp.
**Numb**: CP; Km; SIL.
**Throbbing**: Cp; KS; Nm; SIL.
**Ulcer**: Sil.
**OCCUPATION Amel.**: Cp; Kp.
**OCCUPATIONAL Disorders**: MP; SIL.
**ODONTALGIA, Tooth-ache**: See Pain, Teeth in.
**ODOURS Smells Agg**:
**OEDEMA** (See Dropsy): Cs; Fp; Kp; SIL.
    **Affected** part, around: Nm; Sil.
    **Foot**: Cs; NM; NS.
    **Injury**, After: Fp; Nm; Ns; Sil.
    **Joints of**: Cf; Cs; FP; Kp; NM; Sil.
    **Lungs**: Cs; Km; KP; NM; Ns.
**OESOPHAGUS Burning**: Nm.
    **Choking**; Constriction: NM.
    **Dryness**: Nm.
    **Gurgling**, When drinking: Sil.
    **Heat**: Ns.
    **Paralysis**, Sensation: SIL.
    **Sore** Spot, swallowing as if, over a: NM.
    **Stricture**: NM.
    **Uneasy** feeling: Km.
**OFFENDED Easily**: Cs; KP; KS; Nm; Sil.
**OFFENSIVENESS**: Kp; SIL.
    **Body**, Of: Kp; Sil.
    **Breath**: Cs; KP; Ks; NM; NS; Sil.

**Expectoration**: Fp; KP; Nm; NP; SIL.
**Stools**: CP; Km; KP; Ks; Nm; NP; NS; SIL.
**Urine**: KP; KS; Nm; Np; Ns.
**Vomit**: Ks.
**OILY**: Cp; Kp; NM.
**OLD PEOPLE**: CP; NM.
**ONANISM** (Marturbation): Nm.
    **III** effects: CP; Nm; Np; Sil.
**ONIONS** Smell like: Kp.
**ONYCHIA**: See Nails, Felon.
**OPERATIONS** After: Fp.
    **Adhesions**, After: Cf; Cp.
    **Fistulae**, After: Cp.
**OPISTHOTONUS**: CP; Mp; NM; NS.
**OPHTHALMIA** (Conjunctivitis): See Conjunctiva.
**OPTICAL** illusions: See Vision. Illusions.
**OPTIC NERVE** Paralysis: Kp; SIL.
**ORBITS Caries**: Sil.
    **Cellulitis**: Sil.
    **Itching**: Nm.
    **Pain osteoscopic**: Nm.
        Bowels pain in, extending to chest: Np.
        Supra-orbital (r) Agg 11 a.m.: Mp.
    **Periostitis**: Sil.
    **Pressure** and soreness in: Sil.
    **Prickling**, Left: Nm.
    **Twitching**: Nm.

**ORGASM of Blood**: Cs; Fp; Kp; Ks; Np; Ns; Sil.

**Emotions**, after: KP; Nm; NP.

**ORIFICES**, Affections of: NM; SIL.

**OSCILLATIONS**: Sil.

**OSSICLES, Caries** of: CF; CS; Nm; SIL.

**OSTEOMALACIA**: CF; CP; SIL.

**OSTEOMYELITIS**: Sil.

**OTALGIA**: See Ear, pain in.

**OTORRHOEA**: See Ear, Discharge.

**OVARIES**: Mp.

**Abscess**: SIL.

**Cysts**, Dropsy: Ns.

**Enlarged**, As if: Sil.

Menses, before: Sil.

**Inflammation**: Fp; Mp.

Acute, peritonitis with: Sil.

**Left** Side, lying on Amel: Kp.

**Pain**: Fp; Kp; **MP.**

Left: Kp.

Right: Cs; Mp.

Bending double, Amel: Kp; MP.

Burning: Nm.

Cutting: Cs; Nm.

Lying, back on, Amel: Kp. side, left: Kp.

Menses, during: Kp.

Night: Kp.

Pregnancy, during: Kp.

Sharp: Kp.

Shooting, darting: Mp.

Sleep, on going to agg: Kp.

Stitching: Kp; MP.

Thighs, to: Nm.

Urination, during: Nm.

**OVERLIFTING complaints**

From: Cp; NM.

**OXALURIA**: KS; NP.

**OZAENA**: CF; KP; KS; NM; NM; Np; NS; Sil.

**Syphilitic**: SIL.

**PAIN**: MP; Nm.

**Absence**, of (in usually painful conditions): Kp.

**Aching**: Cp.

Bones, in: CP.

Extending to fingers: Cp.

**Appears** Gradually and disappears gradually: NM.

Disappears suddenly: Mp.

One side on, goes to other and agg there: Nm.

With the sun: Nm.

**Attacks** Of, lasting for days: Km.

**Beaten** As if: Nm; **SIL.**

**Benumbing**: Nm.

**Biting**: Nm; Sil.

**Bones**, In: CP; Cs; Ks; Nm; Sil.

**Boring**: MP.

**Broken** as if: Cp; Nm.

Bones: NM.

**Bruised**, Soreness: **SIL.**

Coition, after: Sil.

**Burning**, externally: CP; Ks; **NM; SIL.**

Blood vessels: Nm.
Bones: Sil.
Glands: Nm; SIL.
Internally: CP; Ks; Nm; SIL.
**Bursting**, Splitting: **NM; SIL.**
**Cannot Stand**: Km; MP; NM.
**Colicky**: See Crampy.
**Compressing**, Squeezing: NM.
**Come** and Go: MP.
**Constrictive** (Constriction)
Externally: Sil.
Glands: Sil.
Internally: Nm; Sil.
**Crampy**: Mp.
Exertion, prolonged on Agg: Mp.
**Cutting**, Externally: KM; KS; NM; SIL.
Bones, in: Km.
Glands, in: Sil
Internally: Cp; KS; **NM; SIL.**
**Darting**: See Shooting.
**Digging**: Nm; Sil.
**Extort**, Cries: Km; Mp.
**Fine**: Nm; **SIL.**
**Fleeting**, Come and Go: MP.
**Glands**, in: Ks; NM; Sil.
**Gnawing**: Ks; Ns; **SIL.**
**Goes** To side lain on: Sil.
**Grinding** Boring: MP.
**Growing** Pains: Cp.
**Jerking** Externally: MP; **NM; SIL.**
Bones, in: NM; Sil.

Glands, in: NM; Sil.
Internally: Nm; **SIL.**
**Labour**: See under Labour.
**Lightning**: See Shooting.
**Maddening** (Besides himself): Km; MP; NM.
**Nail**, Clavus: See Plug.
**Needles**: See Fine.
**Neuralgia**: MP; Nm; Sil.
**Night**, only: **MP.**
**Paralytic**: Kp; Nm; SIL.
Bones, in: SIL.
**Paralysed**, Parts, in: Sil.
**Piercing**: Ns.
**Pinching**: Nm; Sil.
Externally: Sil.
Internally: NM; Sil.
**Places**, Changes, suddenly: Mp.
**Pressing**, Externally: CP; Kp; NM; SIL.
Bones, in: Sil.
Internally: **NM; SIL.**
Inward: Sil.
Load as from: Nm; Sil.
Muscles, In: Nm; Sil.
Together: NM; Sil.
Within outward NM; SIL.
**Prickling**: Nm; Np.
**Pulling**: See Drawing.
**Quick**: See Shooting.
**Radiating**: MP.
**Screwing**: Ns; Sil.
**Shifting**: See Wandering.
**Shooting**, Lightning: Km; Mp.

**Small** spots, in: CP; Mp; NM; Sil.

**Sore**, Bruised: Fp; KM; Nm; **SIL.**

Bones, in: SIL

Coition, after: **SIL.**

Externally: **NM; SIL.**

Internally: SIL.

Spots, in: Cp.

**Splinters**, As from: SIL.

**Squeezing**: NM; Ns.

**Stitching**: CP; Fp; KM; **KP; KS;** Mp; NM; NP; NS; SIL.

Bones, in: Sil.

Glands: NM; Sil.

Internally: Cp; **KS;** NM; NS; **SIL.**

Jerking: Sil.

Muscles: NM; SIL.

Outward: NM; SIL.

Tearing, in muscles: Sil.

Upwards: Ns.

**Stinging**: **SIL.**

**Twisting**: SIL.

**Ulcerative**: **KS;** NM; **SIL.**

Bones, in: Nm.

Glands, in: Nm; **SIL.**

Internally: **SIL.**

**Wakened**, By: Sil.

**Wandering**, Shifting: CP; Km; **KS;** MP; Nm; Ns; SIL.

**PAIN DURING** AGG:

**PAINLESSNESS**: See Pain absence of and Numbness.

**PALATE Burning**: Ns.

Crawling: Sil.

**Dry**: NM.

**Greasy**: Kp.

**Itching**: Kp; Sil.

**Membrane**, False covered with: **NP.**

**Necrosis** Of Hard: Sil.

**Pain**: Ns.

Menses, during: NS.

Sore: Cs; Nm; Ns; Sil.

edge of: Nm.

menses during: Ns.

touched, when: Ns.

**Paralysis**: SIL.

**Sensitive**: Ns.

**Stiff**: Nm.

**Swelling**: Nm; Ns; SIL.

Suppuration, with: Sil.

**Ulcers**: NM; Sil.

Perforating: SIL.

**Vesicles**: Ns.

**White**: NP.

**Yellow**, Creamy: Np.

**PALM Contractions**, in: NM.

**Cracks**, Fissures: Cf.

**Desquamation**: Cf.

**Eruptions**: NS.

Discharges, thin watery: NS.

Dry tetters: NS.

Pimples: Ns.

Psoriasis: Ks; Ns; Sil.

Raw: Ns.

Scabs: Ns.

Scurfy tetters: NS.

Vesicles, between fingers: NM.

between index and thumb: NS.

**Felon**: SIL.
**Heat**: Fp; Sil.
  Chilliness, with: Fp.
  Dry: Fp.
  Sitting, while: Fp.
**Itching**: KP; Nm; Sil.
**Pain**, Aching: Ns.
  Burning: CS; Nm.
  Drawing: Ns.
  Stitching: Ns.
**Perspiration**: Cp; Ks; Nm;
  **SIL.**
**Skin**, Hard: Cf.
**Swelling**: Fp.
**Warts**: Km; NM; Ns.
  flat: Nm.
  Painful, on pressure: Nm.
**PALPITATION**: See under Heart.
**PANARIS**: See Nails, Felon.
**PANCREAS Diseases** of: Cp;
  Ns.
**PAN OPHTHALMITIS**: CS; Ks.
**PARADOXICAL**: Nm.
**PARALYSIS** (Paralytic pain): Kp;
  Nm; Sil.
  **Agitans**: MP.
  **Ascending**: Nm; Sil.
  **Bladder** (urinary), of: Fp; Kp;
    Np; Ns; SIL.
  **Descending**: Nm; Sil.
  **Diphtheritic**: KP; Nm.
  **Emotions**, From: Nm.
  **Facial**: Kp; Nm.
  **Feeling** Of, externally: Nm;
    Sil.
    Internally: Nm; Sil.

**Infantile**: Kp.
  Dentition, during: Kp.
**Intermittent** Fever after: **NM.**
**Internal** Sense of: Nm.
**One sided** (Hemiplegia): Km;
  Kp; Nm.
  Right: Nm; Sil.
**Organs** of: Km; Nm; **SIL.**
**Pain**, From: Nm.
**Painless**: Nm; Sil.
**Paraplegia**: Cs; KP; NM; **SIL.**
  Anger after: NM.
  Grief from: Nm.
**Pollution**, after or Coition after:
  NM; Np; Sil.
**Post-diphtheritic**: Kp; NM; Sil.
**Rheumatic**: Fp.
**Sexual** Excess, from: Kp; Nm;
  Np.
**Sitting** After: Sil.
  While: CP.
**PARAPLEGIA**: See under Pa-
  ralysis.
**PARCHMENT** Like: Cf; Sil.
**PAROTIDS**: Cf.
  **Abscess**: **SIL.**
    Fever, typhus, after: Nm.
  **Enlarged**: Km; Sil.
    Ear affections, in: Sil.
  **Induration**: NM; **SIL.**
  **Inflamed** (Mumps): FP; Km;
    Kp; Mp; NM; SIL.
    Metastasis, testes to: Km;
    Nm.
    Persistent: Sil.
    Suppuration: NM; SIL.

**Pain**, Aching: Cp; Fp; Nm.
Pinching: Nm,
Sore, bruised: Cp; Cs.
right: Cs.
Stitching: Sil.
Tearing, drinking when: Nm.
**Swelling**: CS; FP; Km; Kp;
**SIL.**
**Ulcers**: Cp; Sil.
**PARTURITION**: See Labour.
**PAROXYSMS** Repeated: MP.
**PASSIONATE, Hasty,** temper:
Nm; Ns.
**PAST, Disagreeable** dwells on:
NM.
**PASTY, Sticky,** stringy: Km;
Nm.
**PATCHY Mottled**: Km; Nm.
**PATELLAE Bursa**: Sil.
**Cysts**: Sil.
**PEDICULOSIS**:
**PEELING** of skin
(Desquamation): Fp; Km;
**KS**; Nm; Np; SIL.
**PEMPHIGUS**: NM; NS; SIL.
**PENIS** and **Glans**
**Blenorrhoea** (Glans):NM.
**Cancer**: Sil.
**Chancre** (Hard): Cf.
**Condylomata** (Penis): NS.
**Deadness**, Sense of: Sil.
**Denuded**, Glans, were: Sil.
**Eruptions**, Pimples, (prepuce): Sil.
**Excoriation**, Glans: NM.

**Formication,** Glans: NM.
**Inflammation**, Glans: Km; Kp;
KS; NM; Sil.
**Itching**, Glans: Nm; NS; SIL.
Penis: Nm; NS.
Prepuce: Nm; Np; SIL.
**Moisture**, Glans: Nm.
**Pain**, Aching: Nm.
Biting, glans: Nm.
Burning (prepuce): Sil.
urination after: Ns.
Cutting, urination after (prepuce): Nm.
Stitching: Nm; Sil.
glans: Nm.
root of penis: Cp.
Urination during, agg: Nm.
Urging to urinate agg: Fp.
**Paraphimosis**: Nm.
**Perspiration**: Nm.
**Pulsation**, Glans: Nm.
**Redness**, Glans: Nm.
Prepuce: Sil.
**Retraction**, Prepuce: **NM.**
**Spots**, Red on penis, glans:
Nm; SIL.
**Swelling**: Cp; Np; NS; SIL.
Oedematous: NS; Sil.
Prepuce: NS; Sil.
**Tension**: Cp.
**Throbbing**, Glans: Nm.
**Twitching**: Nm.
**Ulcers**, Chancres: Cf; Km; Sil.
Elevated, lead coloured, sensitive edge: SIL.

Indolent: Sil.
Mercuric, syphilitic: SIL.
Painful: SIL.
Phagedenic: Kp.
Soft chancre: Km.
**PERCEPTION changed**
(Mental or visual): Kp.
**PERFORATION:** Sil.
**PERICARDITIS:** Cs; Fp; Km;
Nm.
**Chronic:** Cf.
**PERINEUM abscess:** SIL.
**Ball** Sensation: Km.
**Itching:** NS.
Mons veneris, and: Ns.
**Pain,** Aching: Cp.
Burning: Sil.
coition, after: Sil.
Stitching, shooting: CP.
penis to: CP.
**Pimples,** on: Nm.
**PERIODICITY, Periodically** in
general AGG: Km; **NM;**
NS; **SIL.**
**After:** Nm.
**Alternate** Days on: NM.
**At the same hour:** Nm; Sil.
**Every** Second day: Nm.
Seventh day: Km; Sil.
Tenth to fourteenth day: Kp.
**Exact:** Nm.
**PERIOSTEUM inflammation:**
SIL.
**Suppuration:** Cf; SIL.
**Swelling:** SIL.

**PERITONITIS:** Fp; Km; Kp; Ks;
SIL.
**PERSECUTION** Ideas of: Sil.
**PERSEVERE Cannot:** SIL.
**PERSPIRATION** in General: FP;
Km; Ks; **NM; N?; SIL.**
**Agg:** Nm.
**Amel: NM.**
**Absent** (See Skin Dry): SIL.
**Acrid:** Np.
**Affected** Parts on: Sil.
**Air,** Open in Agg: SIL.
**Anxiety,** During: Cp; Nm; Np;
Sil.
**Axillae,** Hand and feet: Sil.
**Cannot** Perspire: Ks; Nm;
**SIL.**
**Clammy: FP.**
**Cold:** Cp; Fp; Kp; Nm; Np; Sil.
**Coldness** After Agg: Sil.
**Coryza,** During: NM; **SIL.**
**Coughing** Agg: Nm; Np; Sil.
**Daytime** only: **KM;** NM.
Morning, and: Nm; Sil.
**Drinking,** After Agg: Kp; Sil.
**Drinking,** Water Amel: **SIL.**
**Easy:** Cp; KS; **NM;** Sil.
Coughing on: Cs.
**Eating,** While: Kp; NM; Sil.
After: Nm; Sil.
**Emission,** After: Nm.
**Epileptic** Attacks, after: Sil.
**Evening,** and through entire
night: Km.
**Excoriating:** Kp; Nm; **SIL.**

**Exertion**, During slight: **CS**; Fp; **KP**; KS; NM; NP; **NS**; SIL.
Mental: Nm; Sil.
**Exhausting**: Fp; **NM**; SIL.
**Fever**, After: Nm; Sil.
**Fright**: From: Sil.
**Greasy**, Oily: **NM**.
**Headache**, At start of: Nm.
**Hot**: Sil.
**Intermittent**: Sil.
**Lying**, Bed, in Amel: Sil.
**Menses**, Before: Ns.
During: Ns; Sil.
**Morning**, Agg: SIL.
**Motion**, On Agg: NM; Sil.
**Motion**, Amel: SIL.
**News** Unpleasant, from: CP.
**Night** Agg: **KM**; **NM**; Ns; Sil.
Midnight, after: **SIL**.
**Night,** At Phthisis of: Cp; Fp; Sil.
Weak and anemic persons: Fp.
**Odour**, Offensive: Kp; **SIL**.
Mice of a thousand: Sil.
Onions, garlic, like: Kp.
Sour: Nm; NP; SIL.
Urine like: Nm.
**Periodical**: Sil.
**Profuse**: Cp; Cs; FP; **KP**; KS; **NM**; NP; **SIL**.
Night: **CP**; **KM**; SIL.
midnight, after: **KM**.
Pain, from: Mp.
Rage, during: Nm.

**Putrid**: SIL.
**Rest**, During: Agg: SIL.
When at Amel: NM.
**Room**, In Amel: **SIL**.
**Sleep**, On beginning to: Sil.
**Sleep**, Amel:
**Smoking**: **NM**.
**Stool**; During: Nm.
**Uncovering** Agg: Sil.
Amel: NM.
**Urination**, After: NM.
**Waking**, After: Nm; Sil.
**Walking**, While: Nm; **SIL**.
**PERSPIRATION** Absent fever, in: Kp; KS; Nm; Sil.
**PERSPIRATION**, Complaints, from suppressed: Fp; NM; NS; **SIL**.
**PETECHIAE**: Nm. Sil.
**PHAGEDENA**, Slough: **SIL**.
**PHAGEDENIC Skin**: Nm; Np; **SIL**.
**PHANTASY**, Imaginations: See Fancies. Delusions.
**PHARYNX** Inflammation: CP; CS; FP; NM; NS.
**Chronic**: NM; **SIL**.
**Discolouration** Gray: Cp; Cs; NM.
**PHILOSOPHER**: Kp.
**PHIMOSIS** or
**PARAPHIMOSIS**: Nm.
**PHLEBITIS**: Cf; Fp.
**PHLEGMASIA Alba dolens**: (While milk leg): CF; NS; SIL.
**Contractions** with: SIL.

PHLYCTENAE Conjunctiva: Sil.
 Cornea: CF; Cp.
PHOBIAS, Fears: See Fear.
PHOSPHATURIA Phosphates in urine: CP; Mp.
PHOTOMANIA (Light Desire for): Nm; Sil.
PHOTOPHOBIA: CP; Cs; KP; MP; **NM**; Np; **NS; SIL.**
 Artificial light: Cp; NM.
 Chronic: NS; Sil.
 Coition, After: Kp; Sil.
 Daylight: Ks; Sil.
 Evening: Sil.
 Headache, During: FP; Ks; **NS**.
 Menses, During: Fp.
 Morning: NS; Sil.
PHTHISIS: See Consumption.
 Laryngeal: Cp; Fp; Km; SIL.
PHYSICAL EXERTION Agg: See Exertion physical.
PIANO PLAYING Agg: MP.
PICKING, Carphology: Nm.
PIECES IN, Duality: Cp; Nm; Sil.
PIERCING Pain: Ns.
PILES (Haemorrhoids): CP; CS; Fp; KM; Kp; **KS;** NM; NS; SIL.
 Backache, With: Cp.
 Bleeding: Cf; Fp; KM; Nm; Sil.
 Dark venous blood: Km.
 Stool during: Nm.
 Blind: Cf; CP; KS.

Congested: Sil.
Constipation, With: Ks; Sil.
 External: CP; Cs; KM; Ks; NM; SIL.
 Inflamed: Fp.
 Large: Km; Ks; Nm.
 Motion, Agg: Nm.
 Night: NM.
 Oozing Of moisture: Nm.
 Watery fluid all the time: Cp.
 Yellow fluid, from: Cp.
 Painful: **NM;** Sil.
 Pregnancy, During: NM.
 Protruding, During stool: **CP; SIL.**
 Sphincter, Spasm of with: Sil.
 Standing, AGG: Cp.
 Suppurating: **Sil.**
 Touch Agg: Cp. Sil.
 Ulcerating: **SIL.**
 Walking Agg: Cp; Km; Sil.
PIMPLES: See Eruptions.
PINCHING Pain: NM; Sil.
PINK EYE: See Eye, redness.
PINING: NM.
PINWORMS: Km; Np; Sil.
PITCHY: Cs; Ks; NM.
PLACID Tranquil: Sil.
PLAGUE, Fever zymotic: **KP;** Ks.
PLAINTIVE: Cs; Kp.
PLETHORA: Fp; **NM; SIL.**
PLEURISY: FP; KM; Kp; KS; Nm; Ns; Sil.

**PLEURODYNIA: CP; KP;** Mp; **NM; NS; SIL.**

**PLICA POLONICA**
**Tangling of hair:** Nm.

**PLUG Nail,** Wedge, clavus: Nm.

**PNEMONIA:** See Chest, inflammation.

**POISON,** Fear: See Fear, Poison.

**POLLUTIONS:** See Seminal Emissions.

**POLIOMYELITIS:** Nm; NS; Sil.

**POLYPI: CP;** CS; Ks; Nm; **SIL.**
**Urinary Bladder:** Sil.
**Ear:** Cp; KM; KS; Sil.
**Nasal:** CP; SIL.
Bleeds, easily: Cp.
**Uterine: CF;** CP;; CS; SIL.

**POLYURIA:** See Urine, Profuse.

**POPLITEAL** (Hollow of knee): Cp; NM; Sil.
**Bending** Knee Agg: Cp.
**Bursae:** Sil.
**Contraction,** Hamstrings: **NM;** Sil.
Lying on back, while: Ns.
**Eruptions:** NM.
Red: Nm.
**Fibroids,** Recurrent: Cf.
**Pain:** Cp; Nm.
Drawing: Cp; NM; Ns.
Left: Np.
Stitching: Nm.
inner side, as from nail: Nm.
Tearing: Nm.

**Redness:** Sil.

**Tension: NM.**
Menses, during: Np.
Rising, from a seat: Cp; Nm.
Walking, while: Sil.
continued Amel: CP.

**Tumours:** Cf; Sil.

**PORTAL Congestion:** KM; Nm; Ns.
**Chronic:** Ns.

**POSITION Awkward,** Strange: NS.
**Abdominal,** Sleep in: Cp.
**Back** on, Sleep in Head low, with: Kp; Nm.
**Change of Amel:** NS; Sil.
**Limbs** Drawn up: Nm.
**Wrong** As if in (Awkward): Ns.

**POSTERIOR NARES** Closure of: Cs.
**Discharge,** from: **NM;** NP.
Night, at, must sit up to clear the throat: Kp; Ns.
Thick: Cp; Km; NP; NS.
Tough, viscid: Km; NP.
Yellowish green: Cs; Vm; **NM;** NP; NS.
**Dryness:** Cp; NM; SIL.
**Food,** Sensation of, in: SIL, Swallowing, on: Sil.
**Itching:** Kp.
**Lump** in: Nm.
**Rawness,** Inspiration, agg: Fp.
**Scraping:** KP; **NM;** Ns.

**POST-OPERATIVE Disorders:** Cf; Fp; Ks.

**POST-PARTUM Haemorrhage:**
Cf; Fp.

**POWER, Higher** under as if:
Lack of:
Will, of:
Therefore, powerless:

**PRAYING:** Ns.

**PRECOCIOUS:**
Loquacious (children):

**PREGNANCY Disorders** of: Cf;
Cp; Nm.
Desires Strange things: CP.
Flatulence: Cf.
Heartburn: Nm.
Metrorrhagia: Kp.
Nausea: Fp; Kp; NM; SIL.
Piles: NM.
Toxaemia of: CP; NM; Sil.
Urine, Involuntary: NM.
Vomiting: Fp; Kp; NM; Np;
NS; Sil.

**PREMONITION,** Fear of future:
NM.

**PREPUCE Inflammation:** Sil.
Itching: Nm; Np; SIL.
Pain, Burning: Sil.
urination, after: Nm; Ns.
Cutting, urination after: Nm.
Paraphimosis: Nm.
Pimples: Sil.
Redness: Sil.
Retraction: **NM.**
Swelling: NS; Sil.

**PRESBYOPIA** (Hypermetropia):
NM; **SIL.**

**PRESENTIMENTS** (Fear of Future): NM.

**PRESSING:** See Pain, pressing.

**PRESSURE Agg:** Cp; NM; NS;
**SIL.**
Clothes, Of: NM; Ns.
Hat, Of: **SIL.**
Slight: **MP.**
Spine, on: **SIL.**

**PRESSURE Amel:** Cf; Kp; **MP;**
Nm; Np; NS; **SIL.**
Hard: **MP.**

**PRESSURE** Simple:
Sense of: NM; Sil.

**PRIAPISM (Painful** Erections):
Cp; Km; Kp; Mp; Nm; Np;
SIL.
Burning in urethra with: Cp.

**PRICKLING:** Kp; Sil.

**PRICKLY** Heat (Sudamina): NM.

**PRODROME:** Sil.

**PROFANITY:** Nm.

**PROLAPSE,** Falling: Nm.
Anus, of: See Under Anus.
Uterus, of: See under Uterus.

**PROPHYLACTICS Catheter**
Fever: MP.
Exanthemata: KM.
Small-pox: Km; SIL.

**PROPORTION Sense of** disturbed: Kp.

**PROSOPALGIA:** See Face, pain in.

**PROSTATE GLAND**
Abscess: Sil.

**Emission** of prostatic fluid: NM; SIL.

Erections, without: NM.

Lascivious, thoughts during: NM.

Stools with: NM; Np; **SIL.**

after: SIL.

difficult, with: **SIL.**

Talking, to young lady while: NM.

Urinating, after: Nm; SIL.

Walking, while: Sil.

**Enlarged**: Kp; Np; NS; SIL.

**Hard**, indurated: SIL.

**Inflamed**: Fp; SIL.

Chronic: Sil.

**Pain**: Cp.

Dragging, stitching: Cp.

**Sensation** of Ball, on sitting: Sil.

**Suppuration**: Cs; Sil.

**PROSTATORRHEA**: See Prostate Gland, emission.

**PROSTRATION**: See Weakness.

**Mind of**: Cp; Cs; **KP; NM; NP; SIL.**

Reading from: SIL.

Talking from: CP.

Writing, after: SIL.

**PROTRUSION**, Eyes, Hernia etc: Cf; Cp; FP; NM; SIL.

**PROUD** (Pride):

**PRURIGO, Pruritus**: See Skin, itching.

Anus: See Rectum, itching.

Vulvae: See Vulva, itching.

**PSORA**: Cp; Nm; Sil.

**PSORIASIS**: CS; Kp; KS; Nm; SIL.

Inveterate: SIL.

**PTERYGIUM**: CF; Cp; Sil.

**PTOSIS** (eye-lids of): Kp; Mp; NM; Np; NS; Sil.

**PUBERTY** and **Youth**: CP; FP; KP; Nm.

Slow, Girls in: Cp.

**PUBIC REGION**: Nm; Sil.

Cramp: Nm.

Eruptions, Pimples: Nm.

Bones, over: Cp.

Hair, Falling out from: **NM.**

Itching: Nm.

Pain: Cp.

Blood discharge, vagina from: Cp.

Pressure: Cp.

Pulsation: Cp.

Quivering, Bones over: Cp.

Sticking: Cp.

**PUERPERAL Sepsis**: Fp; Km; KP; Sil.

**PUERPERIUM**: NM; Sil.

**PUFFINESS** (Face): Cs.

**PULMONARY Oedema**: KP; NM.

**PULSATIONS Throbbing**: CP; CS; Fp; Km; Kp; **KS; NM; NP; NS; SIL.**

Bones, In: Sil.

Glands, In: Sil.

Internally: Cp; NM; Np; NS; **SIL.**

**Motion**, Agg: Sil.
**Motion**, Amel: NM.
**Night**: SIL.
**Sitting**, While: SIL.
**Sleep**, During: Nm.
**PULSE ABNORMAL**: NM; SIL.
  **Fast**: See Rapid.
  **Flowing**: FP.
  **Full**: FP; Km; Nm; Sil.
  **Hard**: Km; Sil.
  **Imperceptible**: Kp; Ks; SIL.
  **Intermittent**: Km; Kp; Mp; NM.
    Every third beat: Nm.
    One to two beats: Nm.
  Irregular: NM.
  Irritable: Mp.
  Jerky: Nm.
  Large: FP.
  Rapid, Accelerated: FP; NM; NS; SIL.
    And small: SIL.
    Motion, Agg: NM.
    Vexation, after: NM.
  **Slow**: Km; NM; Sil.
    Than heart beat: NM.
  **Small**: Km; Nm; SIL.
  **Soft**: FP; Km; Nm; SIL.
  **Suppressed** (obliterated): Sil.
  **Tremulous**: Nm.
  **Tumultous**: Nm.
  **Unequal**: NM; Sil.
  **Weak**: NM; Sil.
**PUNCTURED Wounds**: Sil.

**PUPILS, Adherent**: SIL.
  **Beclouded**: Sil.
  **Contracted**: Mp; NM; Sil.
    Chill, during: Sil.
    Perspiration, during: Sil.
  **Dilated**: NP.
    Disease, during: Kp.
    Iregular: Sil.
    One contracted and one: Np.
    Right more than left: Sil.
**PURGING AMEL**: NS.
**PURPLE**: See Bluish.
**PURSUED As if**: Sil.
**PUS** bloody, lumpy: Cs.
  **Burrowing**: Sil.
  **Foul**: CF; Sil.
  **Profuse**: Nm.
  **Scanty**: Cs; Sil.
  **Suppressed**: Sil.
  **Thick**: CS; Ks.
  **Thin**: SIL.
  **Unhealthy**: SIL.
  **Watery**: SIL.
  **Yellow**: Cs.
    Green: Ks.
    Stubborn: SIL.
**PUSHED Forward**: Fp.
**PUSTULES**: See under Eruptions.
**PYEMIA**: Sil.
**PYELITIS**: Cs; Ks.
  **Calculous**: SIL.
  **Chronic**: Sil.

**PYLORUS Constriction**: Km; Nm;

  **Relaxation**: Fp.

  **Wall**, indurated: Sil.

**PYORRHEA**: Ns; **SIL.**

**PYREXIA**: See Fever.

**PYROSIS**: See Heartburn.

**PYURIA** (Pus in Urine): KS; NS; **SIL.**

**QUALMISHNESS**: NS.

**QUARRELSOME** (Abusive): Sil.

**QUARTAN, Chill, fever**: NM.

**QUESTIONS, Speaks**, in Continuously:

**QUICK Pains** (shooting): Km; MP.

**QUININE Abuse** of: **NM.**

**QUINSY** (Tonsil Acute suppuration): FP; Km; Nm; SIL.

**QUIVERING**: Nm; **SIL.**

  **Glands**: Sil.

**QUOTIDIAN Chill**: Ks; **NM; NS.**

  **Fever**: **NM.**

**RADIATING**: Mp; NS; Sil.

**RAGE, Fury**: Nm.

  **Headache**, With: Nm.

**RAINS, When AGG**: Cf.

**RAINY SEASON Amel**: SIL.

**RAISING Arms, Agg**: Cp; Nm.

  **Up Agg**: Nm; Sil.

    **Amel**: SIL.

**RANCID Taste**, odour:

**RANULA**: Cf; Fp; **NM.**

  **Stinging** pain, with: NM.

**RASHNESS Reckless**: Sil.

**RATS, Sees**: Sil.

**RATTLING** (Chest in): Cs; KS; Sil.

**RAW** (Pain, biting): Nm; Np; Sil.

**RAYNAUD'S Disease**: Fp.

**REABSORBENT**: Km.

**REACTION Poor, Lack of**: CF; CS; Km; KS; Nm; Ns.

  **Suppuration**, In: Cf; Sil.

  **Syphilis**, In: Cf.

**READING, Eye strain Agg**: NM; Sil.

  **Averse**, to: Sil.

  **Difficult**, in Artificial light: Nm.

**RECKLESS** (Rashness): Sil.

**RECTUM & ANUS**

  **Abscess** (Peri-rectal): CS; SIL.

  **Boils**, in Anus: Cp.

  **Bubbles** At: Nm.

    Feeling of or escaping as if: Nm.

  **Bug**, Crawling from: Km.

  Stool, after: Km.

  **Burning**: NM.

    Stool, after: CS; NM; NS; Sil.

  **Coition**, Agg: Sil.

  **Coldness**, in Anus: Km; Nm; Sil.

    Walking in open air: Sil.

  **Condylomata**: Km; NS.

  **Congestion**: Nm.

  **Constriction**, Contraction: Cs; NM; Np; Sil.

    Painful: SIL.

Rectum and testes, to: Sil.
Spasmodic: Nm; Sil.
Stool, after: Fp.
before: NM.
during: **NM; SIL.**
preventing: NM.
Urination, on: Nm.
**Cutting**: Sil.
**Dragging**, Heaviness: Kp.
Stool, after: Nm.
**Drawing** In: Np.
**Dryness**: NM.
**Eruptions**, About Anus: **NM;** NS.
Herpetic: NM.
**Excoriation**: Cs; NM; NP.
Nates, between: Nm.
Walking, from: Nm.
**Feces**, Remained in as if: **NM.**
**Fissure**: Cf; CP; Nm; SIL.
Children, in: Cp.
Stool after, agg: Nm.
**Fistula** in Ano: **CP;** Cs; **SIL.**
Abscess, about: Cs.
Alternating with chest disorders: Cp; SIL.
**Foreign** Body: Nm.
**Formication**, Anus in: **CS;** Kp; Sil.
**Fullness** Of: Mp.
**Genitals**, To: Sil.
**Haemorrhages**, From anus: CP; CS; Fp; Km; Kp; KS; **NM;** NS; Sil.

Grief, after: Nm.
Night: FP; KP.
Stool after: CP; Nm.
during: CP; **NM.**
hard, from: **NM.**
**Inactivity** of Rectum: CP; KP; Ks; **NM;** NP; SIL.
**Inflammation**: Fp.
**Itching**: CP; **CS;** Fp; Km; Kp; **KS;** NM; NP; Ns; SIL.
Anus, around: NS.
Ascarides, from: Cf; NP.
Bed, warm in: Cp; Np.
Evening: **CP.**
Night: **NP.**
awakes: Cf.
Pain, worm as from: Cf.
Scratching, agg: Nm; SIL.
Stool, after: KM; NM; SIL.
during: Nm; Sil.
Violent: KS.
Voluptuous: SIL.
Walking, while: Nm.
**Lump**, As of: NM; SIL.
**Moisture**: Cp; Cs; Fp; NM; **SIL.**
Bloody: Sil.
Orange coloured: KP.
Scratching, after: Sil.
Yellow: Cp.
**Motion**, As if, something alive in: Cp.
**Mucous** Discharge: Cp; Sil.
**Narrow**: Nm.

**Pain**. Aching: Cp; Cs; Fp; Kp; Ks; Nm; Np; Sil.

Burning: Cp; CS; Fp; **KS; NM;** Np; NS; **SIL.**

afternoon: Sil.

constant: Nm.

diarrhoea, during: Ks.

night: Kp.

Coition, agg: Sil.

Constrictive, spasmodic: NM.

Cramping, testes to: Sil.

Cutting: Cp; Ks; **SIL.**

stools, during: Np.

Forenoon: Nm.

Genitals, to: Sil.

Griping: Nm.

Lancinating, even after soft stool: Nm.

Morning: Cp.

Pinching: Nm.

Pressing (Pressure): CS; Kp; Ks; Mp; Nm; Sil.

diarrhoea; as in a: Nm.

downward, outward: Cp.

Pulsating, throbbing: Cp; **NM.**

Rasping: Nm.

Scraping: Cp; Nm.

Sore, bruised: CP; Cs; Km; KP; **KS;** NM; Np; Ns; **SIL.**

Splinter, like: Np; SIL.

Sticking: Sil.

Stitching, shooting: CP; Cs; Kp; **KS;** MP; NM; **SIL.**

Stinging: NM; Sil.

stool, amel: Cp; Ns.

stool, after: Cp; CS; KM; Kp; Ks; Nm; Np; Sil.

before: Nm; NS.

during: Cp; Cs; Km; Kp; Ks; Nm; **SIL.**

diarrhoea, after: Nm.

hard, after: Cs; NM; SIL.

long after: NM; Sil.

straining, after: SIL.

Tearing: Nm.

Tenesmus: Cs; Fp; NM; Np; SIL.

menses, during: Nm.

Vexation, agg: Nm.

Walking, while: Km; Nm; Np; SIL.

**Paralysis**: Km; Kp; Nm; **SIL.**

Piles, removal after: Cp; Kp.

**Polypi**: CP.

**Prolapsus**, of: Cf; CS; Fp; Kp; Mp; NM; NS; SIL.

Burning and oozing bloody water: Nm.

Children, in: FP.

Feeling, as if torn: Mp.

Stool, after: NM.

during: Fp.

**Pulsation**: NM; Sil.

Stool, during: Nm.

**Raw**, Anus were: Np.

**Redness** Of anus: Nm.

**Relaxed**: Kp.

**Retraction**: Np.

**Rough** Substance, within as if: Nm.

**Stricture**: NM.

**Swelling** of: Nm.
**Tenesmus**: Cs; Fp; NM; Np; SIL.
  Coffee after: Nm.
  Night: FP.
**Tension**: SIL.
**Testes** to: Sil.
**Tickling**: Nm.
**Ulcerations**: NS; SIL.
**Warts**: NS.
**Weakness**, Feeling, stool before: Np.
**Weight**, And feeling as if plug between pubes and coccyx: Sil.
**Worms**, As if in: Sil.
**Worms**, complaints: Km; Nm; NP; Ns; SIL.
  Ascaria (round): **NM**; NP; SIL.
  Oxyuris (thread worms): Km; Np; Sil.
  Taenia (tapeworm): Sil.
**RECURRING** (Relapses): MP; NM.
**RED**, Redness (Skin, Discharges): Fp; NM; Sil.
  **Pale**: SIL.
  **Rosy**: Sil.
  **Spots**: Ks; Nm; Np; SIL.
  **Streaks**: Sil.
**REELING Tottering**, staggering: Nm; SIL.
**REGURGITATION**: FP.
  **Bitter**: Ns.
  **Eating**, Immediately, after: Mp.

**Fluids**, Of: Sil.
**Ingesta**, Of: Km; NM.
**Salty**: Nm.
**Sour**: Np.
**Vexation** After: Fp; Nm.
**RELAPSES Recurrences**: MP; NM.
**RELAPSING Fever**: Fp.
**RELAXATION**: Nm.
  **Abdomen** (Flabby): **CP**; SIL.
  **Anus**, and Rectum: Kp.
  **Male** Sex organs: Mp; Sil.
  **Muscles**: Km; Sil.
  **Pylorus**: FP.
  **Scrotum**: Cp; NM; SIL.
  **Sphincter**, Urinary: Sil.
    Vaginal: Nm; Sil.
**RELIGIOUS** Affections: KP; Nm; Sil.
**REMITTENCY**: Ns.
**REMITTENT** Fever: Ns.
**REMORSE**: See Guilt.
  **Trifles**, about: Sil.
**RENAL** Colic: See pain, under Kidneys.
**RENDING** (shooting pain): Km; MP.
**REPRIMANDS agg**: Nm.
**REPROACHES Himself**: Cp; NM.
  **Others**: Cp; Nm.
**REPULSIVE Mood**: Sil.
**RESERVED**: Nm.
  **Displeasure**: Nm.
**RESPIRATION**: CP; Km; KS; NS.

**Abdominal**: Ks; Nm.

**Accelerated**: CP; NM; SIL.

**Air, Open Agg:**

 **Amel**: KS; **NM.**

**Anxious**: **NM.**

**Arms** Exertion Agg: NM; SIL.

**Arrested** (Difficult): Nm; Ns; Sil.

 Children, lifted, on being: CP.

 Cough, during: Nm.

 Evening, grasping in inguinal region with: Nm.

 Night, cough, during: Nm; SIL.

**Ascending Agg**: Cs; NM; Nm.

**Asthmatic**: See Asthma.

**Breath** Again cannot: Nm; SIL.

**Catching**: **SIL.**

**Chill**, During Agg: NM.

**Cough**, With: Cp; Cs; Fp; KS; Nm; NS; SIL.

**Deep**: Cp; Km; Nm; NS; SIL.

 Desire to breath: CP; Mp; NS; Sil.

 constant: Ns.

 impossible: Cp.

**Difficult** (Dyspnoea): CF; Cp; CS; FP; KM; KP; KS; NM; Np; **NS; SIL.**

 Back, stitches in with: Kp.

 Children, in: Cp; **NS.**

 Dust, as from: **SIL.**

 Periodical attacks: CP.

**Drinking**, When agg: Nm.

**Dust** Agg: SIL.

**Eating**, After Agg: Kp; Nm; Ns.

**Epigastrium** or Stomach from: NM.

**Eructations**, Amel: Ks.

**Exertion** Agg: **NM;** NS; SIL.

 Least Agg: NS.

 With hands and arms: NM; SIL.

**Flatulence** Agg: NS.

**Heat**, With: Nm; SIL.

**Hot** Breath: Cp; Nm.

**Humid**, Air Agg: NS.

**Impeded**: See Oppressed

**Kyphosis**, In: SIL.

**Light**: See shallow.

**Loud**: NM; NS; SIL.

**Lying**, While Agg: Cs; Fp; Ks; Nm; SIL.

 Back, on Agg: Nm; SIL.

**Lying**, Amel: CP; NS.

**Manual** Labour Agg: NM; SIL.

**Menses** After Agg: Nm.

 Before Agg: Ns.

**Morning** Agg: Ns.

**Motion** Agg: Fp; Nm; NS.

 Amel: Nm; Sil.

**Neck**, Draft of air Agg: Sil.

**Oppressed** (Impeded): Cp; Km; Nm; SIL.

 Sensation, as if, during sleep: Sil.

**Pain**, During Agg: NM; Ns; SIL.

Periodically Agg: Ns.
Raising Up Agg: Cp.
Rapid: Km; NM; SIL.
Rattling: CP; CS; Fp; Km; Kp; KS; NM; NS; SIL.
Expectoration, without: Ks.
Rising, When: Cp.
Running, After: SIL.
Shallow: FP; MP; NS; Sil.
Short: NM; Sil.
Stools, before: NS.
Sighing: CP; Np; SIL.
Menses, during: Np.
Takes deep breath: Sil.
Sitting Up amel: Mp.
Sitting, While Agg: Ns.
Snoring: Km; NM; SIL.
Adenoids removal after: Ks.
Sobbing: MP; Sil.
Paroxysmal: MP.
Standing Agg: Nm.
Amel: Sil.
Stormy Weather Agg: NS.
Suffocative Attack: CP; Nm; Sil.
Suffocation, Threatened: Kp.
Talking, After Agg: SIL.
Thunder-Storm Agg: SIL.
Tight: NM; NS; SIL.
Tremulous, As if were: Mp.
Waking, On Agg: Sil.
Walking, Agg: Ks; Nm; NS.
Rapidly: NM; NS; SIL.
Warm Room Agg: KS; Sil.
Wet Weather Agg: NS.

Wheezing: KS; NM; NS.
Expiration, when: Nm.
Whistling: Ks; Nm; SIL.
Expiration on: Nm.
Working, When Agg: SIL.
REPONSIBILITY Inability to realise:
Unusual Agg: Sil.
REST Agg: See Motion, amel.
Cannot in any Position: Fp; Nm; Sil.
RESTLESSNESS, Nervousness: CP; Cs; Fp; KP; KS; Mp; NM; Np; Ns; SIL.
Anxious: Cp; NM; Np; SIL.
Backache With when tired: Cf.
Bed, Driving out of: Fp; Nm; Sil.
Tossing about, in: Fp; Nm.
Evening: Cs; Np.
Extremities, Upper: Km; KP; SIL.
Lower: CP; KP; NM; SIL.
sitting, while: Nm.
sleep, before: NM.
Headache During: Sil.
Heat, During: Fp.
Internal: Nm; SIL.
Lying on back, Agg: Kp.
on side Amel: Cp.
Menses, During: Kp; Ks.
Mental Labour, during: KP.
Midnight, At: Nm.
Sitting, While: Nm.
Sleep, Before going to: NM.

**RETCHING and GAGGING**: Kp; Ks; NM; Np; NS; Sil.
  **Constant**: Ns.
  **Cough**, With: KS; Mp; NM; SIL.
  **Eating**, After: Ns.
  **Expectorating**, When: Sil.
  **Hawking**, Agg: CP.
  **Ineffectual**: Sil.
  **Warm** Drinks, from: NM.
**RETENTION** Sense, of: Sil.
**RETENTION** of urine: See Under Bladder.
**RETICENT Taciturn**: See Silent.
**RETINA Anemia**: Fp; Nm.
  **Detachment** Of:
  **Exudation**: Km.
  **Haemorrhage**: Fp; Kp; Nm.
  **Haziness**: Sil.
  **Hyperaesthesia**: **NM.**
  **Images**, Retained too long: Nm.
  **Inflammation**: Kp.
  Leukaemic: Ns.
  **Irritable**: Km.
  **Paralysis** of: Cp; KP.
**RETRACTION**, Drawn back: Nm; Sil.
**RETROVERSION** of Uterus: Cf; CP; **NM**; Np; Sil.
**REVENGE** and Hatred: NM.
**REVERBERATIONS**: See Noises in Head, also hearing, Illusory sounds.
**REVERY**: See Dreaminess.

**RHEUMATISM**: CP; CS; FP; Km; Ks; NM; Mp; NS.
  **Acute**: Cs.
  **Alternating** With: CP; FP; NM.
  **Asthma**, With: Ks; NS.
  **Chronic**, Diarrhoea, in: Sil.
  Rigidity, with: Cs; Sil.
  **Heat**, Hot weather Agg: Ks.
  **Recurrent** : Ns.
**RHINITIS** Cold in Head: Fp; NM; Sil.
**RIBS Border** of: Ns.
  **Costal cartilages**: Cp.
  **Lower**: Sil.
**RICKETS, rachitis**: CP; Fp; SIL.
**RIDING Horse** back, on AGG.: Sil.
  **After**: **SIL.**
  **Cars or wagon**, in: Nm; SIL.
**RIGIDITY**: See Stiffness.
**RINGING noises**: See Hearing Illusory.
**RINGWORM**: See Eruptions, herpetic
**RISING Agg**: NM; **SIL.**
  **After**: **NM**; SIL.
  **From** a seat: Km; **NM; NS;** SIL.
**RISING Amel**: Nm; SIL.
**RIVET feeling**: Nm.
**ROARING**: See Head, Noises in, and Hearing Illusory.
**ROBUST Habit**: Fp; NM; SIL.
  **Emaciation** suddenly: Nm.

ROCKING Agg: Sil.
  To and fro: Nm; Sil.
ROLLING or Turning over as
    if: Nm.
ROMANTIC: CP; Kp; Sil.
ROOM in Agg: Ks; NM.
  Full of people: Nm.
ROOM in Amel: Nm; SIL.
ROSE Cold: Kp; Ks; NM; Sil.
ROSE Rash: Km; Np; Sil.
ROSEOLA: Km; Np; Sil.
ROTATION Agg: Nm; Sil.
ROUGH, Scratchy: Cf; Nm.
RUBBING, Stroking Agg: SIL.
  Amel. C; Km; MP; NS; Sil.
    Abdomen: Ns.
RUBELLA (German measles):
    FP; Km; Ks; Sil.
RUDE (impertinent): Nm.
RUMBLING: See under Abdo-
    men.
RUNNING Agg: NM; SIL.
  Amel: Nm; SIL.
RUNNING Creeping: SIL.
  Better, than walking:
  Forwards, trying to walk when:
    Kp.
  Impulse, for: Fp.
RUNS about (Escape):Fp.
RUN-ROUND: See Fingers:
    Felon.
RUPIA: NM; NS; Sil.
RUSTY (Brownish): Cp; Cs; Np;
    Sil.
SACRUM and Region: CP; Cs;
    Nm; SIL.

Aching: CP; CS; Nm; SIL.
Boring: Nm.
Broken as if: Nm.
Burning: Sil.
Crampy: Sil.
Crushed, As though: Sil.
Cutting: CP; Nm; Np; Ns.
Drawing: Nm; Sil.
Eruptions, Scabs: SIL.
Feet, To: Km.
Lameness: CP; SIL.
Lying After, not able to rise:
    Sil.
  Compels: CP.
Numbness: CP.
  Legs, and: CP.
Pain: CP; CS; KM; KP; Ks;
    NM; Np; Ns; SIL.
  Night: NS.
    Frequently, during: Cp.
  Pressing: Nm.
Pulsating: NM; SIL.
Sore, Bruised: NM; NS; Sil.
Stiffness, Tension: Nm; Sil.
Stitching, Shooting: CP; Cs;
    Nm; Ns; Sil.
  Compels to lie on back: Cp.
Weak: Sil.
SACRO-ILIAC region
  Pain, Aching: CP; Np; Sil.
    Cutting: Np.
    Dislocated, as if: Cp.
    Sore, bruised, beaten: CP.
SADNESS, Despondency: CP;
    CP; CS; FP; KP; Ks; NM;
    NP; NS; SIL.

**Afternoon**: Cs.
**Alone**, when: NM; Sil.
**Causeless**: Nm; Sil.
**Coition**, Agg: Nm.
**Emissions**, After: Np.
**Enjoys**: Nm.
**Evening**: Km.
　Chilliness, with: Km.
**Girls**, in, before Puberty: Cp.
**Head** Injuries, from: NS.
**Heat**, During: **NM**; Np; Ns; **SIL.**
**Labour**, During: Nm.
**Life**, Tired, of, but fears death: Kp.
**Light**, Subdued Agg: Ns.
**Masturbation**, From: Nm; Sil.
**Menses** Before: Fp; NM.
　After: Sil.
　During: NM; Sil.
　Suppressed: Nm; Sil.
**Morning**, Mirthful in evening: Cs.
　Walking on: Kp.
**Music**, From: Np; NS.
**Night**: Kp; **NM.**
**Periodical** Attacks of mania with: Ns.
**Perspiration**, During: Cs; NM.
**Pregnancy**, In: Nm.
**Unusual** Tendency to look on dark sides of things with: Cf.
**Walking**, on: Cp; KP.
**Weep**, cannot: **NM.**

**SALIVA Bitter**: Ks.
**Bloody**: NM.
　Menses, before: NM.
**Brown**: Np.
**Cottony** (Frothy); Km; **NM; Sil.**
**Diminished**, Scanty: Nm; Sil.
　Thirst, with: Sil.
**Expectoration** Of: Nm.
**Frothy**: Km; NM; Sil.
**Green**: Nm; Ns.
**Gushes** of: NM.
　Suddenly: Nm.
**Increased** (Salivation): **CP;** Cs; FP; Kp; Ks; NM; Np; NS; SIL.
　Cough, with: Nm.
　Dentition, during: CP.
　Dryness, with: Nm.
　Eating, after: Kp; NS.
　Evening, in bed: Nm.
　Headache, during: NS.
　Mercury, from: Nm.
　Night: Nm.
　Pain with: Nm.
　Pregnancy, in: Ns.
　Sleep, during: Nm.
**Salty**: Kp; NM.
**Slimy**: Cs.
**Soapy**: See Frothy.
**Sour**: CP; Nm; NS.
**Sticky**: Mp.
**Thick**, viscid: Kp.
**Tough**, Stringy: Km.
**Watery**: Nm.

**SALIVARY GLANDS**: Cf.

**SALIVATION**: See Saliva, increased.

**SALPINGITIS** (Fallopian tubes): Fp; Km; Sil.

   **Serum or pus** escaps from uterus: SIL.

**SALT Agg**: **NM;** SIL.

   AMEL: Nm.

**SALT Abuse** of (Halophagia): Nm.

**SALTY, Saltiness**: Nm.

**SALVATION**: KP.

**SAND As** if: Km; Nm; Sil.

**SARCOCELE** (Testis of): Sil.

**SARCOMA**: Sil.

   **Cutis**: Cp; Sil.

   **Osteo**: Cf.

**SATYRIASIS**: **CP;** Fp; Kp; **NM;** NP; NS; **SIL.**

**SAWING As** if: Cf.

**SCABIES**: KS; SIL.

**SCABS** (See Crusts): **KS; SIL.**

**SCALDED**: Cs; KM; Ns.

   **As if**: Mp; Nm.

**SCALES, Scaly**: Cs; Km; KS; SIL.

   **Bran-like**: Km; Nm; **SIL.**

   **Ichthyosis**: Sil.

   **Spots**: Sil.

   **Yellow**: **KS.**

**SCALP Abscess**: SIL.

   **Itching**: **CS;** Fp; Kp; KS; **NM;** SIL.

**SCAPULAE** (And Region):

   **Buzzing** Under Left: Km.

**Coldness**, Between: Nm; SIL.

**Heaviness**: Sil.

**Itching**: Sil.

   Between: Cs.

**Pain**: Cp; Kp; Nm; Sil.

   Aching: Cp.

     between: Km; Kp.

     under: Nm.

   Between: Cp; Cs; Fp; KP; Ks; Nm; Np; **NS;** SIL.

   Broken as if: Sil.

   Bruised, beaten as if: Nm; Sil.

   Burning: Nm; SIL.

     left: Nm; Sil.

     right: Ns.

     between: SIL.

     nape to: NS.

     spine to: SIL.

   Cutting in or between: **NS.**

   Drawing: Nm; Sil.

     between: Nm; NS; SIL.

     under: Ns.

   Jerking: Cp.

     under: Cp.

   Left: Np.

     under, morning: Kp; Nm; Ns.

   Pressing: Nm; Ns; Sil.

     between: Sil.

     under: Cp.

   Right then left: Kp.

     under: Nm.

   Sore, bruised: Cp; Nm; Sil.

     between: Sil.

right: SIL.
under: Nm.
Tearing: Nm; Ns.
below: SIL.
walking on: SIL.
between: NS; SIL.
under: CP; Ns.
**Quivering**: Sil.
**Swollen** Feeling: Sil.
**Tension**, Stiffness: Sil.
Between: NM.
**Twitching**: Cp.
**Weak**: NM.
**SCARLATINA** Scarlet fever: Fp;
Km; Kp; Ks; Nm; Sil.
**SCARS**: See Cicatrices.
**SCIATICA**: CP; Fp; KP; **MP**;
NM; NS; SIL.
**Bed**, Turning in, Agg: Ns.
**Coldness** of Painful parts with:
Sil.
**Feet**, Tender, with: Mp.
**Heat** Amel: MP.
**Hips** To feet: Sil.
**Mental** Exertion Agg: Kp; Mp.
**Pressure** Amel: MP.
**Rising** From sitting Agg: Ns.
**Standing** Amel: Mp.
**Suddenly** Comes and goes:
MP.
**Tonic** Contraction, chronic:
NM.
**Uncovering** Agg: MP; **SIL.**
**Vertebral** Origin: NM; Sil.
**SCIRRHUS Carcinoma**: **SIL.**

**SCLERODERMA**: Cf; SIL.
**SCLEROSIS**: Km; Nm; SIL.
**Arterio-sclerosis**: Cf; Np; Ns;
Sil.
**Multiple**: Sil.
**SCLEROTITIS**: CP; **CS**; Fp;
Km; Sil.
**SCOLDING**: SIL.
**Herself**: Cp; Nm.
**SCORBUTIC symptoms**: FP;
Km; **KP**; NM; SIL.
**SCORN** (contempt): NM.
**SCORPIONS, Sees**: Sil.
**SCRAPED**, As if:
**SCRATCHES Hands**, with:
**Desire** to: Cp.
**Himself**, Raw: Sil.
**Lime** of the walls: Cf; CP; Fp.
**SCRATCHING Agg**: Kp; KS;
NM; Ns; **SIL**.
Amel: Cs; KM; Ks; Np.
**SCRAWNY**: Cp.
**SCREAMS** (Cries): See Shriek-
ing.
**SCREWED together**: NS.
**SCROFULA** (Psora of child):
Cp; SIL.
**Erethistic**: Cp.
**SCROTUM Condylomata**: Sil.
**Elephantiasis**: Sil.
**Eruptions**: Nm.
Itching: Nm; NS.
moist spots: SIL.
Moist: **NM**; Sil.
Pimples: CP.

Vesicles, thighs, between: Nm.

**Excoriation:** CP; Sil.

**Formication:** Sil.

**Inflamed:** Nm.

Erysipelatous: Nm.

**Itching:** CP; KS; **NM;** Np; Ns; SIL

Spots: Sil.

**Moisture:** CP; SIL.

Serum running with: CP.

**Pain,** Burning: Sil.

Scratching after: NS.

Sore: CP.

oozing fluid: Cp.

Stitching: Ks.

**Perspiration:** CP; NS; SIL.

**Relaxed:** Cp; NM; SIL.

**Sensitive:** Nm.

**Skin** Thickened: Sil.

**Spots,** Red: SIL.

**Swelling:** NM.

Oedematous: Cf; NM; Ns.

Oozing: Cp.

**Thighs,** between and excoriation, itching moisture etc.: NM.

**SCURFS:** See Scaly.

**SCURVY** (Scorbutic): FP; Km; **KP;** NM; SIL.

**SEA Agg:** NM; NS.

**Air amel.:**

**Bathing:**

**SEARCHING** On the **floor:** Nm.

**SEA-SICKNESS:** Nm; SIL.

**Feeling** of:

**Nausea** without: Kp.

**SEASONS, change** of: See Change of temperature.

**Autumn, summer:** See different headings.

**SEBACEOUS Cysts:** SIL.

**SEBORRHOEA:** Ks; NM.

**SECRETIONS,** Discharges

**Increased** in general: Km; Nm; NS; SIL.

AGG: Cp.

AMEL: Nm; NS; SIL.

**Acrid,** Excoriating: SIL.

**Albuminous:** Cp; NM.

**Bland:** Sil.

**Blood-streaked:** Fp; Sil.

**Checked,** Ill effects of: SIL.

**Fibrinous:** Km.

**Foamy,** frothy: Ns.

**Greenish:** NS.

**Gushing:** Nm; NS.

**Hair,** Destroying: Nm; Sil.

**Lumpy:** CS; Km; SIL.

**Meat** Water like: Fp.

**Milky:** KM; Kp; Ns.

**Mucous** Altered: Cs; **NM;** Sil.

**Slimy:** Km; Nm.

**Stain** Indelibly: Mp; Sil.

**Sticky,** Stringy: Km; Ks; Nm.

**Thick:** Cs; KM; Nm; Sil.

**Turn** Grass green: CF; NS.

**Urinous** Odour: Nm.

**Watery,** Thin: Ks; Ns; Sil.

**White:** KM.

**SECRETIVE**: NM.
**SEDENTARY** Living AGG: Kp; Sil.
**SEEING**: See Looking.
**SELF Accusation:** Cp; NM.
　Centered:
　Criticism: Sil.
　Loathing: Kp; NM; SIL.
　Pity: Cs.
　Torture: Nm.
**SELFISH:**
**SEMEN Bloody**: Fp.
　Cold, Coition, during: Nm.
　Urine, Stale, like: Np.
　Watery: Np.
**SEMINAL Discharge**: Mp; Nm; SIL.
　Absent, Coition during: Nm.
　Cold, Coition, during: Nm.
　Convulsions, with: Np.
　Copious: Nm; Sil.
　Deficient, Scanty: Nm.
　Feeble: Nm.
　Night, Every: NM; NP.
　Pleasure, Without: NP.
　Smells Like stale urine: Np.
　Too late: NM.
　Too quick: NM.
　Voluptuous Dreams, with: Sil.
　Watery: Np.
　Weakening: Np.
**SEMINAL Emission**
　(Nightly): Cp; Fp; Km; **KP; NM; NP;** SIL.
　Amel: Cp.

Coition, after: **NM**; NP.
Debility, Backache, with: Cp; Np.
Dreams, Absent, with: Np.
　vivid, with: Np.
Dribbling in sleep: Sil.
Erections, Without: Kp; Nm; Np.
Frequent: Kp; Nm; Np.
Impotency, With: Cs.
Insensible: NP.
Involuntary: Np.
Morning, Stool, during: Nm.
Night, Every: NM; **NP.**
Scrotum, Itching of, with: Km.
Spasms, With: NP.
Stool, During: Nm; Sil.
Thin, Watery: Np.
Unconsciousness of: NP.
**SEMINAL VESICLES**: FP; Sil.
**SENILITY** (old age): CP; NM.
**SENSES, Special** dulled: NM; SIL.
**SENSITIVENESS**: Fp; Km; Kp; Ks; NM; **NP; SIL.**
　Bones: SIL.
　Everything To: Kp; Nm.
　Glands: Sil.
　Internally: Kp; **NM; SIL.**
　Morbidly: Kp.
　Pain To: Cp; Fp; KP; MP; Np; SIL.
　　Not too much: Nm.
　Periosteum: Sil.
　Skin Of: CS; FP; KP; KS; NM; Np; **SIL.**

**Want** Of: Mp; Nm.
**What** Others say about her, to: Cp; Kp; NP.
**SENSORIUM Depressed**: Cp; Kp.
**SENTIMENTAL**: CP; Sil.
**SEPARATED** As if: Cp.
**SEPSIS, Septicaemia**: KP; Sil.
**SEROUS Membranes**: Km; Nm; Sil.
**SEWING Agg**: **NM.**
**SEXUAL Affections** (General): CP; Fp; KP; NM; NP; SIL.
**Desire**, Decreased (Male): Cp; **KP**; Ns; NM; Np; **SIL.**
Chilliness and apathy: Km.
**Desire**, Decreased (Female): Fp; NM; Sil.
**Enjoyment** Absent (Male): Nm.
**Increased**, Desire (Male): **CP;** Fp; Kp; **NM;** NP; NS; **SIL.**
Emissions, after: Nm.
Erections without: NM; NP; SIL.
Excessive: NM; SIL.
Paralytic disease, in: Kp; SIL.
Power, weak, with: Fp.
Priapism, with: **NM; SIL.**
Violent: **SIL.**
**Increased**, Desire (Female): CP; KP; Nm; Np; SIL.
Insatiable: CP.
menses, after: Kp.
before: CP.

Plethora, from: Sil.
Violent: CP; SIL.
involuntary orgasm with: Nm.
spinal irritation, from: Sil.
**SEXUAL Excess** Agg: Cp; CS; **KP; NM; NP; SIL.**
**SEXUAL Excitement**
**Indulged** or suppressed: Kp.
**Irregularities** of: Cp.
**SHADE in Agg** and Amel: See Twilight.
**SHAKING Agg**: SIL.
**SHALLOW**: See Respiration and Ulcers.
**SHAMELESS**: Nm.
**SHATTERED** Flying into pieces, explosions: Sil.
**SHIFTING**: See Wandering.
**SHINGLES** (Herpes Zoster): Km; NM; SIL.
**SHINING**: See Glistening.
**SHIVERING**: MP.
**SHOCKS**, (Through body): Sil.
**Electric-like**: CP; NM; Np.
Sleep, during: NM; Np.
Wide awake, when: Np.
**Injury**, from: Fp; Ns.
Mental:
Nervous: KP.
Sudden:
Surgical: NS.
Traumatic: FP.
**SHOOTING**, Pain: Km; MP.

---

**SHORT as if:** Nm; Sil.
**SHOULDERS** (And Region): FP.
 **Right**: KM.
 **Left**: FP.
 **Abducting** Arm Agg:
 **Ankylosis**:
 **Arm**, behind him Agg:
 **Caries**: SIL.
 **Chest**, To: FP.
 **Cold**: Sil.
 **Heaviness**: NM; Ns.
 **Jerking**: Sil.
 **Joint**: FP; Nm.
  Cracking, in: Nm.
 **Lameness**: NM.
 **Pain**: CP; CS; FP; Kp; Nm;
  Ns; Sil.
  Aching: Cp; NM; Sil.
  Air open Amel: Cs.
  Bed in Agg: Nm.
  Boring: Ns.
  Broken as if: Nm.
  Cold, on becoming: Cp; **SIL.**
  Cutting: Sil.
  Drawing: Fp; NM; Np; Ns;
   SIL.
   right: Fp.
  Extending to chest or wrist:
   Fp.
   fingers to: CP.
  Left: Fp; Km; Nm.
   right, to: CP.
  Lying, painful side on: Nm.
  Motion Agg: Fp; Nm; Sil.
   Amel: FP; Kp.

 slow, Amel: FP.
 Night Agg: FP.
 Paralytic: NM.
 Pressing: Km; Kp; Nm; Np;
  NS; Sil.
 Raising arm Agg: CP; Nm.
 Rheumatic: CP; FP; NM;
  Np.
  left: Km.
 Shooting: Cp.
 Sore, bruised: Cp; Cs; Nm.
 Sprained, as if: NM.
 Stitching: Cp; Cs; Fp; Kp;
  Nm; Np; Ns; SIL.
  extending downward: Sil.
 Tearing: Cp; FP; Kp; NM;
  Np; NS; Sil.
  arms to: Cp.
  right: FP.
 Walking, Agg: Ns.
  Amel: Cs.
 Wandering: KS.
 Warm wrapping Amel: Sil.
 **Paralysis**, Sensation of: Nm.
 **Raise**, Impossible to: Nm.
 **Stiffness**: CS; Ns; Sil.
 **Swelling**: Cp.
 **Tension**: Nm; Np.
 **Twitching**: Sil.
 **Weakness**: Nm; Sil.
**SHRIEKING**: CP; Kp; Ks; Sil.
 **Cause**, Slight from: Nm.
 **Children**, in: CP.
 **Convulsions**, Before: Sil.
 **Feels**, That she must: Cp; Sil.

**Grasping**, Hand, with: Cp.
**Pain**, With: Mp.
**Sensitiveness**, From, undue: Kp.
**Sleep**, During: CP; Nm; Sil.
**SHUDDERING** (Nervous): NM; SIL.
**SHUT PLACES Agg**: NS.
**SHY Timid**, Bashful: CS; Kp; Sil.
**SICK feeling**: Nm.
  **Says**, he is not:
  **Suddenly**: Ns.
**SICKLY**, See Expression under face.
**SIDE Lain** on, Pain goes to: Nm; Sil.
  **Symptoms** on one: KP; Nm; Sil.
    Left: Cf; Fp; Ns; SIL.
    Right: CP; Fp; MP; SIL.
    to left: Cp.
**SIGHS Groans**: Cp; Nm.
**SILENT, Taciturn**: Cp; Cs; Fp; Km; Kp; Ks; NM; Np; NS; Sil.
  **Morning**: Ns.
**SILLY** (Childish): Sil.
**SINGING Trilling**: Nm.
  **After Agg**: Fp; SIL.
**SINGLE PARTS** Effects: Kp; Nm; Sil.
**SINGULTUS**: See Hiccough.
**SINKING** Down: See Prolapse.
  **Hollow feeling**: See Empty.
  **Sensation**: Nm.
**SINUS Affections** of: See Sinus under Nose.

**SIT Aversion**, To:
  **Inclination**, To: Kp; NM; Np; Sil.
  Complete silence in: Km.
**SITS, Bed** in, will not lie down:
  **Bent** forward:
  **Elbows** and knees on:
  **Legs** crossed, cannot uncross:
  **Meditating**: Cs.
  Misfortunes, imaginary over: Cs.
  **Quite**, Stiff: Km.
  For a long time: Np.
  **Still**, in Moody silence: Km; Mp.
**SITTING Agg**: Km; Kp; Ks; NM; Np; SIL.
  **Erect**: Nm.
**SITTING Amel**: Nm; SIL.
  **Erect**: Nm; Ns.
  **On first**, down: Nm; Sil.
**SIZE** (Proportion disturbed): Kp.
**SKIN**: Cp; CS; Fp; Kp; KS; NM; SIL.
  **Adherent**, Bones, to: SIL.
  **Alternating**, With digestive symptoms:
  Internal symptoms:
  Joint pains, with:
  **Anaesthesia** Of: Nm.
  **Barber's** Itch (Sycosis): Km; Mp; Ns; Sil.
  **Biting Sensation**: Nm; Np; Sil.
  Spots, in: Nm.

**Bleeds**, Scratching on:
**Bluish**: Nm; Sil.
 Spots: Sil.
**Branny**: Cp.
**Brownish**: Cp; Cs; Np; Sil.
**Burning**: Cs; Fp; Kp; KS; NM; Np; **SIL.**
 Nettles, as from: Cp.
 Sparks, as from: CP; Nm.
 Spots: Np.
**Burnt**, Scorched as if:
**Chafed**, infants, in: Nm; Np; NS.
**Chapping**: Nm; Sil.
**Cheloid**: CF; Sil.
 Itches, when warm: Sil.
**Chilblains**: Fp; Km; Kp; Sil.
**Cicatrices**: See Cicatrices.
**Coldness**: CP; Fp; Km; Kp; KS; Nm; Np; **SIL.**
 Exercise, during: SIL.
 Icy: NM.
 Left side: SIL.
  before epilepsy: SIL.
 Menses, before: SIL.
 One-sided: Kp.
  during convulsions: SIL.
 Painful nerves, along: Sil.
 Suffering parts of: SIL.
**Contraction**: Nm; Sil.
**Corns**: See Corns.
**Cracks**: Cs; KS; NM; SIL.
 Washing, after: CS.
 Winter, in: CS.
**Cutting**: Sil.

**Dirty** colour: Cp; NM.
**Dry**: Cs; Fp; Kp; Ks; NM; Np; **SIL.**
 Burning: Ks; Nm; Np; SIL.
 Inability to perspire: Ks; Nm; **SIL.**
 exercising, when: NM.
**Dusky**: Cp.
**Edges**: Np.
**Elephantiasis**: Sil.
**Eruptions**: See Eruptions.
**Excoriation**: **CS**; Ks; NM; Np.
**Filthy**: Nm; Sil.
**Flabby**: Sil.
**Folds**, Flexures: NM; Sil.
**Formication**: Cp; Cs; Fp; Ks; Nm; Np; SIL.
**Fragile**: See Cracks.
**Freckles**: Cp; Np; Sil.
**Friction** Agg:
**Hairy**:
**Hard**: Cf; SIL.
**Heal** won't, Vulnerable, sup-purates, unhealthy: Cs; SIL.
**Heat**, Fever without: Sil.
**Inactive**: KP; Ks; Nm; NP; SIL.
**Indented**: Nm.
**Inelastic:** Nm.
**Inflammation**: Fp; KS; Nm; SIL.
 Inclination, to: Ns; **SIL.**
**Injury**, Slight Agg: Ns.
**Intertrigo**: CS; Ks; NM; SIL.
**Irritable**: Fp; Kp; SIL.

**Itching**: See Itching.
**Jumping** out as if:
**Loose**: See Loose and Loose as if.
**Menses**, Agg: Km; NM.
**Moist**: Nm; Sil.
   Spots, in: SIL.
**Moles**: Sil.
**Naevus**: Cf; Nm.
**Nodes**, hard: Ns; Sil.
**Numb** (insensitive): Nm.
**Oily**: Sil.
**Oozing**: Km; Sil.
**Pain**: Nm; **SIL.**
**Parchment** like: Cf; Sil.
**Peeling** Off: See Desquamation.
**Prickling**: Nm.
**Prurigo** (Pruritus): See Itching.
**Puffed**, Bloated.
**Quivering**, Twitching: Nm; Sil.
**Rough**, Ragged: NM.
**Scaly**, Scurfy, mealy: Km; SIL.
**Seborrhea**: Ks; NM.
**Sensitive**: CS; FP; KP; KS; NM; Np; **SIL.**
**Shiny**: Nm; Sil.
**Shrivelled**: Sil.
**Soft**, Boggy: Sil.
**Sore**; Becomes: CP; Nm; **SIL.**
   Children, in: Sil.
   Feeling: Fp; Ks; NM; NP; Sil.

**Sticking**: Fp; Ks; Nm; Np; SIL.
**Stiff:** Cs; SIL.
**Stinging**: SIL.
**Stings** of insects: NM; Sil.
**Stripes**, Streaks: SIL.
**Swelling**: See Swelling.
**Swollen** Sensation: Sil.
**Tanned**: Cp; Np; Sil.
**Tense**: Nm; Ns; Sil.
**Thick**: Sil.
**Under**: Km.
**Ulcerative** Pain: Ks; NM; Np; Sil.
**Ulcers**: See Ulcers.
**Unhealthy** (would not heal): CS; Np; SIL.
**Urinary** affections with:
**Warts**: See Warts.
**Washing**, Bathing Agg: MP; NS; Sil.
**Waxy**: SIL.
**Wens** (Sebaceous cysts): SIL.
**Whitlow**: Cf; Cs; Ns; Sil.
**Wine** coloured:
**Winter** Agg: Kp; Sil.
**Withered**, Shrivelled: Sil.
**Worms**: Sil.
**Wrinkled**: Kp; Nm; SIL.
**SLEEP at** Beginning of **Agg:** Nm; Sil.
   **Before Agg: SIL.**
   **During Agg**: Cp; Kp; KS; NM; Np; **SIL.**
   **Falling asleep,** on **Agg**: Cp; Ks; NM; Np; NS; SIL.

**SLEEP Amel,** loss of Agg: Nm.
　**After Amel**: Fp.
**SLEEP Anxious**:
　**Broken**: See Unrefreshing.
　**Comatose**: NM.
　**Deep**: Kp; NM; Np.
　　Morning: **CP.**
　**Disturbed**: CP; Nm.
　　Dreams, by: Cp; Nm.
　　　dreadful and vicious: Sil.
　**Dozing**: Sil.
　**Erections**, with: Nm.
　**Expectoration** with: Nm.
　**Interrupted**: Nm; Sil.
　　Thirst, by Nm.
　**Jerks**, Starts, on falling to: Sil.
　　Air, wanting, as if from: Cs.
　**Light**, Wakes from slightest
　　noise: Np.
　**Position**, in, Abdominal: Cp.
　　Back, on: Kp; Nm.
　　Head, low with: Sil.
　　Limbs, drawn up: Mp; Nm.
　**Restless**: Cp; Cs; Fp; Km;
　　Kp; NM; Np; NS; **SIL.**
　　Menses, during and after:
　　　Np.
　　Pain in limbs, with: Sil.
　　Worm, from: Cp; Np.
　**Saliva** Runs from mouth: NM.
　**Screams**, and Shrieking, with:
　　Nm; Sil.
　**Sinking** Down, in bed: Nm.
　**Sobbing**, With: Nm.
　**Starting** Up, as in fright: Nm;
　　SIL.

**Talking**: NM; **SIL.**
**Thirst**: SIL.
**Tossing**, About: Nm; Sil.
**Twitching**: Nm; Ns; Sil.
**Unrefreshing**: Cf; NM; Np;
　SIL.
　Abdominal pain, with: Nm;
　　Sil.
　Anger from: Kp.
　Blood ebullitions, from: Nm;
　　Sil.
　Chest symptoms, with: Sil.
**Waking**, Anus itching, with
　Cp.
　Cough, from: Sil.
　Difficult: CP; Nm.
　　morning: CP.
　Dreams, from: Nm; Sil.
　　convulsions, of, with: Cs.
　　on falling, asleep: Sil.
　Early: Cp; Km; Kp; Ks; NM;
　　NP; **SIL.**
　　hunger, with 2 a.m. to 3
　　　a.m.: Km.
　　too early: Cp; Km.
　　1 a.m.: Nm.
　　2 a.m.: Ns.
　　3 a.m.: Km; Nm; Sil.
　　4 a.m.: Km; NM.
　cough with stitching in chest:
　　**KM.**
　Erections, with desire to
　　urinate: Sil.
　Frequent: Ks; NM; Np; Ns;
　　SIL.

Fright, as from: Kp; NM; Np; Sil.

Gastric symptoms, with: Nm; Sil.

Headache, with: Ns.

Heat from: Nm; Sil.

Impression, as if someone in the room with: Mp.

Late: CP; Nm; NP.

Nightmares in: Sil.

Pain in limbs from: Sil.

Palpitation, from: Nm.

Restlessness with: Nm; Sil.

Shrieking: Cp.

Starts from sleep as if wanting air: Cs.

Vomiting, with: Sil.

SLEEPINESS (by day): CP; Cs; FP; Km; KP; Ks; NM; Np; Ns; SIL.

Afternoon, 3 p.m. unconquerable: Nm.

But sleep, cannot: Nm; Sil.

Day, During: CP; Mp; NM; SIL.

Night sleeplessness with: Nm.

Eating, after: Cp; Nm.

Forenoon: Cp; Ns.

Headache, During: Ns.

Hectic Fever with: Cs; NM.

Jaundice, Before: Ns.

Menses, Before: Cp.

Mental Exertion, least from: Ns.

Morning: CP; Nm; NS; SIL.

Motion, during: Sil.

Musing (when unoccupied): Nm.

Night: Cs.

Overpowering: Nm.

Pregnancy, During: Cp.

Reading, While: CP; NM; Ns; Sil.

Rising, After: Nm.

Sitting, While: CP; NM; Np.

Stools, After: FP.

Student, In: Mp.

Study, During: Mp.

Thunderstorm: Sil.

Walking In open air: Sil.
 After: Nm.

Warm Room, in: Sil.

Washing, When: CP; Ns.

SLEEPLESSNESS (Insomnia): CP; Cs; Fp; Kp; KS; NM; NP; NS; SIL.

Abdomen, Pain in from: Sil.

Anxiety, From: Nm; Sil.

Chest symptoms with upto 1 a.m: NS.

Coition, After: Sil.

Coldness, After: Nm; Ns.
 Feet of, from: Sil.

Eating After: NM; SIL.

Excitement, From: Kp; NS.

Frightened Easily: Nm.

Grief, From: NM.

Heat, During: Nm; Fp.

Indigestion, From: Mp.

Late, (After midnight): Km; Nm; SIL.

1 a.m. to 2 a.m.: Km.
2 a.m.: Nm; Sil.
3 a.m.: Np.
**Menses**, During: N .
**Mental** Exertion, after: KP.
**Midnight**, Before: CP; Cs; Fp; Ks; NM; NP; Sil.
**Morning**: Nm; Sil.
**Noise**, From slightest: Np.
**Orgasm** of Blood, from: **SIL.**
**Overtired**, When: Sil.
**Palpitation**, From: NM; Sil.
**Pulsation**, Body in, abdomen; ear, head: Sil.
**Restlessness**, With: Ns.
**Rush** of Ideas, from: Sil.
**Shocks**, From: NM.
**Sleepiness**, With: Fp; Kp; NM; Np; Sil.
**Thoughts**, From, activity of mind: CS; NM; Np; SIL.
**Thunderstorm**, Before: Sil.
**Trembling**, In body, from: Sil.
**Twitching**, In limbs from: Nm.
**Vertigo**, From: Nm.
**Vexation**, After: Kp.
**Vivacity**, from: Sil.
**Waking**, after: Fp; NM; SIL.
**SLEEPS** abdomen on: See Position, under sleep.
**SLIDES**, Down in bed: Nm.
**SLIGHT** Causes, AGG: KP.
**SLIMY**: Nm.
**SLOUGH** (Phagedena): **SIL.**
**SLOVENLY**: Sil.

**SLOW** (Comprehension, thinking, etc.): Km; KP.
**Repair** of broken bones: Cf; **CP; SIL.**
**SLUGGISH**: Km; Kp; Nm.
**Processes**: Sil.
**SMALL-POX**: CS; Km; Kp; NM; Sil.
**Black**: Sil.
**SMEGMA Increased**: Km.
**SMELL** In General: Nm; Sil.
**Acute**: Kp; Ks; Np; Sil.
Strong odours: Nm.
**Diminished**: Cs; **NM; SIL.**
**Perversion** of: Mp.
**Taste** And, lost: NM; Sil.
**Wanting**, Lost: CS; Kp; KS; Mp; NM; **SIL.**
Paralysis of nerves, from: Kp; Nm.
**SMILE Does** not: Nm; Ns.
**SMOKE Agg**: Nm.
**SMOKE as of**:
**SMOKING Agg**: Nm.
**SMOOTH**: Nm; Ns.
**SMUTTINESS**: Sil.
**SNEEZING Agg**: Kp; Ks; NM; Sil.
**Amel**: Cp.
**SNEEZING**: CP; CS; FP; Kp; Ks; NM; NP; NS; SIL.
**Air open**, Amel: Cs.
**Combing** or brushing hair Agg: Sil.
**Chronic** Tendency: Sil.
**Continuous**: Nm; Sil.

**Coryza**, Without: Sil.
**Discharge** from Nose, with: Cp.
**Excessive**: Ns; **SIL.**
**Frequent**: Cp; Kp; Nm; SIL.
**Hay asthma**: NS.
**Ineffectual** efforts: **CF;** Nm; **SIL.**
**Morning** Agg: Nm; Sil.
**Paroxysmal**: Sil.
**Salivation**, With: Cp.
**Tension** and Tensive drawing in cheeks inducing desire to: Km.
**Uncovering** From: Nm; Sil.
**Urging**, To: SIL.
**Violent**: Kp; Nm; Sil.
**Worms** Quivering in, as from: Kp.
2 a.m.: Kp.
**SNOW Air Agg**: CP; SIL.
**Exposure** to or melting: CP.
**Light Agg**:
**SNUFFLES Stuffy** cold: See Obstruction, Nose.
**SOCIETY, Social** functions AGG: Cp; **NM; SIL.**
AMEL: Cp; KP.
**SOFTENING of Bones:** Cf; CP; **SIL.**
**SOLES**
**Blue** Spots: Kp.
**Callosities**: SIL.
Tender: NS; Sil.
**Corns**: Sil.
**Eruptions**: Nm.

Vesicles: Nm; Ns.
bloody serum with: Nm.
**Formication**: Cp; Nm.
**Heat**: Fp; Nm; SIL.
Evening: Sil.
**Itching**: Cs; KP; Nm; Ns; SIL.
Voluptuous, after scratching: Sil.
**Lameness**: Kp.
**Pain**: Kp; Np; SIL.
Burning: CS; Km; Kp; KS; Nm; NS; SIL.
Crampy: Kp; Nm; SIL.
walking, while: SIL.
Cutting: Sil.
Drawing: KP; Sil.
Eating, after: Sil.
Knees, extending to: KP.
Shooting: Cp.
Sitting while: Ns.
Sore, bruised: KP; SIL.
Stitching: Cp; Np; Ns; Sil.
Tearing: NS; Sil.
knee above extends: Sil.
Ulcerative: NS.
Walking, while: Sil.
**Perspiration**: NM; **SIL.**
Acrid: Sil.
Cold: Cp; Km.
Destroys shoes: Sil.
Itching: SIL.
Offensive: Cs; SIL.
**Tingling**, Prickling: Kp; SIL.
Scratching, after: Sil.
Voluptuous: SIL.
**Weakness** in a.m. Nm.

Suddenly, while walking as if paralyzed: Np.

**SOMEONE ELSE:** See Duality.

**SOMNAMBULISM** (Walks in sleep): Kp; Ks; NM; SIL.

**Gets up, walks** about and lies down again: Sil.

**SOOTY:**

**SORE:** See Sore under Pain.

**SORROW:** See Grief.

**SOUR, Acidity:** Nm; Np; Ns; Sil.

**SPARKS Sensation:** See Electric sparks.

**SPEAKING** (Talking) **Agg:** CP; Fp; NM; NS; SIL.

**By others:** Nm; NS; Sil.

**Hearing**, Others: Nm.

**SPEECH Difficult:** CS; MP; NM; Np; Sil.

**Begins** To speak with teeth closed: MP.

**Chorea**, From: Mp.

**Heaviness** Of tongue from: Mp.

**Slow:** Kp.

**Stammering:** MP.

**Thick:** MP; NM.

**Throat**, As if closed: Np.

**Wanting:** Kp.

**Weakness**, Of Organs of speech: NM.

**SPERMATIC CORD**

**Coition**, Emission Agg: NP.

**Pain**, Aching: Np; Sil.

cough, during: NM.

emission, after: NP.

left: Np.

Drawing: Nm; Np.

morning: Cs.

Pressing: Sil.

Rending, tearing asunder: Nm.

Stitching: Nm.

**Tubercles:** SIL.

**Varicocele:** FP; SIL.

**SPHINCTER:** Sil.

**SPINA BIFIDA:** Cp; CS; SIL.

**SPINAL CORD** Degeneration (Multiple sclerosis): Sil.

**Inflammation** (Myelitis): Nm; NS; Sil.

Membrane of (Spinal meningitis): NM; NS.

**Pain**, Burning: Kp.

**Softening** of: Kp.

**Tabes Dorsalis:** Mp; Nm; Sil.

**Wasting** of: Km.

**SPINE Absent** vertebrae as if: Mp.

**Caries** (Pott's Disease): CP; Sil.

**Curvature** of: **CF**; CP; **CS; Sil.**

Lumbar region: Cs.

Pain, in: **SIL.**

**Heat:** NM; SIL.

**Injuries: NS;** SIL.

**Necrosis** of Vertebrae: Nm; Sil.

Pain in General: Kp; **NM; SIL.**
Aching: SIL.
Burning: NP; SIL.
Cutting, up: Ns.
Dorsal spine, in: Nm; **NS;
SIL.**
Drawing: NM.
Relieving the headache: Kp.
Sore; bruised (Spinal irrita-
tion): **KP; NM; NP;** NS;
**SIL.**
  cervical spine of: NS.
    dorsal spine of: SIL.
    lumbo-sacral spine of:
      Np.
    sacral: Sil.
    vertebrae: Kp.
  Tearing: Nm; NS.
    extending downward: Nm.
**Weakness,** Tired feeling: Cp;
Cs; Kp; **NM;** Np; SIL.
Eating Agg: NM.
Emissions, after: Np.
Evening: Np.
Lying down, Amel: NM.
Manual labour Agg: **NM.**
Motion of arms Agg: SIL.
Riding on: Cs.
Sexual excess, after: NM.
Sitting, after: SIL.
**SPITEFUL** (Revengeful): NM.
**SPITTING spits:** NM.
  **Agg:**
  **In face of people:**
**SPLASHING Swashing** ˆs of
  water: Nm.

**SPLEEN** (Left Hypochondria):
Cp; NM; NS; Sil.
**Enlarged:** Fp; Km; NM.
**Inflammation:** Fp; NM.
**Pain,** Aching: Kp; NM; Ns.
  Cutting: Cp.
  Heat, during: Nm.
  Lancinating: Nm.
  Motion, Agg: Kp.
  Pressing: Km; NM.
  Pressure, clothes of Agg:
    Nm.
  Stitching, sticking: Kp; NM;
    Ns; Sil.
    walking while: Nm.
  Throbbing, beating: Ns.
  Thrusting: Nm.
  Walking, Agg: Kp; Nm.
**Sensitive:** Nm.
**Stretched,** Strained, sensa-
tion: Nm.
**Swelling:** Nm.
  Heat, during: NM.
**SPLINTER:** See Pain, stitching.
**SPLITTING:** See Pain, Burst-
ing.
**SPOKEN TO Aversion:** Kp;
Nm; NS; Sil.
  **Morning:** Ns.
**SPONDYLITIS Cervical:** Cp;
Kp; NM; Sil.
**SPOONERISM:** Kp; Nm.
**SPOTS symptoms,** in General:
CP; NM; Sil.
  **Cold:** Cp.
  **Hectic:** Nm.

**Moist**: Km.
**Painful**: CP; Mp; NM; Sil.
**SPRAINS Strains** (See Lifting Agg): Cf; CS; Fp; Km; Nm; Ns; SIL.
**As if**: Nm.
**Chronic**: Nm.
**Easy**: Nm; SIL.
**Lameness**, After: Kp; Np; Ns.
**Old**: Nm.
**Tendency** To: Nm; SIL.
**SPRING Agg**: Cp; Ks; NM; NS; SIL.
**SQUATTING** AGG:
**SQUINT**: See Strabismus.
**STAGE FRIGHT**: KP; NM; Sil.
**STAGGERING**: See Reeling.
**STAINS**: See under, Secretions, Menses, Leucorrhoea, urine, Stool.
**STAMMERING Speech**: MP.
**STANDING Agg**: Cs; Fp; Kp; NM; NS; SIL.
**Amel**: Nm.
erect amel: Kp.
**Eyes**, closed with Agg:
**Inability** to remain:
**Legs**, keeps wide apart:
**STAPHYLOMA**: Sil.
**STARTING** Startled: Cs; Km; KP; KS; **NM**; NP; SIL.
**Convulsive**: Cp.
**Easily**: Cs; **KP**; Ks; **NM; NP;** SIL.
**Electric** Shocks through body, while wide awake: Np.
Sleep, during: **NM**.

**Feet**, As if coming from, waking her: NM.
**Lying** on Back: Cp.
**Night**: Ns; Sil.
**Sleep**, From: SIL.
As if wanting air: Cs.
**Touched**, When: KP; SIL.
**Trifles**, At: NM; SIL.
**STARTS**: See Jerks.
**Noise**, least from: Sil.
**STARVE** he must: Km.
**STEAM Agg**:
**Amel**.
**STEPPING Backwards**: Sil.
**Hard Agg: SIL.**
**High**: Nm.
**Persons**, are, as if:
**STERILITY**: See Conception, Difficult, under females.
**STERNUM**: CP; Cs; KM; NM; Sil.
**Behind**: SIL.
**Doubling** Up amel: Cs.
**Lower** Third, as if torn into two: Np.
**Scapula**, Extending to: Nm.
**Throbbing**: Sil.
**Under**: Cp; Sil.
Burning:
Food, lodged as if:
Lump: Sil.
**STERTOR**:
**STICKY, Stringy**: Km; Nm.
**STIFFENING Out** (Body of):
**STIFFNESS**: Cs; Sil.
**Paralytic**: Nm.

**STIFLING** (Pain): Cp; Mp; Nm.
**STINGING: SIL.**
**STINGS** (of Bees, insects): NM; Sil.
**STITCHES**: See Stitching, under Pain.
  **Painful**: Ns.
**STOMACH**: CP; Cs; Fp; NM; NP; Sil.
  **Acidity**: Nm; Np; Ns; Sil.
  **Afternoon**, Agg: Cs.
  **Alternation**, with Headache: Cp.
  **Anxiety** Felt in: CP; Ks; Nm; SIL.
    Menses, during: Sil.
    Rises to head: Nm.
  **Bandaging** Abdomen Amel: Nm.
  **Being** Heated Agg: SIL.
  **Bending** Double Amel: MP; Sil.
  **Burning**: CP; Cs; Fp; Km; Kp; Ks; NM; Ns; SIL.
    Eructations, after: CP.
    Evening 8 P.M.: Cp.
    Extending, upwards: Sil.
    Hours after eating: NM.
  **Chill**, During: Sil.
  **Clawing**: NM; Sil.
  **Clothes** Tight Agg: NM.
  **Clothes** Tightening Amel: Nm.
  **Cold** Drinks Agg: CP; Mp.
    Amel: CS; Fp.
    From: CP; Sil.
  **Coldness**: Kp; Ks; NM; SIL.
    Diarrhoea during: Nm.

**Coughing** From: Sil.
**Croaking**, Like frogs: Nm.
  On turning in bed: Nm.
**Diarrhoea** With: Cp.
**Digestion**, Disordered: See Indigestion.
**Distension**: CS; Fp; Kp; Ks; NM; NS.
  Eating after: Cs; Fp, **NS.**
  Eructations Amel: NS.
  Feeling of: Cp.
  Flatulent: Cf; Sil.
**Drinking,** from: Ks; NM; Sil.
  Quickly, Agg: Sil.
**Eating**, while Agg: CP.
  2 or 3 hours after: Np.
**Eating,** After Amel: Cp; Kp; MP; NS; Sil.
  When: Ns.
**Empty,** Faintness, goneness: CP; Cs; KP; KS; NM; NP; NS; Sil.
  Aversion to food with: NM; SIL.
  Daytime: Np.
  Eating, not relieved by: Cp; Km; Nm; Sil.
    after: Np; Sil.
    an hour before causing headache: Sil.
  Evening: Cp.
  Fatigue Agg: NM.
  Forenoon 11 a.m.: Nm; Np.
  Headache, during: NM; Sil.
  Hunger without: NM; SIL.
  Menses, during: Kp.

Morning: Nm; Np.
  anxiety, with: Nm.
  breakfast before: Cp.
  rising on: Np.
  Nausea, during: Cp; Kp; SIL.
  Throbbing, with: Nm.
**Enlarged**: Sil.
**Epileptic** Aura: Sil.
**Eructations**, Agg During: Sil.
**Eructations**, Amel: CP.
**Extending** To other parts: Nm.
  Upwards: Km.
**Fainting**: See Empty.
**Fats**, From: Np.
**Foreign** Body, as if in: Nm.
**Fullness**, of: CP; Cs; FP; KP; Ks; NM; Np; NS; Sil.
  Eating, so little After: KS; NM; SIL.
  Eructation, Amel: Sil.
  Evening, bed in: NS.
  Menses, during: KP.
  Oppressed breathing with: NS.
**Gagging** (See Retching): Cp.
  Breakfast, after: Cp.
  Mucus, white, gulping with: Km.
**Hanging** Down, relaxed as if: CP; Nm.
**Headache** With: Cp.
**Heat**, Flushes of: Fp; Ks; NM; Np; Ns.
  Extending over chest: Nm.

**Heat**, During Agg: NM.
**Heat** Amel: Mp; SiL.
**Heaviness**; Weight, oppression of: Cs; Km; Kp; KS; NM; Np; NS; SIL.
  Damp weather: Ns; Sil.
  Eating after: KP; SIL.
  Menses, during: Np.
  Morning: Cs.
**Hot** Drinks or food Amel: Mp.
**Hyperacidity**: Cp; Np.
**Ice Cream** Agg: Cp.
**Inactivity**: Sil.
**Indigestion**: CS; FP' Kp; Ks; NM; NP; NS.
  Bread after: NM.
  Debauchery, in general: Ns.
  Fatigue, Brain-fag in children: Cf.
  Farinaceous food: Nm; NS.
  Fat food, after: KM; NP.
  Ice cream: CP.
  Meat, after: FP; Sil.
  Milk, after: Np.
  Pastry: Km.
  Pregnancy during: Nm.
  Wine, liquors: Ns.
**Inflammation**: Fp; Ks.
  chronic: Sil.
  Hot drinks from: Km.
**Jar** On walking Agg: Ks.
**Jerking**: Nm.
**Lifting** AGG: Sil.
**Lump** Sensation: Nm; Sil.
  Eating, after: Nm.

**Lying** Amel: Sil.
Knees drawn up with: Sil.
**Menses** After Agg: Np.
Before Agg: Nm.
During Agg: Kp; Np.
**Morning** Agg: NM; Ns.
Rising on: Ns.
**Motion**, On Agg: CP.
**Movement**, In, sensation: Nm.
**Nausea** With: NM.
**Night**, In bed: Ns.
**Pain**: CP; CS; Fp; Kp; KS; MP; NM; NP; NS; SIL.
Clawing: NM; Sil.
Cramping, griping: CP; Cs; Fp; Kp; Ks; MP; NM; NP; Ns; **SIL.**
Cutting: CP; Cs; Kp; Ks; SIL.
convulsive, before stool: Cs.
Gnawing, digging: Cs; Kp; Np; NS; Sil.
5 a.m.: Kp.
Pinching: Ns.
Pressing: CP; Cs; Fp; Kp; Ks; **NM;** NP; Ns; SIL.
Weight as from: Sil.
Scraping: Nm.
Sore, bruised: CP; Cs; Fp; KP; Ks; NM; NP; NS; SIL.
Stitching: Cs; Kp; Nm; Np; Sil.
hip joint to: Sil.
lying down after: Sil.
Ulcerative: NM.

**Paroxysmal**: NM.
**Pressure** Amel: Mp.
**Pulsations**: Cs; Ks.
Cough, with: Nm.
Eating, after: NM.
while: Nm.
**Pylorus**, Induration of: Cf; SIL.
Relaxation of: FP.
**Riding**, Rocking Agg: Sil.
**Satiety**, He had eaten to: Sil.
**Sinking**: See Empty.
**Sitting**, While Agg: Ns.
**Sour** Food Agg: NM.
**Stepping** On Agg: Ks; Sil.
**Stone**, As if in: Cs; Kp; Nm; Sil.
Cold, after vomiting: Sil.
Eating, after: Nm; Sil.
**Stool**, After Agg: CP; Cs.
Before: Cs.
**Swallowing**, on Agg: CP.
**Sweets** Agg: Np.
**Tenderness** to contact, pressure, jars: Nm; Sil.
**Tension**: Nm; Sil.
**Tickling**: Nm.
**Tingling**: Nm; Ns.
**Touch** Agg: NM; Sil.
**Turning**: Nm.
**Twisting**: **NM.**
**Twitching**: Sil.
**Walking**, Open air in Agg: Sil.
While, in Agg: Ks.
**Warm** Application Amel: MP; SIL.

**Weak**, (Relaxed, flabby): NM; Sil.

**Weakness** feeling: See Empty.

**Weakness** With: Cp; Nm.

    Seem to come from head: Cs.

**Weight**: See Heaviness.

**Yawning** Amel: Nm.

**STOMATITIS**: See Mouth, Aphthae.

**STONE** Cutter's phthisis: SIL.

**STOOLS Before**, during and After **Agg:** Nm; Sil.

**STOOLS, After Amel:** Cp; **NM;** NS.

    **Loose Amel**: NS.

**STOOLS Acrid,** Corrosive: Fp; Km; Kp; Ks; **NM.**

    **Albuminous** (See Mucus): NM.

    **Balls** (See sheep Dung): CP; NM.

    **Bilious**: Cp; NS.

    **Black**: Cs; KS; NM.

    **Bloody:** Cp; Cs; FP; KP; Ks; NM; Np; Ns; SIL.

        Covered with: Nm; Ns.

        Oily: Km; Kp.

        Water: FP.

    **Breakfast** Agg: NS.

    **Brown**: Fp; Kp; Nm; NS.

    **Burning**, Hot: Kp.

    **Changeable**: Sil.

        Consistence: Nm.

    **Chopped**, hacked: Np.

    **Clay** Coloured: Km; Kp; NS.

        Like: SIL.

**Colours**, Several: Kp.

**Crumbling**: **NM;** Np.

**Curdled**: Nm; Np.

**Dark**: Kp; Mp; NS.

**Difficult:** Cp; CS; Fp; Kp; **KS; NM;** Np; NS; **SIL.**

    Although soft: CP; KS; NM; NS; SIL.

    Natural: **SIL.**

    Recedes: Ks; NM; **SIL.**

**Dry**: Cs; Km; KS; **NM;** SiL.

**Expel**, Inability, to: Cf.

**Fibrous**: Cp.

**Flaky**: Cp.

**Flat** (Ribbon shaped): Mp.

**Flatulent**: Cp; NS.

**Flocculent**: Km.

**Foul**: See Under Odour.

**Forcible** (Gushing): Cf; Cp; Mp; **NM; NS;** Sil.

**Frequent:** Fp; NM; Np; Ns; SIL.

**Frothy**, Foamy: NM; Ns; SIL.

**Granular**: Nm.

**Gray**: NM; NS.

    Whitish, in part: Nm.

**Green**: CP; Km; **NM;** NP· **NS.**

    Turns, blue: Cp.

        green: Cf; NS.

**Gushing** (Forcible): Cf; Cp; Mp; **NM; NS;** Sil.

**Hacked** (Chopped): Np.

**Hard**: CP; CS; Fp; KM; Kp; KS; **NM;** Np; NS; **SIL.**

    First, then fluid: Cf; Cp; NM; Ns.

        then soft: Mp.

Menses, during: NM; Ns; Sil.

**Heavy**, And tearing anus: Nm.

**Holds**, Back: Sil.

**Impacted**: Nm; Sil.

**Insufficient**, Incomplete unsatisfactory: Cs; Ks; **NM; SIL.**

**Involuntary**: Cs; Fp; Km; Kp; Ks; **NM; NP.**

Flatus, on passing: Km; NM; **NP**; NS.

Sleep, during: Nm; Ns.

Urination, during: Ns.

and stool: Nm.

**Irregular** (now hard now soft): Nm.

**Knotty**, Nodular: Cp; CS; Kp; KS; Nm; NS; **SIL.**

Liquid, with: NS; Sil.

**Large**: Cs; Km; **KS;** NM; NS; SIL.

**Lienteric**: CP; Cs; FP; Kp; SIL.

**Light** coloured: KP; KS; Np; NS; **SIL.**

**Membranous**: Sil.

**Mis-shapen**, Angular: Nm.

**Mucous** (Slimy): CP; Fp; Km; Kp; **KS**; NS; SIL.

Bloody: Fp; Km; Sil.

Coated, with: Nm.

Discharge of, stool after: Cp.

Green: CP.

Jelly-like masses: Np.

Red: Sil.

Transparent: Nm.

White: Km; NM.

Yellow: KS.

**Muddy**, Dirty water: Fp.

**Mushy**: Cp; Sil.

White: CP.

**Natural** first, then Fluid or loose: Cf; Np.

Constipation, with: **SIL.**

**Odour**, Cadaveric: **KP;** SIL.

Foul, offensive: CP; Km; KP; Ks; Nm; NP; **NS; SIL.**

Putrid: Cf; **KP**; NS; SIL.

Sour: NP; Sil.

**Odourless: FP.**

**Oily:** : Nm; Ns..

**Painless**: Sil.

**Pale**: Km.

**Pasty**: Cp; NM; Np; **SIL.**

**Pepper**, Looking as if in: NM.

**Purulent**: CP; CS; KP; Ks; **SIL.**

**Recedes**: Ks; NM; **SIL.**

Fear of pain, from: Sil.

**Reddish** (Bloody): NS; SIL.

**Retained**: Sil.

**Ribbon-shaped** (Flat): Mp.

**Rough**, As if: Nm.

**Scanty**: Cp; Cs; Ks; NM; Ns; SIL.

Normal, but: NS.

**Sheep** Dung like: : KS; NM; NS; **SIL.**

**R.&M.M.-14**

**Shooting**, out: Cp; Np; NS; Sil.
**Small**: Cp; Fp; Ks; Nm; **SIL.**
**Soft**: CP; Cs; Fp; KS; NM; NS; SIL.
  passed, difficulty, with: Cp; Ns; Sil..
**Sour: NP.**
**Sputtering**, Noisy: Cp; **NS.**
**Strain** Must, at: Nm; Sil.
**Tearing**, Anus: Nm.
**Tenacious**: Nm; Sil.
**Thin** Liquid: Fp; NP; **NS;** SIL.
  Black: Ks.
  Brown: Ns.
  Dark: Ns.
  Fecal: **NS.**
  Formed, then: Cf; Ns.
  Lumpy, and liquid: NS; Sil.
  Pouring, out: CP; NS; Sil.
  Yellow: **NS.**
**Triangular**: Nm.
**Undigested**: Cp.
**Urging**, Desire to: Cp; Nm; Np; Ns; **SIL.**
  Abortive: Sil.
  But passes only wind: Ns.
  Coffee, after: Nm.
  Coition, after: Nm.
  Constant: Km; Nm; NS.
  Frequent: NM; Ns.
  Ineffectual: **NM; SIL.**
  Rising, after Amel: CP; Ns.
  Stool, after: Kp; Np.
    before: Cf.
    during: Np; Sil.

Sudden: NP; NS.
Urination, Amel: Nm.
With normal stools: Km.
**Watery**: Cf; CP; Fp; Km; Kp; KS; **NM;** NP. **NS;** SIL.
  Black: Ns.
  Bloody: Fp.
  Clay coloured: Kp.
  Green: Fp; Nm; Ns.
  Morning: **Ns.**
  Rice water: KP; NM; NP.
  White: Km; NM.
  Yellow: Ns.
**White**: Cp; Cs; Nm; Ns.
  Chalk like: SIL.
  Fecal: CP; SIL.
**Yellow**: Cs; Kp; Ks; Nm; Np; Ns.
  Bright: KP.
  Brownish: Np.
  Fecal: NP; NS.
  Greenish: Kp; Ns.
  Orange: Nm.
  Pale ochre coloured: Km.
**STOOP Inability**, to: NM; SIL.
  **Coccyx,** fall on, from: Ns.
  **Shouldered**: Cp; Kp; Np.
**STOOPING Agg**: CP; Cs; Fp; Kp; Ks; NM; Np; Ns; **SIL.**
  AMEL:
  **Easy,** Stretching difficult: Nm.
**Prolonged** Agg: SIL.
**STORM Approach of Agg**: Nm; Np; NS; Sil.
  **After Agg:** Cp.
  **During Agg**: Nm; Np; SIL.

STOVE Heat Amel: MP; **SIL.**

**STRABISMUS Squint**: CP; Kp; MP; NM; Np; Sil.

Convergent: Mp.

Diphtheria, After: Kp.

Divergent: **NM.**

Sense of: NM.

Worms, Due to: Np.

**STRAINING**: See Pain, Pressing.

**STRAINS Sprains**: Cf; CS; Fp; Km; Nm; Ns; **SIL.**

**STRANGE** Position in Amel: NM.

Everything, Seems: Kp.

Motions, in Pregnancy: Cp.

**STRANGER**, in Presence of **Agg:**

As if one were: Nm.

**STRANGLING Sensation**: Cs; KS; MP; NM.

**STRANGURY, Difficult**

Urination: CP; Kp; Ks; NM; Np.

**STREAKS Stripes**: SIL.

**STRENGTH Increased or Sense of**: NP.

**STREPTOCOCCUS infection**:

**STRETCH Impulse**, to: Cp; NM; Ns; Sil.

Chill, Before: Nm.

During: Ns.

Coldness, During: NS.

**STRETCHES**, Twists, turns: Cp; Sil.

Convulsions before: Cp.

**STRETCHING Agg**: See Bending

AMEL: See Bending

**STRICTURE Oesophagus: NM.**

Rectum: NM.

Urethra: NM; Ns; **SIL.**

**STRINGY Sticky**: Km; Nm.

**STROPHULUS** (Skin): Ks; Sil.

**STUBBING Toe** Agg:

**STUBBORN, Obstinate:** Cs; Fp; Km; KP; Ks; SIL.

**STUDY Agg**: Mp; (See Mental exertion.)

**STUFFED Up:** CS; KP; **NM;** NS; **SIL.**

**STUMBLING**: MP; NM; Sil.

AGG:

**STUMPS, Pain,** in: FP; KP; NS.

**STUNNED**: See Stupefaction.

**STUPEFACTION**: Cp; Cs; Kp; NM; Np; .Ns SIL.

Vertigo, During: Sil.

**STUPIDITY**: Cp; NM; SIL.

**STYES** (See eye lids): Cf; Fp; Kp; SIL.

**SUBARACHNOID**:

**SUBINVOLUTION** (Uterus): Ns; Sil.

**SUBMAXILLARY Glands**

Abscess: SIL.

Contraction: Sil.

Enlarged: Sil.

Induration: Nm.

Inflammation: Km; Ks; Mp; Nm; SIL.

**Pain**, Aching: Nm; SIL.
  Boring: Nm.
  Drawing: SIL.
  Sore, bruised: Nm; SIL.
  Stitching: Sil.
  **Swelling:** CP; CS; Km; Kp;
    Ks; NM; Np; NS; **SIL.**
  Painful: SIL.
**SUBSULTUS Tendinum**:
**SUCCEEDS, Never:** Sil.
**SUCKLING Children**: Cp.
  AGG: Sil.
**SUDDEN Effects**: Mp; Ns.
  **Ailing persons,** in: Ns.
  **Continuing** and Going: Mp.
**SUFFOCATION: CP;** Nm; Sil.
  **Threatened**: Kp.
**SUGAR Abuse** of: Np.
**SUICIDAL Disposition**: NS; Sil.
  **Drowning**, By: Sil.
  **Hanging**, By: Ns.
  **Menses**, During: Sil.
  **Perspiration**, During: Sil.
  **Shooting**, By: Ns.
  **Thoughts**: NS.
  **Tired** of life: Ns.
**SULCI Membranes** of: Cp.
**SULLEN** (Morose): Cs; Fp; KP;
  SIL.
**SUMMER Agg:** Km; Nm.
  AMEL: Cp; Sil..
**SUNBURN** (Freckles): Cp; Np;
  Sil.
**SUN Exposure to Agg: NM.**
  **Amel:** Km.

**SUNSET Agg**:
  **amel:** Kp; Nm.
**SUNSTROKE**: NM.
**SUPERSTITIOUS**: Cp; Kp; Nm.
**SUPPORT Amel:** Nm.
**SUPPRESSIONS** (Discharges
  etc.)
  **Amel:** Sil.
**SUPPURATION**: See Abscess.
  **Bones:** Cf; Cp; Nm; SIL.
  **Glands**: Cs; SIL.
  **Periosteum**: Cf; SIL.
  **Pus**, Bloody, lumpy: Cs.
  Burrowing: Sil.
  Foul: CF; Sil.
  Profuse: Nm.
  Scanty: Cs; Sil.
  Suppressed: Sil.
  Thick: CS; Ks.
  Thin: Sil.
  Unhealthy: SIL.
  Watery: SIL.
  Yellow, green-yellow: Ks.
  **Stubborn**: SIL.
**SURGINGS** (Waves): Nm; SIL.
**SUSPENDED, Hanging** down:
  CP; Kp; Mp; Nm; Sil.
**SUSPENSE Agg:** Kp; NM.
**SUSPICIOUS**: CP; Cs; Kp; Np;
  Ns; Sil.
  **Foolishly**: Cp.
  **People** are talking about her:
**SUTURES**: See Fontanelles,
  under Children.
  **Painful**: Cp.

**SWALLOW Constant** Disposition to: Mp; NM; Ns.

**Drink** must, to: Nm.

**Larynx**, Tickling in, from: Cf.

**Lump**, in throat from: NM.

**SWALLOWING Difficult**: Cp; Cs; Km; Ks; Nm; Np; SIL.

**Agg**: CP; Cs; Fp; Kp; Ks; Nm; NP; NS; SIL.

**Empty, Agg**: Cp; Fp.

**Food**, Goes wrong way: Nm.
enters naso-pharynx: Sil.

**Hasty Agg**: SIL.

**Impeded**: NS.
For liquids, only: SIL.

**Liquids**, Can swallow: NM; Np; SIL.
Agg: Nm.
Warm drinks, Amel: Cf; Cp.

**Lump**, As of a: Fp.

**Must** Drink at every mouthful to swallow: Nm.
Twist his neck to get it down: Km.

**Noisy**: Sil.

**Pain** in back of head, with: Mp.

**Paralysis**, from: NM; Sil.

**Solids**, Can swallow: Cp; Mp; Nm.
Amel: Np.
Food, gags: SIL.
Reach a certain point and are violently rejected: Nm.

**SWASHING, Splashing**: Mp; Nm.

**SWAYING Agg**: See Car sickness.

**As if**: See Vertigo, Swinging.

**SWEAT** in **General**: See Perspiration.

**Debility** from: Nm.

**Sadness** from: Cp.

**Salty** Deposit: Nm.

**Scanty**: Sil.

**Sleep** Amel: Sil.

**Sleep**, On beginning to: Sil.
During Agg: FP; KP; Nm; **SIL.**

**Stiffens**, Hose, linen: Nm.

**SWELLED** As if: CP; Sil.

**SWELLING**: Nm; SIL.

**Affected parts** of: Fp; Nm; SIL.

**Bones**: CP; Nm; **SIL.**

**Glands**: Cp; **CS**; KM; Nm; SIL.
Bluish: Sil.
Hard: Sil.
Hot: Sil.
Inflammatory: NM; SIL.
Lymphatic: Np.
Knotted like cord: SIL.
Painful: SIL.
Painless: Sil.

**Inflammatory**: Fp; NM; SIL.

**Oedematous**, Smooth: Ns.

**Periosteum**: SIL.

**Receding**: Sil.

SWIMMING or Falling, into water Agg: Mp.

While Agg: Mp.

SWINGING Agg: See Car sickness.

SWOLLEN Sensation: CP; Sil.

SYCOSIS: KS; Nm; NS; SIL.

SYMMETRICAL:

SYMPATHETIC: Nm.

SYMPATHY Agg: NM; SIL.

AMEL:

Resents: Nm.

SYMPTOMS Alternate: Cp; Fp.

Ascend: Fp; Nm; Sil.

Backward: Nm.

Crosswise: Km; Sil.

Forwards: Sil.

Groups, recurring, in: Sil.

Here and there: Mp.

Left upper, right lower: Nm.

Outward: Km; SIL.

Radiating: MP; Sil.

Distant parts, to: Mp.

Right: Fp; Mp.

Upper, left lower: SIL.

SYNCOPE: See Faintness.

SYNOVITIS: Cf; Sil.

Chronic: Cf.

Crepitation: Np.

SYPHILIDAE: SIL.

SYPHILIS: Cf; CS; Km; KS; SIL.

Congenital: Cf.

TABES DORSALIS: Sil.

TABES MESENTERICA: CP; Cs; NS.

Diarrhoea, with: Cp.

TACHYCARDIA: See Pulse, Rapid.

TACITURN, Reticent: See Silent.

TALK, indisposed, to: See Silent.

TALKING Speaking Agg: CP; Fp; NM; SIL.

By others: Nm; NS; Sil.

Pleasure, takes in his own: Nm.

TALKS Always, about her pain: MP.

Dead People, with: Nm.

Excitedly: CP; KP; NM.

Fast: Kp; NM; NP.

Himself To or sits in moody silence: Mp.

Nose, Through: NM.

Persons, Imaginary, with: Nm; Ns; Sil.

Senseless: Sil.

Sleep, In: Km.

Loudly: Sil.

Slow Learning, to: Cp; NM.

Troubles, of her: Mp.

TALL: Cp; Mp.

TAPE WORMS: SIL.

TARRY: Km; Mp.

TARSI (Edges of eyelids):

Burning: Kp; Ns.

Eruptions, Scaly, herpes: KS.

Inflammation: NM.

**Itching**: Np; NS.
**Nodules**: Np; NS.
**Red**: KS; NM.
**Thick**, Swelled: NM.
**Tumours**: Sil.
**Ulcers**: NM.
**TASTE Acrid**: Cs.
  **After** Taste of food eaten: Nm.
  **Altered**, Eating, after: Nm.
  **Bad**: CP; CS; KM; Kp; Nm; Np; **NS;** Sil.
    Morning: Cp; NM; **NS.**
    awakening on: CP; Np.
    Water, tastes: NM; SIL.
  **Bananas** Like: Mp.
  **Bitter**: Cs; KM; Kp; MP; **NM;** Np; **NS;** SIL.
    Bread, tastes: CP.
    Breakfast or dinner after: Km.
    Eating, during and after: NS.
    Food, tastes: NM; SIL.
      Intermittents, in: Nm.
      swallowing, after: SIL.
    Menses, beginning of: CP.
    Morning: CP; Kp; Nm; SIL.
      disgusting: Cp.
    Tobacco tastes: Nm.
    Tongue, cold, with: Km.
    Water, tastes: Cp.
  **Bloody**: Sil.
    Morning: Sil.
  **Clammy**: NM.

**Clay like**: Sil.
**Eggs**, Like rotten: Sil.
  Morning: Sil.
**Fatty**, Greasy: Kp; SIL.
**Inky**: Nm.
**Insipid**: Cp; Fp; Kp; Ks; NM.
**Lost** (Wanting): Ks; **NM;** Ns; **SIL.**
  Coryza, in: Nm.
  Morning: NS.
    tastelessness of food: **NM;** Sil.
**Metallic**: Cs; Km; Nm; Np; Sil.
**Oily**: See fatty.
**Putrid**: Cp; Fp; KM; Kp; Ks; NM; Sil.
  Water tastes: Nm.
**Salty**: KM; Nm; Np.
**Slimy**: NS; Sil.
  Morning: Sil.
**Soapy**: Cs; Sil.
**Sour**: Cs; KM; Kp; Ks; NM; NP; SIL.
  Eating, after: NM; SIL.
  before: NM.
  morning: Nm.
  **Sweet**: Cp; Cs; Fp; KM; Ks.
**TEARING**: See Under Pain.
**TEARS**: See Lachrymation.
  **Things**: Kp.
**TEETH**: Cf; CP; NM; SIL.
  **Alternating**, Between upper and lower: Nm.

**Changing,** About: Mp; Nm; Sil.

**Radiating:** Mp.

**Row,** In a whole: Mp; Nm.

**Upper**: NM; Sil.

**Lower**: SIL.

**Incisors:** NM; Sil.

**Molars:** Nm; Sil.

**Roots:**

Abscess: **SIL.**

**Air,** Cold Agg: SIL.

Draft: Cp; Nm.

Drawn, in: Cp; NM; SIL.

**Alternating,** With Headache: Kp.

**Bed,** In Agg: MP.

**Benumbed,** Deadened: Nm.

**Biting,** Chewing, when Agg: Nm; SIL.

**Black** Film cannot be brushed off: Sil.

**Blunt**: NM; SIL.

**Boring**: CP; NM; MP; SIL.

**Broken** As if: Nm.

**Brushing** Agg: Nm.

**Burning**: NM; Sil.

**Caries,** Decayed, Hollow: Cf; CP; CS; Kp; Nm; Np; Ns; SIL.

Preventive, in children: CF; Cp.

Rapid: CP.

**Chatter**: Kp; Nm; Ns.

**Coffee** Agg: Sil.

**Cold,** From a: Kp.

Damp weather, Agg: NS; SIL.

Drinks, Agg: Kp; Mp; **NM;** Sil.

Anything, from Agg: Cp; Kp; MP; **NM;** Sil.

Or, warm things Agg: **NM;** Sil.

**Cold,** Amel: Fp; Ks; Ns.

Anything, from Amel: FP.

Water Amel: FP; NS.

**Contracted,** As if: Cp.

**Crumbling**: CF; CP.

**Cutting**: Nm.

**Dentition,** Difficult: **CP; SIL.**

Diarrhoea, with: CP; Fp; SIL.

Slow: **CP; SIL.**

**Digging**: Sil.

**Drawing**: Cp; NM; Ns; Sil.

**Drinking,** from: MP; Sil.

Warm things, Agg: FP; NS; Sil.

**Eating,** During Agg: Mp; SIL.

After: Fp; NM; SIL.

Fruits, after: NS.

Warm food: NM; SIL.

**Eating,** Amel: Sil;.

After: Sil.

**Edge** On, As if: NM; Sil.

Vomit, from: Np.

**Elongated,** as if: NM; Ns; SIL.

**Enamel,** Deficient: CF; Sil.

**Evening** Agg: Km; Kp; Ks.

**Extending** to, Cheek bone: SIL.
Ear: NM.
Eyes: CP; Nm.
Face: Sil.
Forehead: Sil.
Oesophagus: Nm.
Temples: Nm; Sil.
Throat: Nm.
**Filling** Teeth, after Agg: Mp..
**Fistulae** Dentalis: Cf; Nm; SIL.
**Fit,** do not: Nm.
**Foreign** Substance in as if: Cp; Nm.
**Forenoon,** Agg: Kp; Nm.
**Fruits,** Agg: Ns.
**Gums,** Bleeding, with: Kp.
Swelling, with: Km.
**Head,** Wrapping, Amel: SIL.
**Inflammatory,** Pain: Fp; Mp.
**Intermittent,** Pain: Sil.
**Jerking:** Kp; Ns; Sil.
**Lachrymation,** Involuntary: Nm.
**Large** and Swollen, as if: Sil.
**Loose:** CF; SIL.
**Lying** Down, after Agg: Nm.
**Masticating** Agg: CP; Kp; **NM; SIL.**
Food, after: Nm.
**Menses,** After Agg: Mp.
Beginning, before, during Agg: NM.
**Midnight:** NM.
After: Nm.

**Nervous** Patient: MP.
**Night:** Fp; MP; NM; Ns; SIL.
**Nose-bleeding,** With: Ns.
**Neuralgia:** KP; **MP;** SIL.
**Periodically:** Nm.
Every other day: Nm.
**Periostitis:** SIL.
**Piercing:** Sil.
**Pregnancy,** During Agg: Cf; Cp.
**Pressing:** Kp; NM; SIL.
As if held in grip: SIL.
**Pressure** Agg: Nm.
**Pulled,** Torn out, as if: NM.
**Pulsating:** Kp; NM; Np; NS; SIL.
**Racing:** Ns.
**Saliva,** Involuntary, with: Nm.
**Sensitive,** Tender: MP; NM; SIL.
Air to: Cp; Cs; Mp; **NM.**
Cold: Cp; Nm; **SIL.**
Brushing: Nm.
Chewing when: Cp; Sil.
Touch to: NM.
Warmth, to: NM.
**Sleep,** After Agg: Kp; Sil.
**Soft,** Feel: Cp.
**Sordes:** KP.
Brown: Kp.
**Sore,** Bruised: Kp; NM.
**Spring,** in: NM.
**Stitching,** Stinging: Cp; Km; Kp; MP; NM; SIL.
**Sucking,** Teeth: Sil.

**Summer,** in: NM.
**Suppressed** Foot sweat from: **SIL.**
**Tearing:** Cp; KP; NM; Ns; SIL.
**Tension,** In: Nm.
**Tongue,** Swelling with: Mp.
**Tossing,** About in bed: Ns.
**Touch,** Agg: Cf; NM.
　Tongue of: Mp.
**Touch,** Amel: Nm.
**Trembling,** With: Cp.
**Ulcerative** Pain: Sil.
　Root, at: Sil.
**Ulceration of Roots:** Cs; Mp.
**Walking** in Open air, Amel: KS.
**Wandering:** Mp.
**Warm** Drinks, Amel: MP; Sil.
**Warm** Things Agg: Cp; FP; Nm; SIL.
**Warmth,** External Agg: FP.
　Room, of: Ks.
**Warmth,** External Amel: **MP;** Np; SIL.
　Bed of: SIL.
**Wisdom** tooth, eruption
　Complaints, and Agg: Sil.
**Yellow:** Sil.
**TEMPERATURE change of Agg:** CP; Sil.
**Extreme of Agg:**
**TEMPLES:** FP; Kp; **NM;** Np; Ns; SIL.
**Left:** Sil.
**Right:** CP; Nm; Ns.

**Backwards** Over ears: Np.
**Eyes,** To: Np.
**Forehead,** Over: Sil.
**Hammering:** Nm.
**Holds,** Coughing, while: Ns.
**Throbbing:** Sil.
**Veins:** Cf; FP.
**TEMPESTUOUS Action:** Kp; Nm.
**TENACIOUS, Sticky:** Km; Nm.
**TENDER, Delicate:** See Pain, Sore.
**TENDO ACHILLES:** Np; Ns.
　**Contracted:** Cp; Nm.
　**Painful:** Cp; Nm; Sil.
　**Short** As if: Nm.
　**Stiff:** Mp; Nm; Np.
**TENDONS Cracking** in: Km.
　**Injured,** inflamed: Cp; Ns; Sil.
　**Rice** Bodies, in: Cf.
　**Shortened:** Nm.
　**Stiff:** Np.
　**Swollen,** hard: Cf.
**TENESMUS, Bladder,** urinary: Fp; SIL.
　**Rectum:** Cs; Fp; NM; Np; SIL.
　Menses, during: Ns.
**TENSION, Tightness:** Km; Mp; NM; Np; Sil.
　**Glands:** Sil.
　**Internally:** Nm; Sil.
　**Muscles:** Km; NM; Sil.
**TERROR:** Kp; Nm; SIL.
　**Sudden:** Ns.

**TESTES:**
  **Empyocele**: KS; **SIL.**
  **Flaccidity**: Sil.
  **Heat, In**: Nm; Sil.
  **Hydrocele**: See Hydrocele.
  **Induration**: CF; Cp; Km; Ks;
    SIL.
    Right: Sil.
    Small: Sil.
  **Inflamed** (Orchitis): Cp; Fp;
    Km; KS; NM.
    Epididymitis: Fp.
    Gonorrhoea, suppressed
    from: Cp; Km; KS; Nm.
  **Pain:** NM; Np; Sil.
    Aching: Fp; NM.
      right: Fp; Nm.
    Boring: Sil.
    Cramping, rectum, to: Sil.
    Drawing: Cs; Km; Ks; Nm;
    Np.
      morning: Cs.
    Erection, before: Np.
    Neuralgic: MP.
    Pinching: Nm.
    Pressing: Nm; Np; SIL.
    Sore: NM.
      afternoon: Cs.
    Squeezing: SIL.
  **Retraction**: Sil.
  **Sensitive**: Sil.
  **Suppuration**: Cs; SIL.
  **Swelling**: CP; Ks; NM; Np;
    SIL.
  **Tubercles**: NM; **SIL.**

  **Tumours** (Sarcocele): Sil.
  **Twitching**: Sil.
  **Undescended** (children): Cp.
**TETANUS** (Lock-jaw): Mp; Siol.
  **Opisthotonus**: Cp; Mp; Ns.
  **Spasms** (Back): CP; NM; NS.
**TETANY**: NM.
**TETTERY** (Eruptions): NM; Sil.
**THERMIC FEVER**: NM; **SIL.**
**THICK, Thickness:** Cs; KM;
  Nm; Sil.
**THIGHS**: NM.
  **Anterior**: Ns.
  **Front** Part: Np.
  **Inner**: Cp; Np; Sil.
  **Knee** above: Sil.
  **Lower** CP.
  **Posterior** (Sciatics): NM; Sil.
  **Abscess**: SIL.
  **Brown** Spots, inside: Ns.
  **Bubbling** Sensation: SIL.
  **Caries: SIL.**
  **Contraction** of
    Hamstrings: CP; **NM;** Np.
    Menses, after: Np.
  **Cramps:** Fp; Km; Kp.
  **Eruptions**: Nm; SIL.
    Boils: **SIL.**
    Herpes: **NM.**
    Itching: NM.
    Moist: Nm.
    Pimples: NM.
    Vesicles between: Nm; Ns.
      Inside, menses, during:Sil.
  **Heaviness:** Ns.

**Inflammation**: **SIL.**
**Itching**: Nm; Sil.
  Between: Nm.
**Jerking**: Nm.
**Numbness**, Sitting while: Sil.
**Pain**: Cp; Cs; Fp; NM; Sil.
  Aching: Cp; Np.
  Alternating with convulsive pain in arms: Sil.
  Ascending, stairs: Np.
  Bed in, warm Agg: Nm.
  Bones, in: Nm; Ns; SIL.
  Burning of bend: Ns.
  Chill, during: Nm.
  Drawing: CP; Kp; NM; Ns; Sil.
    extends downwards: CP; Sil.
    feet, to: SIL.
  Jerking: Sil.
  Lying, while Agg: Nm.
  Motion, Agg: Nm; Sil.
  Paralytic: Sil.
  Pressing: Kp; Sil.
  Riding, after Agg: Nm.
  Shooting: CP; Np.
    downwards: Cp.
  Sitting, while Agg: KS; Nm; Sil.
  Sore, bruised: CP; Ns; SIL.
    male genitals, near: Nm.
  Stitching: CP; KS; Nm; Np; SIL.
    downwards: Cp; SIL.
  Tearing: Ks; NM; **NS;** SIL.
    back and forth: Sil.
  Thrusting: Nm.
  Walking Agg: Cp; Nm; Ns; SIL.
    amel: KS.
  Weather, cold damp, in: **CP.**
**Pulsation**: SIL.
**Redness**: Sil.
  Itching: Nm.
**Softening** of Femur: Sil.
**Stiffness**: Cs; NM.
**Swelling** Femur: **SIL.**
**Tension**: NM.
  Ascending steps: Nm.
  Extends downwards: NM.
  Hamstrings: CP; Nm; Np.
  Menses, during: Nm.
  Walking while: Nm.
**Tingling,** prickling: Sil.
  Sitting, while: Sil.
**Twitching**: KM; KS; NM; Sil.
**Ulcers**: NS; Sil.
  Outer side: NS.
**Weakness:** Nm; Np; **NS;** Sil.
**THIN**: See Secretions, Watery.
**THINNESS Spare habit:** Cp; Mp; NM.
**THINGS LOOK Strange**: See Confusion.
**THINKING Affected:** Nm; **SIL.**
  See Thoughts.
  **Aversion** to: Fp; Nm.
  **Difficult**: **NM; SIL.**
  **Inability** of: Kp; Mp; Nm; NS; SIL.
**THINKING** of it, AGG: **CP;** Fp; Nm; Ns.

**THIRST**: CS; FP; KP; KS; **NM;** NP; Ns; SIL.

**Appetite,** Lack of with: Sil.

**Burning,** Vehement: Ks; NS; SIL.

**Chill,** After: NM; Ns.

Before: Nm.

During: Km; **NM;** Ns; **SIL.**

**Cold** Drinks, for: Mp; NS.

**Dread** Of liquids, with: Nm.

**Eating,** After: Sil.

**Extreme: CS;** Km; KP; **NM;** Np; NS; SIL.

Headache with: NM.

after: Ns.

Heat, during: Kp; **NM;** SIL.

Large quantities for: FP; NM.

and often: NM.

Menses, before: Nm.

Mouth and tongue dry with: Cp.

Perspiration, during: **NM.**

Small quantities for: NM; SIL.

Unquenchable: KP; NM.

Urge to urinate, with: NM.

Walking, after: Nm.

Without desire to drink: Nm; NS.

**Fever,** At start, only: Ns.

**Forenoon:** Cs; Ns.

**Morning:** Nm; Ns.

Milk, after: Nm.

**Night:** Fp; NM; SIL.

Waking, on: NM; NS.

**THIRSTLESS:** Kp; Ks; Nm; Ns.

**THOUGHTS Changing** suddenly from pleasant to unpleasant: Fp.

**Diseases** of: Nm; Np.

**Evening:** Np; Sil..

**Persistent:** Cs; Kp; NM.

Evening: NM.

Unpleasant subject haunted by: **NM.**

**Sleep,** Before going to: Sil.

**Slow:** Fp; Nm.

**Tormenting: NM.**

**Vanishing** of: Cs; Kp; Nm.

Mental exertion, on: Nm.

**Wandering:** Nm; Np.

One subject to another: Cp.

**What** would become of him: Nm.

**THREAD Sensation:** NM; Np; **SIL.**

**THREAD Worms:** Km; Np; Sil.

**THREATENING:** Kp.

**THROAT** (Inner Mouth included): Km; SIL.

Left: SIL.

Right: Km.

**Abscess,** Retropharyngeal: Sil.

Predisposition to: Fp; Sil.

**Adenoids:** CF; CP; Ks.

**Angina:** See Raw, Sore.

**Awns** of barley as if in: KP.

**Bitter:** Sil.

**Blood** Oozing: FP.

**Catarrh: NM.**

**Choking**, Constriction: Km; Kp; KS; MP; NM; NS.

Clearing the throat when: Cp.

Convulsive: MP.

Day time: Ns.

Drinking when: **NM.**

warm amel: Cf.

Oesophagus, to: NS.

Swallowing, on: Mp; NM.

liquids: MP; Ns.

Walking, while: Ns.

Water, from: Nm.

**Closed** as if: Cf.

Something by, preventing speech: Np; Ns.

**Cold** Agg: Sil.

**Cold** Amel: Km.

**Cold** Drinks, from: Cf; Sil.

on becoming: CP; **SIL.**

**Coldness**, Sensation: Km.

Swallowing, on: Ns.

Warm drinks seem cold: Nm.

**Contraction**: Cp.

**Corn** Husk, lodged as if: Mp.

**Coughing**, On: Nm; Sil.

**Crawling**: Km.

**Diphtheria** (Exudation of membrane): Cp; KM; Kp; NM.

Croup, with: Km.

Tonsils, to: Kp.

Trachea, involving: Cf.

Yellow: **NP.**

**Discharge,** Pus, tonsils were about to: Cs.

**Drinks** Warm Amel: Cf; Cp.

Cold, seem warm: Nm.

**Dry**: Cp; Cs; KM; Ks; **NM;** NP; NS; SIL.

Cough, with: Km.

Eating, after: Nm.

Evening: Kp.

Night: Cp; NM; Sil.

Oesophagus, to: Ns.

Saliva, with flow of: Ns.

Thirst without: Ns.

**Ear,** Extending to: Km.

**Egg**, white of, dried up and causing tension: Mp.

**Empty**, Hollow: Cp.

**Food**, lodges in: NM; Sil.

Passes into choanae: SIL.

Swallowing, solid amel: Np.

**Fullness** of: Kp; SIL.

Eructation, Amel: Kp.

**Gangrene**: Kp; SIL.

**Glistening**, Glazed: NM.

**Grayish** white: KM.

**Hair,** Thread, sensation: Cs; **NM;** SIL.

**Hawking:** See Hawk, Hawking.

**Heat**: Fp; Km; Ks; Nm; Ns.

**Inflammation**: CP; CS; **FP;** Km; Kp; Ks; NM; Np; NS.

Chronic: NM; SIL.

tobacco, from: Nm.

Follicular, acute: FP; KM; **NM.**

chronic: Cf; Cp; Km; Nm.
Herpetic: NS;
Pharynx, chronic: NM; **SIL.**
Septic: Sil.
**Itching**: CS.
**Jerking**: Nm.
**Lifting** Agg: SIL.
**Liquids**, are forced into nose:
NM.
**Lump**, Ball, Plug, as of: Cs;
FP; Kp; Ks; **NM**; Np; SIL.
Left or right: Sil.
Rising up: Kp; **NM.**
Soreness, with: Nm.
Speech, preventing: Np.
Swallowing, on: NM; Ns; Sil.
not amel, by: NM.
when not: NM.
**Marble**, Hot, near palate as if:
Kp.
**Menses**, Before and during
Agg: Ns.
**Morning** Agg: Cp.
**Mucous**: Cp; CS; Km; Kp;
**KS; NM;** NP; NS; SIL.
Albuminous: NM. NS.
Bitter: Nm.
Drawn from posterior nares:
Cs; **NM;** Np.
Frothy: Sil.
Grayish: SIL.
Greenish: Sil.
Morning: Ks; NM; Ns; SIL.
Night: Np; **NS;** Sil.
Offensive: SIL.

Saltish: Kp; NM; NS; Sil.
Sweetish: Mp.
Tenacious: KM; Mp; Np;
**NS; SIL.**
Thick: Km; Nm; Np; Sil.
morning: SIL.
White: KM; NM; Np; Ns.
Yellow: CS; Np; SIL.
**Narrow**, As if closing: Nm.
**Obstruction**, Swallowing
when: Ns.
**Pain** (See Raw, sore): CP;
Cs; Fp; Kp; Ks; NM; **SIL**
Burning: Cp; Cs; Fp; Kp;
**NM;** Np; Ns; Sil.
Itching, smarting, swallow-
ing, when: Sil.
left upper, Cp; Nm.
Drawing: Cp; Nm.
Ear, to: Km; Kp; Mp; Nm;
Sil.
Oesophagus to swallowing:
NM.
Pressing: Cs; Kp; NM.
back of: Nm.
into other parts, from: Cp.
**Pinching**: Nm.
**Pins**, As if: Np.
**Pricking**, Prickly: Cf.
**Raw**, Sore, in: CP; CS; Fp;
Kp. Ks; Mp; Np; Ns; SIL.
Aching in body and chilli-
ness, with: Mp.
Chronic: Cp; Km.
Clergyman's, Singer's: Cp;
Fp.
Cold, Agg: Sil.

Dry spot: NM; SIL.
Evening: Cp; Nm; SIL.
Lump: SIL.
Morning: CP; Nm; Sil.
  'waking, on: Cp.
Nervous: Mp.
Operations, after: Fp; Ns;
Right: Cp.
Smoker's: Nm,
**Relaxation**: Cf; CP.
**Roughness**: NS.
  Coughing, on: Ns.
  Swallowing, on: Cp.
**Scraped**, As of: Mp.
**Scraping**: Cp; Cs; Km; Kp;
  Np; Sil.
  Forenoon, evening and
    night: Sil.
  Lying on side, while: Sil.
**Singing**, Agg: Fp.
**Smoking**, While agg: Nm.
**Spasms**, of Glottis: Cp, MP;
  NM.
**Splinters**, Sticking: Nm.
  Coughing, when: Sil.
**Stiffness**: Km; Mp.
**Suffocative**: Cf.
  Night: Cf.
  Warm drink. amel: Cf'; Cp.
**Swallowing** Agg: Km; Kp.
  Nm; Sil.
  Empty, on: Cp.
  Liquid on: NM.
  Solid food, amel: Np.
  Warm drinks, amel: Cf; Cp.

**Swelling**: Cp; CS; Km; Kp;
  Ks; NM; Sil.
  Oedematous: Mp.
**Swollen**, As if: Sil.
**Taste** in or bitter: Sil.
**Ulcers**: CS; Kml Nm; SIL.
  Fauces: NS.
  Gangrenous: Sil..
  Soreness, from: Km.
**Upward**, through: Nm.
**Walking** Agg: Nm.
**Warm** Drinks, Amel: Cf; Cp.
**Weakness** in: Cp; Ks.
**Yawning** Agg: Cp; Nm; Sil.
**THROAT EXTERNAL**: Nm; Sil.
  **Air** Sensitive to: SIL.
  **Alternating** Sides: Cp.
  **Brown** Discolouration: Ks.
  **Carotid** Arteries, throbbing:
    Cp.
  **Eruptions**, Blotches: Nm.
    Boils, pimples: Nm.
    Pustules: Sil.
  **Fistulae**: SIL.
  **Fullness**, Sense of: Sil.
  **Glands**, Induration of: Cf; CP;
    NM; **SIL.**
    Like knotted cords: Sil.
  **Pain:** NM.
    Burning sides: Ns.
      left: Ns.
    Cervical glands in: NM; **SIL.**
      coughing Agg: Nm.
      sticking: Sil.
      soreness: Nm.
      sticking: Sil.

Drawing, sides: Ns.
 left: Ns.
Pressing sides: Ns.
 behind the ears to: Ns,
Rheumatic sides: Cp; Cs;
 Ns.
**Pressure**, Sense of: Sil.
**Stiffness** of Sides: Nm; Ns;
 **SIL.**
Right: Nm.
**Swelling** Cervical glands:
Chest, to: np.
Hard: **SIL.**
Suppurative: SIL.
**Tension**, Sides: Nm.
Walking, after: Nm.
**Tumours** Recurrent fibroid:Sil.
**Ulcers**: SIL.
**Warts**: Ns; Sil.
**Uncovering** Agg: Sil.
**THROAT PIT Irritation**: SIL.
**Tickling**: SIL.
**THROBBING**: See Pulsation.
**THROMBOSIS**: Fp; KM.
**THRUSH**: See Aphthae (Mouth).
**THRUSTS**, Stings, as of: NM;
 Sil.
**THUMB Clenching**: MP.
**Convulsions**: Nm.
**Cramps**: Nm.
**Drawn** Inwards: Mp.
**Eruptions**, Vesicles: NS.
**Formications**, Tip: Nm.
**Lameness**: Cp; Km.
**Numbness**: Nm.

**Pain**: Cp; Cs.
Ball of: Cp.
Digging, tip of: Nm.
Dislocated as if, thumb: Cp.
Drawing: Nm; Ns.
 Joint, of: Ns.
Elbow to: Cs.
Gnawing, tip: Nm.
Joints of: Nm.
Sore, bruised: Cp.
Sprained, as if: Cp; Nm.
Stitching: Nm; Ns; Sil.
Tearing: Nm; Ns.
 ball of: SIL.
 joints, of: Nm; Ns; **SIL.**
**Pulsation**: Nm.
**Stiffness**: CS.
**Sucking**: CP; NM; Ns; SIL.
**Weakness**: Nm; Sil.
**THUNDERSTORM** AGG: See
 Storm.
**THYROID Cartilage**
Swelling of: SIL.
**Gland**, Hard: Cf.
Lumpy: Cf.
Pressed in as if: Np.
Thickened: Nm.
**Goitre**: See Goitre.
**TIBIAE Caries: SIL.**
**Discolouration**: SIL.
**Exostosis**: Cf; CP; Sil.
**Inflammation**: SIL.
**Nodes**: Cf.
**Pain**: Nm; Sil.
Drawing: CP; Ns; SIL.

Pressing: Sil.
Sore, bruised: KS; Nm; Sil.
Tearing: Ns; SIL.
  Swelling: CP.
TIC: Mp.
  Doulourex: See Face, pain.
TICKLING: SIL.
TIGHTNESS: See Tension.
TIME Agg and Amel.
  Morning (4 A.M. to 9 A.M.)
  Agg: CP; FP; Kp; NM; NP;
    NS; SIL.
    4 a.m.: Nm; Ns; SIL.
    4 a.m. to 5 a.m.: Ns.
    4 a.m. to 5 p.m.: Ns.
    5 a.m.: Kp; NM; NP; SIL.
    5 a.m. : Cp; Nm; SIL.
    5 a.m. to 7 a.m.: Cp.
    6 a.m. to 8 a.m.: Sil.
    6 a.m. to 6 p.m.:Cp.
    7 a.m.: Nm; Sil.
    7 a.m. to 9 a.m.: Nm.
    7 a.m. to 10 a.m.: Sil.
    8 a.m.: Nm; Sil.
    8 a.m. to 9 a.m.: Nm.
    8 a.m. to 12 noon: Nm.
  MORNING AMEL:
  Forenoon (9 a.m. to 12 noon)
    Agg: Kp; NM; Np; Ns;
      SIL.
    9 a.m.: NM; NS; Sil.
    9 a.m. to 11 a.m.: NM.
    9 a.m. to 2 p.m.: Nm.
    9 a.m. to 4 p.m.: Nm.

10 a.m.: NM; Np; Ns; Sil.
10 a.m. to 11 a.m.: NM.
10 a.m. to 12 noon Cs; Nm.
10 a.m. to 3 p.m.: Nm; Sil.
10 a.m. to 4 p.m.: Nm.
11 a.m.: MP; NM; NP; Sil.
11 a.m. to 12 noon: Km.
NOON Agg: NM; SIL.
Afternoon (12 noon to 6 p.m.:
  CP; Fp; Kp; Nm; SIL.
  12 to 1 p.m.: Sil.
  12 to 2 p.m.: Sil.
  12 to 6 p.m.: Sil.
  1 p.m.: FP; Ns; Sil.
  1 p.m. to 10 p.m.: Sil.
  2 p.m.: MP; Nm; Ns; Sil.
  2 p.m. to 5 p.m.: Kp; Sil.
  3 p.m.: Cf; Cp; NM; Ns; Sil.
  3 p.m. to 7 p.m.: Nm.
  3 p.m. to 9 p.m.: Ns; Sil.
  4 p.m.: Cf; Cp; NM; NS; Sil.
  4 p.m. to 6 p.m.: Nm.
  4 p.m. to 7 p.m.: Nm; Sil.
  4 p.m. to 8 p.m.: NS.
  5 p.m.: KM; Ks; NM; Ns; Sil.
  5 p.m. to 8 p.m.: NM; Ns.
Evening (6 p.m. to 9 p.m.)
  Agg: Cp; CS; FP; Kp; KS;
    NM; NP; SIL.
  6 p.m.: Cp; Fp; Kp; Ks; NM;
    Ns; SIL.
  7 p.m.: NM; NS; Sil.
  8 p.m.: Cf; Cp; Nm; Ns; Sil.
  8 p.m. to 11 p.m.: Nm; SIL.

**Night** (9 p.m. to 4 a.m.) **Agg:**
**CP; CS;** FP; KM; KP; MP;
**NM;** NP; NS; **SIL.**
9 p.m.: Cp; Ns; Sil.
9 p.m. to 4 a.m.: Sil.
10 p.m.: Mp; Nm.
11 p.m.: Nm; Ns; Sil.
**Midnight** 12 p.m. **Agg:** Km;
NM; Sil.
**Midnight**
After Agg: Fp; **KM;** Kp; Nm;
Np; **NS; SIL.**
1 a.m.: Nm; Np; Sil.
2 a.m.: Kp; NM; NS; **SIL.**
2 a.m. to 3 a.m.: Cp.
2 a.m. to 5 a.m.: Kp.
2 a.m. to 2 p.m.: Ns.
2-30 a.m.: Kp.
3 a.m.: Cs; **NM;** Np; SIL.
3 a.m. to 4 a.m.: Nm.
3 a.m. to 11 a.m.: Nm.
3 a.m. to 2 p.m.: Ns.
4 a.m. to 10 a.m.: Fp.
**TIME SENSE changed:**
**Passes** Too slowly:
Too quickly:
**TIMID:** See Bashful.
**Appearing** in Public: **SIL.**
**TINGLING** (Itching internal): Km;
Nm.
**TINNITUS:** See Illusory sounds,
under Hearing.
**TIRED:** See Weakness.
**Acts**, as if born: KP.
**Of life**: See Death desires.

**TOBACCO** Abuse of: Cp; Nm;
SIL.
**Aversion** to: Nm.
**Smoking**, Craving for: Cp.
**TOES Alternating** Sides: Ns.
**Caries**, Left big toe: **SIL.**
**Cracked** Skin between toes:
NM; **SIL.**
Violent itching with: NM.
**Eruptions**: SIL.
Scabs: **SIL.**
Vesicles: Sil.
walking from: Sil.
**Excoriation** Between: Nm;
SIL.
**Formication**: Nm.
**Great**: Ns; Sil.
**Itching**: Nm; Ns; Sil.
Ball of: NS.
Between: NM; NS.
Frozen toes, of: SIL.
Undressing, Agg: NS.
**Jerking**: Cp.
**Numbness**: NM; Ns.
Sitting, while: Ns.
**Pain**: Cp; Kp; Nm; SIL.
Aching in joints: Ns.
nails, root of: Cp.
Boring, first toe: SIL.
itching, with: Cs.
joint: Ns.
Burning: FP.
Constant in first: Sil.
Crampy: FP; Sil.
first toe: Cp.
walking while: SIL.

Cutting: SIL.

Drawing: Ns; Sil.

  first toe: Nm.

    joints: Ns.

  joints: Sil.

First toe: Cp; Np; Ns; SIL.

  alternating with pain in heart: Np.

Fourth toe: Cs.

Gouty, in joint: CP; SIL.

Nails, as from splinter: SIL.

  under: Sil.

Pressing in joints and toes: Ns.

Pressure Agg: Ns.

Second: Ns.

Shooting: Cp.

  ball of: Cp.

Sore, bruised: NM.

  ball of: Sil.

  between: NM.

Sprained, as if: Sil.

Standing agg: Nm; Sil.

Stepping agg: Sil.

Stitchig: Cp; Nm; Ns; SIL.

  ball of: Cp.

  joints: Ns; Sil.

  nails: SIL.

  sudden: Nm.

  tip: Ns.

Tearing: Nm; Np; Ns; Sil.

Ulcerative: SIL.

Waking on: Ns.

Walking, while: Cp; Ns; SIL.

**Perspiration: SIL.**

Between: **SIL.**

Offensive: **SIL.**

Rawness, causing: SIL.

**Stiffness**: SIL.

**Swelling**: Ns.

**Tingling**, Prickling tips: NM.

**Twitching**: Cp.

**Ulcers**: SIL.

  Nails: **SIL.**

**TONGUE Across**: Kp.

  **Aphthae**: Km; Ks; NM.

  **Asleep**, As if: Nm.

  **Biting**: NM.

  **Black**: Fp.

  **Bleeding**: Nm; Np.

  **Blue**:

  **Broad**: Nm.

    As if: Nm.

  **Burning**, Burnt: Cp; Ns.

  **Cancer**: SIL.

  **Clean**: Fp; Mp; Nm.

    Dry, and: Mp.

    Moist, and: Np.

    Red, and: Fp.

  **Cleave** To roof of mouth, as if would: Kp.

  **Coated**, Brown: **KP**; Mp; SIL.

    centre: Np.

    sides, white: Np.

    Green: **NS.**

    Greenish brown: Ns.

    grey: **NS.**

    yellow: Ns.

    White: Cp; Fp; Km; KP; NM; NS; SIL.

    base, at: **KM**; Nm.

centre, dark brown: Np.

dirty: Np.

edges, on: **KS.**

patches, red insular with: **NM.**

Yellow: Kp; KS; Nm; NP.

base: Cs; Ks; NM; Ns.

dirty: Km.

golden: Kp; NP.

greenish: Kp.

looks like half-dried clay: Cs.

mustard were spread on: Kp.

slimy: Ks.

**Cold**: NM.

Eating amel: Km.

**Cracked**: Cf; Cp; Cs.

**Dirty**: Ns.

As if: **NM.**

Brown: NS.

**Dry**: CP; Cs; Km; Kp; NM; Sil.

Morning: Kp.

Thirst, without: NM.

**Edges,** Of: Nm.

Beads, form on: NM.

Ulcer, right: Sil.

Vesicles: Sil.

**Enlarged**, as if: Nm.

**Eruptions** on: Nm.

Ringworm: Nm.

**Flabby**: Cs; Nm; Sil.

**Glistening**: Nm.

**Gray**: Km.

**Hair**, on: **NM; NP; SIL.**

Anterior part: **SIL.**

Trachea to: Sil.

**Hangs** Out of mouth: Sil.

**Heaviness: NM.**

**Herpes**: NM.

**Indurated**: Km; Sil.

**Inflammation**: CS; Fp; NM; SIL.

Induration, after: Cf; SIL.

Suppuration threatens: Cs; Sil.

**Mapped**: Km; NM.

**Moist**: Nm; Np.

**Nodes,** on: SIL.

**Numbness**: CF; NM; Np; Sil.

One sided: NM.

**Obtrusion**: Nm.

**Oscillating**, Spasms during: Sil.

**Pain**, Burning: CS; Fp; Kp; Ks; Ns.

Eating, while: NM.

Edges: Ns.

Raw: Sil.

Smarting: Nm; Ns.

Sore: Kp; Ks; Sil.

near tip: CP.

spot: Sil.

Swallowing, on: CP.

**Palate**, Sticks to: Kp.

**Pale**: NM.

**Papillae**, Blunt as if: Nm.

**Paralysis**, Creeping: Kp

**Patchy**, Mapped, spot: **NM.**

**Protruding** Agg:
**Protrusion**, Difficult: NM.
**Raw**: Sil.
**Red**: CS; FP; Nm; NS.
  Dark: Fp.
  Fiery: CS.
  Lines: Cs.
**Root**, Of: Ns.
  Green yellow: Ns.
  Puckered as if: Cs.
  Stitching: NS.
  White: Km; Nm.
  Yellow: NP; Ns.
**Rough**: Nm.
**Sensitive**, To touch: Nm.
**Smooth**, Shiny: NM.
**Soft**:
**Stiff**: CP; Kp; NM; Ns.
**Swelling**: CP; Fp; KM; Kp; Mp; NM; Sil.
  Chronic: Cf.
  One sided: Sil.
  Stings of insects after: Nm.
  Under (See Ranula): Cf; Fp; NM.
    stinging pain, with: NM.
**Thick**, As if: Kp.
**Tip**, Of: Sil.
  Blisters: Cp; NM.
  Burnt: Cp; Ns.
  Hair, on: Np; Sil.
  Pain: **CP**; NM; **NS.**
    pepper, as from: NS.
  Pimples: CP.
  Sore: Cp; SIL.

Stitching: Np; Ns.
Swelling: NM.
Trembling: Nm.
Vesicles: CP; **NM;** NP; Ns.
**Trembling**: Nm; Sil.
**Tumour**, Were forming: Km.
**Ulcers**: Km; NM; Sil.
  Phagedenic: Sil.
  Right edge: Sil.
**Vesicles**: NM; Np; Ns.
  Burning: Ns.
**Wrinkled**: Cp.
  Morning: Cp.
**Yellow**: See Coated.
**TONSILS**: CP; Sil.
  **Caseous** Deposit on: KM.
  **Chronicity**: Nm.
  **Crypts**, Mucus, plugs, of constantly form: Cf.
  **Diphtheritic** Membrane on: Kp.
  **Enlarged**: **CF; CP;** Fp; Km; NM; **SIL.**
    Mouth, opening Agg: Cp.
    Pus, plugs of, with: Cf.
  **Exudation**, Tuft like: Fp.
  **Gray**: Km.
  **Inflammation:** Fp; KM; NS; **SIL.**
    Acute (quinsy): Fp; **Km;** Nm; SIL.
    Chronic tendency: Cp; Sil.
    Recurrent: SIL.
  **Pain**: Cp; Kp;
    Drawing: Nm.
    Yawning, on: Cp.

**Pricking**: Np.
**Pulsation**, Left: Np.
**Red**: Fp.
**Rough**, Ragged: Cf.
**Suppuration**: CS; **SIL.**
Predisposition, to: Fp; SIL.
**Swelling**: CP; CS; Km; Kp; Ks; NS; **SIL.**
Abscess (Peritonsillar): Cs.
Left: Kp.
**Ulcers**: Ns; SIL.
Grey: Km.
**Yellow**, Creamy: Np.
**TOPER**: Km; Nm; SIL.
**TORMENTS Everybody** with her complaints: Kp; Mp; Nm.
**TORN, Loose**, As if: Km; Nm; Ns; Sil.
**Flesh** From bones, as if: Nm.
**Out**, Feeling: Nm.
**Pieces**, To (Shattered): Sil.
**TORPID**: Nm; Sil.
**TORTICOLLIS** (Wry, Neck): Sil.
**TOSSING About** (Restless): Fp; Nm.
**TOUCH Agg**: Cp; Fp; Km; KP; Ks; Mp; NM; Ns; **SIL.**
**Amel**: Nm.
**Illusions** of: Nm; Sil.
**TOUCHED Aversion** to, being: SIL.
**TOUCHING Anything Agg**: SIL.
**Cold** Things: NM; SIL.
**TOUCHY**, Mentally and Physically: Kp; Nm; Sil.

**TOURIST**: CP.
**TOUSY**: Nm.
**TOXAEMIA** (Blood Sepsis): Fp; Km; **KP;** Sil.
**Pregnancy** Of: Cf; Cp; Nm.
**Puerperal**: Fp; Km; KP; Sil.
**TRACHEA Crawling**: Sil.
**Dryness**: Nm.
**Hair**, In, sensation: Sil.
**Inflammation** (Tracheitis): NM.
**Irritation**: KP; NM; **SIL.**
**Mucus**, In: Fp; Ks; NM; NS; SIL.
**Pain**: Nm.
Coughing on: Kp.
Rawness: CS; NM.
Soreness: NM; Np; SIL.
**Tickling**: Kp; Nm; Ns; Sil.
**TRAIN SICKNESS**: Nm; SIL.
**TRANQUIL, Placid**: NM; Np; Sil.
**TRAUMATISM**: See Injury, Shock.
**TRAVEL Desire** to: CP.
**TREMBLING, Tremors**: CP; Fp; Mp; NM; NS; SIL.
**Breakfast**, Before: Nm.
**Concomitant** As a: Cp.
**Delirium**, With: Nm.
**Direction**, Upward: Sil.
**Emissions**, After: **Np.**
**Emotions**, From: Nm.
**Epilepsy**, Before: **SIL.**
**Evening:** SIL.
Walking, after: **SIL.**

Exertion Agg: NM; Sil.

Fright, As from: Np.

Headache With: Cp.

Holding Object, on: SIL.

Internally: NM; Sil.

Menses, during: Cp.

Motion On, slight: MP.

Nervous: Mp.

Night: SIL.

Noon, Sleep after: Nm

Senile: Sil.

Smoking, From: Nm.

Upward: Sil.

Spasmodic movements with: Nm.

Uterine Affections, in: Cp.

Weakness, From: Nm.

Writing, When: Mp; Sil.

TRENCH MOUTH: KP; Sil.

TRICKLING: Nm.

TRIFLES Vexed over: NM.

Seem Important: Nm; Sil.

TRISMUS (Lock-jaw): Mp; Sil.

TUBERCULOUS: See Consumption.

TUMID: See Swelling, Swollen.

TUMOURS Acuminate: Sil.

Cheloid: Cf; Sil.

Cystic: Cp; CS; Sil.

Enchondroma: Cf; Sil.

Encysted: Cf.

Fibroid: CF; CS; SIL.

Malignant, Suspected: Kp;

Sarcoma: Cf.

TURGIDITY: See Swelling, swollen.

TURNING Around Agg: Nm.

Affected part: Nm.

Over In bed: NM; SIL.

Twisting, and: NS.

TWILIGHT Agg: NM; Ns.

TWINGES, Nips: Np; Sil.

TWISTING: SIL.

TWITCHING (See Convulsions): CS; Km; Kp; KS; Mp; Np; SIL.

Here and there: Nm.

Hysterical, Menses before: Nm.

Menses, during: Cs; Nm.

TYMPANUM, Tympanic membrane:

Calcareous deposit: CF.

Dark Beefy red: Fp.

Granular: Km.

Perforation: Sil.

Proliferous Inflammation: Km; Mp.

Red, Bulging: Fp.

Retracted: Km.

Thickened: Fp.

Ulceration: KP; SIL.

TYPHLITIS (Caecal inflammation): FP; Km; NS; SIL.

TYPHOID Fever: Fp; Km; Nm; KP; Ks; SIL.

ULCERATION Ulcers: Cp; CS; KM; Kp; KS; NM; Np; SIL.

**Aching**: Sil.
**Areola**: SIL.
 Hard, indurated: Sil.
**Atonic**, Indolent, painless: SIL.
**Biting**: Np; Sil.
**Black**, Base, margins: SIL.
**Bleeding**: Cs; KS; NM; SIL.
 Edges: Sil.
 Night: Km.
**Bluish**: SIL.
 Edges: Ks.
**Boils** from:
**Boring** Pain, with: Nm; SIL.
**Bruised** Pain with: Nm.
**Burning**: Cs; Km; Kp; Ks; Nm; Np; **SIL.**
 Around, about: SIL.
 Margins: **SIL.**
 Touched, when: Sil.
**Cancerous**: CS; **SIL.**
**Cold** Feeling, with: SIL.
**Crawling**, With: Nm; Np.
**Cutting**: SIL.
**Deep**: **CS**; Nm; Np; **SIL.**
**Discharges**, Bloody: Cs; Ks; Nm; SIL.
 Bony fragments: Cf; SIL.
 Brownish: SIL.
 Copious: SIL.
 Corrosive: Nm; **SIL.**
 Flowing: Ks; Ns.
 Gray: SIL.
 Green: NS; SIL.
 Ichorous: KP; **SIL.**
 Maggots, with: SIL.

Offensive: Cp; CS; KP; NM; SIL.
Putrid: CS; SIL.
Scanty: **SIL.**
Tenacious: Sil.
Thin, Watery: KS; SIL.
Whitish: Sil.
Yellow: Cs; KP; KS; Nm; Np; **SIL.**
**Elevated**, Indurated margins with: **SIL.**
**Fistulous**: **CF**; CP; Cs; NM; Np; **SIL.**
**Flat**: SIL.
**Foul**: CS; SIL.
**Fungus**: **SIL.**
**Gangrenous**: Kp; SIL.
**Glands**: Kp; **SIL.**
**Indolent**: Cf; CP; Cs; Ks; **SIL.**
**Indurated**: Cs; **SIL.**
 Areola: Sil.
 Margins: SIL.
 shining: Sil.
**Inflamed**: NM; Np; **SIL.**
**Itching**: Nm; **SIL.**
 Around about: SIL.
**Jagged**, Margins: SIL.
**Jerking** pain: SIL.
**Mercurial**: SIL.
**Mustard** Poultice, from: Cp.
**Painful**: Nm; SIL.
 Margins: SIL.
**Phagedenic**: KP; NM; SIL.
**Pimples**, Surrounded by: Sil.

**Pressing**: SIL.
**Pulsating**: Cs; Ks; Nm; SIL.
**Red**, Areola: Np; SIL.
**Reopening** Of old: Sil.
**Salt** Rheum: SIL.
**Sensitive**: Nm; Np; SIL.
Around about: Sil.
Margins: SIL.
**Serpigenous**: SIL.
**Shining**: Sil.
**Smarting**: NM; SIL.
**Spongy**: SIL.
Margins: SIL.
**Stinging**, Stitching: Nm; Np.
Areola, in: SIL.
Margins: SIL.
**Superficial**: NM; SIL.
**Suppurating**: Kml KS; Nm;
Np; SIL.
**Swollen**: NM; Np; SIL.
Areola: Sil.
Margins: SIL.
**Tearing**: Sil.
Tense, areola: Sil.
**Unhealthy**: Np; SIL.
**Varicose**: SIL.
**Vesicles**: Surrounded by NM.
**White**, Spots with: SIL.
**ULNAR NERVE along**:
**UMBILICUS**: See Navel.
**UNATTRACTIVE, Things,**
seem:
**UNCERTAIN, execution**, of: Sil.
**Gait**, etc.: Np.
**UNCLEAN**, Dirty: Sil.

**UNCONSCIOUS, Uncon-
sciousness**: NM; Np; Sil.
**Advanced** states, of brain
and meningeal diseases:
Km.
**Cold**, After taking: SIL.
**Conduct**, Automatic during:
Nm; SIL.
**Convulsions**, After:
**Emotions**, From:
**Fever**, During: Fp; Nm.
**Head** On moving: Nm.
**Odours**, From:
**Pain**, During:
**Pregnancy**, During:
**Riding.**, While: Sil.
**Sitting**, While: Nm; Sil.
**Sudden**: Cs.
**Trance**, As if in:
**Transient**: NM; Sil.
**Vertigo**, During: Nm; Sil.
**UNCOUTH**:
**UNCOVERING Agg**: Kp; MP;
NM; Np; SIL.
**Least**: SIL.
**Single** Part: NM; SIL.
**Throat**: Nm; NS; SIL.
**UNCOVERING Amel**: Cs; Ks.
**UNDERTAKES, Nothing** lest
he fail: Sil.
**UNDRESSING Agg**: NS; SIL.
**UNDULATIONS Waves**: Sil.
**UNEASY Feeling**: Nm.
**Knows** Not what to do with
himself:
**Sexual** Desire, with:

**UNHAPPY**: See Sadness.
**UNLUCKY**:
**UNSOCIAL**: Nm.
**UNSTEADY** As if: Np; Sil..
**UNSUCCESSFUL, Thinks**, him-
self: Sil.
**UNSYMPATHETIC**: Nm.
**UNTIDY**: Sil.
**UNUSUAL THINGS** From any:
**UP AND DOWN**: See Direc-
tions.
**UPPER LIMBS**: See Arms.
**UREMIA**: KS.
**URETERS**: CP; Fp; Nm; NS;
Sil.
**Burning**: FP; Np; Nm.
**Cramp**; CP; MP; Nm; Sil.
**URETHRA Agglutination**
of Meatus: Cp; NM.
**Contraction**, Stool and urina-
tion, before: NM.
Urging to urinate: NM.
**Discharges**, Acrid: NM.
Bloody: **CS; Kp.**
Clear, colourless: NM.
Foetid: SIL.
Gleety: CP; Cs; Fp; Km;
NM; NS; Sil.
eczema, with: Km.
painless: **NM;** NS.
Gonorrhoeal: **CS;** FP; KS;
NM; **NS;** SIL.
chronic: **CP; CS;** KS; NM;
SIL.
Greenish: Ks; NM; NS.
chronic: **Ns.**

thick: **NS.**
priapism with: NS.
yellow: Ks; **NS.**
Milky: Km; **NM.**
sticky: NM.
urination, after: Nm.
Mucous: Fp; Ks; Mp; NM.
gelatinous: Nm.
Painless: NS.
Purulent: **CS;** KS; NM; SIL.
Spotting, linen: NM.
Thick: NS; Sil.
Thin: NM.
Urination after Agg: NM.
Watery: KS; NM.
White: KS; NM.
anemic subjects, in: **CP.**
chronic: **NM.**
Yellow: CS; NM; SIL.
chronic: CS; Ks; NM; SIL.
spots on linen: NM.
**Haemorrhage**: Fp; Ks; Nm.
**Induration**, Chronic: Cp; SIL.
**Inflammation**, Meatus: Nm.
**Itching**: Km; Kp; NM; Sil.
Coition, after: Np.
Gleet, with: NM.
Gonorrhoea, with: NM.
Meatus: Nm.
**Jerking**: Nm.
**Moisture**, Meatus: Nm.
**Pain**, Biting: Nm.
Burning: Cf; Cs; Km; Kp;
Nm; Np; NS; SIL.
fossa navicularis: Nm.

meatus: Cf; KS; NM.

morning: **NM.**

night: **NM.**

Coition, after: Nm; Np.

Cutting: CP; Km; Ks; NM.

anterior part and

meatus: Ns.

Erection, after morning: NM.

during: Cp; Nm.

Menses, during: NM.

Pinching: Nm.

Semen, discharge, during: Nm.

Sore: Nm.

Stitching: Kp; Nm; Sil.

anterior part: Sil.

fine: Nm.

fossa navicularis: Nm.

Walking, while: Nm.

When not urinating: CP; NM.

**Sensitive**: Nm.

**Stricture**: NM; Ns; SIL.

**URGING** (Pain, Pressing):

to urinate: Fp; Kp; Ks; **NM;** Np; Ns; Sil.

**URIC ACID DIATHESIS**: Ns.

**URINARY ORGANS** in General: CP; Cs; FP; MP; **NM;** Np; NS; SIL.

**URINATION Before Agg**: Cp; Nm; Sil.

**During**: CP; Km; NM; Ns; SIL.

**At** Close of: NM.

**After**: Cp; **NM;** Ns.

**When not**: CP; NM.

**URINATION, Amel**: Fp; SIL.

**URINATION**: Cp; NM; SIL.

**Abortion**, after Agg: Cp; SIL.

**Cutting**: Cp.

**Desire** Morbid (urging): Fp; Kp; Ks; **NM;** Np; Ns; Sil.

Coition, after: NP.

Constant: Fp; Kp; Ks; NM; Np; SIL.

Day and night: Nm; Sil.

Day time only: Fp.

Frequent: CP; Fp; KM; KP; Ks; **NM;** Np; Sil.

Ineffectual: Km; KP; Ks; Nm; Sil.

night: Nm.

stool, urging to, with: Nm.

Labour, after: Kp; Nm; Ns; SIL.

Married Women, newly:

Night: Fp; **NM;** Ns; **SIL.**

painful: Fp; Kp; NM; Ns.

Painful, with urging to stool: Nm.

Sudden: FP; NM.

hasten to urinate must, or urine will escape: FP.

menses, during: Nm.

Violent: Nm,

**Difficult**, Dysuria: CP; Kp; Ks; NM; Np.

**Dribbling** (by drops): Km; Kp; Ks; NM; Sil.

Involuntary: Mp.

Stools, after: Nm.

Urination, after: Kp; NM; Sil.

**Drinks**, Every after: FP.

**Dysuria**: See Difficult.

**Feeble**, Stream slow: CP; Km; KP; Sil.

Retention, long from: Cp.

Violent pain in bladder: Cp.

**Frequent**: FP; Kp; Ks; MP; NM; Np; Sil.

Children, in: Mp.

Day and night: Kp; NM.

Evening: Cp.

Exposure, to cold wet from: Cp.

Menses, during: Mp.

Nervous: Sil.

Night: CP; Km; Ns.

Perspiration, during: Np.

Prostate, enlarged: KP.

Stool, during: NM.

**Incomplete**: NP; Sil..

**Interrupted**, Intermittent: Kp.

**Involuntary**: CP; FP; Km; KP; Mp; **NM;** Np; Sil.

Blowing nose, when Nm.

Blow on head, from: Sil.

Catheterization, from: Mp.

Cough, during: FP; NM.

Day time (diurnal): FP.

lying down amel: Fp.

Desire, if resisted: Nm.

Laughing: FP; NM.

Nervous prostration, from: Kp.

Night (See Bed wetting): Fp; Km; KP; **MP;** NM; NP; **SIL.**

worms from: Sil.

Old people, in: Kp.

prostate, enlarged: Kp.

Pregnancy, during: NM.

Sitting, while: NM.

Sneezing, when: FP; NM.

Standing, while: NM.

Stool, after: Nm.

Typhoid, in: Kp.

Walking, while: Fp; **NM.**

**Irresistible**, Hurried: NM.

**Nightly**: Cf.

**Retarded**, Must wait for urine to start (feeble): NM; Np; SIL.

Can only pass, when alone: NM.

Pressing at stools: Np.

Must press a long time: Np.

**Seldom**: Ns.

**Spurts**: Cp.

**Stops** and **starts**: KP.

**Unsatisfactory**: Kp; Np; Sil.

**URINE Acrid**: NM; NS.

Menses, during: Nm.

**Albuminous**: CP; Fp; Km; Kp; NM; **NP;** NS.

Heart disease, consecutive to: Kp.

Pregnancy, during: Cp; Km; NM.

Scarlet fever, after: KS; **NS.**

**Alkaline**: Mp; NM.

**Bile** Containing: NS.

**Black**: Km; NM.

**Bloody** (Haematuria): Fp; KM; NM; Sil.

Last part: FP.

**Brown**: Nm.

Dark, during menses: Nm.

**Burning** (Hot): CP; Fp; Kp, Ks; NM; Np; **NS;** SIL.

**Clay**: Nm.

**Cloudy**: Cf; Km; KP; KS; NM; Np; Sil.

Passing, soon after: Sil.

Standing, on: Fp.

While, clouds: Nm.

**Coffee** like: NM.

**Colourless**: MP; **NM;** SIL.

**Copious** (Profuse): Cf; CP; Fp; KM; KP; KS; Mp; NM; NP; **NS;** SIL.

Afternoon: Nm; Np.

Amel: Sil.

Amenorrhoea, with: Nm.

Exhausting: CP.

Headache, with: Fp; Sil.

Morning: NP.

8 a.m. to 3 p.m.: Cf.

Night: **CF;** FP; **KP;** NM; NS; **SIL.**

Perspiration, with: Nm.

**Dark**: Cf; CP; Fp; Kp; NM; Np; Ns.

**Frothy**: Nm; NS.

**Greenish**: Nm.

Black: Km.

Dark: Nm.

**Milky**: Kp; Nm.

Menses after and during: Nm.

**Muddy**: NM.

**Odour**, Acrid, pungent: Cf.

Ammoniacal: Fp; Sil.

Offensive: KP; KS; Nm; Np; Ns.

Strong: Cf; Cp; Nm.

**Pale**: CF; Fp; Km; **NM;** Np; NS.

**Red:** Fp; Km; Ks; NM; Np; SIL.

Dark: Ns.

Whitish: Nm.

**Scanty**: Cf; Fp; Km; Kp; KS; Nm; Np; **NS;** Sil.

Fever, during: Nm.

Menses before: Sil.

during: Nm.

Night: Fp; **NM.**

**Sediment**: KP; KS; Nm; SIL.

Adherent: Nm.

Bright: Nm.

Chalk (like flour): Nm.

Flocculent: Cp; Kp.

Gelatinous: Km.

Hemoglobin: Fp.

Lithic acid: Ns.

Mealy: Km; NM.

Mucus: Fp; Kp; **NM;** Np; NS.

tenacious: Sil.

Oxalate of lime: KS; NP; Ns.

Phosphates: CP; Kp; Mp.

Purulent: KS; NS; **SIL.**

Red: Kp; Ks; **NM;** Ns; Sil.

  brick colour: **NM;** Ns.

  reddish white: NS.

Sand, (gravel): Cp; Kp; NM; NS; **SIL.**

  red (brick dust): NM. NS; SIL.

  white: Ns.

  yellow: **SIL.**

Slimy: **NM.**

White: Nm; Ns.

  yellow: NS; Sil.

**Specific** gravity, increased: CP; Fp; Kp; Ns.

Decreased: Nm.

**Sugar**: See Diabetes mellitus.

**Suppressed**: Fp; Km; **SIL.**

  Heat, from: Fp.

**Viscid**: NS.

**Watery,** Clear water: Cf; Cp; Kp; NM; NS.

**URINOUS Odour** (of breath, secretions, etc.): Fp; Nm; Sil.

**URTICARIA**: CS; Kp; KS; NM; NP; ·Sil.

**Asthma,** Alternating with: Kp; KS.

**Ascarides,** With: NM; NP; Sil.

**Cold Air,** in: NS.

  Bath after: CP.

**Exercise,** Violent after: NM.

**itching,** without:

**Night:**

**Nodular:** Ks; NM; Np; SIL.

**Rosy** (Erythema): Km; Np; SIL.

**Undressing,** Agg: Ns; SIL.

**Warmth,** from: **NM.**

**UTERUS:**

**Cancer:** Cs; Kp; Ks; Mp; NM; **SIL.**

**Contractions,** In: ᴄP; NM.

**Displacement** (Anteverted): Cf; CP; **NM;** Np; Sil.

  Adherent, to rectum: Sil.

**Enlarged**: Sil.

**Fibroids,** Polypi: **CF;** CP; CS; SIL.

**Flabby,** Relaxed: Cf.

**Foetus,** Movements, painful: Sil.

  violent: Sil.

**Heaviness**: Cp; Sil.

**Induration**: Cf.

**Infantile**: CP.

**Inflammation,** Acute: Sil.

  Chronic: Kp; Ks; Nm; SIL.

  Peri and para metritis: Sil.

**Moles**: SIL.

**Nursing,** Agg: Sil.

**Pain**: CP; Cs; Fp; Kp; NM.

  Aching: CP.

  After-pains: CF; Fp; Kp; Mp; NM.

  child nurses, when: Sil.

  Bearing down, in region of: Cp; Ks; **NM; SIL.**

  everything would come out, as if: **NM.**

  ovarian pain, with: Fp.

Bed in Agg: Ns.

Burning: CP; **NM.**

Coition during, Agg: Fp.

Cold, damp weather Agg: CP.

Coughing agg: NM.

Crampy: CP; MP; Nm.

Drawing: Cp.

menses would appear as if: Cp; Nm.

Driving: Cp.

Extending downward: Cp; Nm.

sacrum, to: Cp.

thighs, to: CP; Nm.

reading and writing Agg: Nm.

Labour like: Cp; Kp; Nm; SIL.

Menses beginning Agg: CP.

before Agg **CP;** MP; Nm; SIL.

several hours: Cp.

during Agg: CP; Cs; KP; Ks; MP; Sil.

Menses, established Amel: Cp.

Morning, agg: CP; **NM.**

Music Amel: MP.

Nurses child when: **SIL.**

Pregnancy, during Agg: Kp; SIL.

Pressing: Cp.

Pressure amel: MP.

Pulsating: Cp.

Raising up, Agg: Cp.

Rest, agg: Sil.

Rubbing agg: Nm.

Sexual desire, during: Cp.

Sharp, while nursing: **SIL.**

Sitting agg: Cp; Ns; Sil.

Sleep, during and after: Nm.

Sleep, back on, amel: Nm.

Sore, tender: Cp; SIL.

Standing agg: Nm; Sil.

Stitching: Kp.

Stool, after agg: Cp.

during, agg: Cp; NM.

Touch agg: Nm.

Urination agg: Nm; Sil.

Waking, on: Cp; Nm; Sil.

Walking, amel: Nm.

**Prolapse**: CP; Cs; Fp; Kp; Ks; NM; Np; SIL.

Lifting, agg: Sil.

Lumbar backache, with: Nm.

Lying down, amel: NM; Sil.

back on: Nm.

Menses, during: CP.

Morning: **NM.**

Stool, during: CP.

Urination, during: CP.

**UVULA Adheres** to tonsils: Nm.

**Elongated**: Cf; NM; Sil.

**Hangs** to one side: Nm.

**Inflammation**: Nm; NS.

**Pain**, in: Cp.

**Stitching**, Shooting: Nm.

Tonsils, to: Nm.

**Swelling**: CP; Ns; **SIL.**

Oedematous: Km.

**VACCINATION, III effects:** KM; SIL.

**VACILLATING:** See Fickle.

**VAGINA Cold:** NM.

**Cutting:** Sil.

Urinating, Agg: Sil.

**Cysts:** Sil.

**Dry:** Fp; **NM.**

Menses, after: Nm.

**Fistula:** SIL.

**Hot:** FP.

**Induration:** SIL.

**Inflammation**, Acute and Chronic: Km.

**Itching:** CS; Sil.

**Orange** coloured fluid from: Kp.

**Pain:** CP.

Aching: Cp.

epistaxis, after: Cp.

Burning: CP; FP; Kp; NM.

Centres in, from other parts: CP.

Coition, during: CP; FP; **NM;** Sil.

Crampy: Fp; Mp.

Cutting: Sil.

Upwards: Sil.

Faintness and flushes with: Cp.

Menses, before Agg: Nm.

Pressing: Sil.

Sore, tender: Cp; NM; SIL.

digital examination Agg: Fp.

Stitching: Ns.

Urination, after agg: Nm; Sil.

**Relaxation** of sphincters: Nm; Sil.

**Sensitive:** Fp; NM; SIL.

**Spasms** (Vaginismus): FP; MP; NM; SIL.

**Swollen:** Cp.

**Tumours** (Cysts): SIL.

**Vaginismus:** FP; MP; NM; SIL.

**Weakness**, after urination: Nm.

**VAGINISMUS:** See under Vagina.

**VALVE, leaf**, skin as of: Ns.

**VALVULAR Disease** (Heart): Cf.

**VANITY** (pride):

**VARICELLA Chicken-pox:** Fp; Km; Nm; Ns; Sil.

**VARICOCELE:** FP; SIL.

**VARICOSES:** See under Veins.

**VARIOLA Small-pox:** Cs; Km; Kp; NM; Sil.

**VARNISH** like: Nm.

**VAULTS Agg:** Ns.

**VEINS Burst** as if would: Cf.

**Inflammation** (Phlebitis): Cf; Fp.

**Vascular** tumours, of: Cf.

**Varicose:** CF; Cp; Fp; NM; Sil.

Young persons, in: Fp.

**Varicose** ulcer: Cf; Sil.

**VENOSITY:** Cf; Fp.

**VERMIN**:
**VERSES MAKES**, After falling asleep: Nm.
**VERTEBRA Absent**, as if: Mp.
  **Cracking** in: Nm.
  **Gliding** Over each other as if: Sil.
  **Loose** As if: Nm; Sil.
  **Slipping** (Dislocation): Nm.
**VERTEX**: CP; Cs; FP; NM; Np; SIL.
  **Across** (Ear to Ear): Km; Sil.
  **Bursting**: SIL.
  **Cold**: CP.
  **Eyes**, to: Sil.
  **Fly** Off, as if: Sil.
  **Forehead**, and: Nm; Np; Sil.
  **Menses**, Agg: Fp.
  **Neck** and Occiput, to: Cp.
  **Open**, Would, as if: Np.
  **Palate**, To: Nm.
  **Pressure**, Heavy, Crushing: Fp; Nm; SIL.
  **Sides**, Down: Fp.
  **Throbbing**: SIL.
**VERTIGO**: CP; **CS;** FP; Km; Kp; KS; NM; NP; NS; SIL.
  **Agg During**:
  **Air** open in Agg: Fp; Kp; Nm; Sil.
    Amel: CS; Kp; KS; NS.
  **Alcoholic** Liquors, from: Km; **NM.**
    As from: **NM.**
  **Anemia** of Brain, from: Kp.
  **Ascending** Agg: Nm.

**Aural**: Sil.
**Back** Comes up, the: SIL.
**Bathing** Agg: Nm.
**Bed**, Going to: Nm.
**Blindness**, Blackness before eyes with: Nm.
**Bones** Aching in, with: Cp.
**Breakfast**, During: Sil.
**Chill,** Before: Nm.
  During: Fp; Nm.
**Chronic**: Nm.
  One side headache, with: NM.
**Closing** Eyes, on: Fp; Mp; Nm; SIL.
**Coffee**: NM.
**Cold** Applications, Amel: Nm.
**Concussion** of Brain: Kp.
**Constipation** Agg: Cp.
**Continuous**: Sil.
**Descending** Spire Agg: Sil.
**Dinner**, During Agg: Sil.
  After Agg: Nm.
**Driving**: Sil.
**Dulled** Mind, with: Nm.
  Senses: NM; SIL.
**Ear**, Noises buzzing in with: Sil.
**Eating**, While: Sil.
  After: Kp; Ks; Nm; NS.
  Forehead becomes moist: Amel: Ns.
**Elevated**, As if: Sil.
**Epileptic**: Cs; NM; SIL.
**Eructations**, During Agg: **NM;** Np; Sil.

**Evening** Agg: Km; Sil.
**Exertion**, Mental Agg: NM; Np; Sil.
  Physical Agg: Mp; Nm; Sil.
  After, violent headache with: Km; Ks.
  Vision, of: MP; **NM;** SIL.
**Exhaustion**, From: FP; Ks.
**Fainting**, With: KP; KS; Nm.
**Fall**, Tendency to with: Cs; Kp; Ks; Nm; Np; Sil.
  Backward: Ks; MP; SIL.
  Forward: CP; Fp; Kp; MP; **NM;** SIL.
  Left, to: **NM;** Sil.
  Sideways: Sil.
**Feeling, peculiar**, in cervical muscles: Km.
**Flickering,** Before, the eye: Nm.
**Floating**, As if: Cs.
**Gastric Derangement**: Np.
**Going back**, As if: Sil.
**Haemorrhoids**, flow suppressed, from: Nm.
**Headache,** With: SIL.
  Throbbing, face flushed: Fp.
  During: CP; Fp; Kp; Ks; NM; NS; SIL.
**Head,** Congestion with: Sil.
  Injuries, after: NS.
  Moving, Agg: Fp; Nm.
  Pushed, forward, as if: Fp.
**High** places: NM.
**House**, in: Sil.
  Entering, on: Sil.

**Intoxicated**, As if: Fp; Nm; Ns; SIL.
**Lie** Down must: NS.
**Live** Things, head as if full of: Sil.
**Looking**, About Agg: Sil.
  Downward Agg: Fp.
  Moving objects, at: Nm.
  Steadily: **NM;** SIL.
  Up: Kp; Ks; SIL.
  Window, out of: **NM.**
**Lying** Down Agg: Fp; KM; Kp.
  Back, on: SIL.
  Left side, on: Sil.
  Head low with: Nm.
**Lying**, while Amel: Kp; Nm; Sil.
  Head high, with, amel: Nm.
**Meditating**. Agg: Sil.
  Walking, in open air while, Agg: Sil.
**Memory**, Thinking, affected: NM; Sil.
**Menier's** Disease, from: Fp; Km; Sil.
**Menses** Before Agg: Cp.
  During Agg: Cp; Fp.
  After agg: Nm.
  Suppressed, from: Sil.
**Mental**, Exertion, from: **NM;** Np; Sil.
**Morning** Agg: Km; NM; SIL.
**Motion**, Agg: CP; Fp; Nm; SIL.
**Moving** Agg: KP; Mp; Nm.
  Head agg: Nm.

**Nausea**, With: CP; CS; Fp; Kp; Ks; NM; NS; SIL.
Periodic: **NM.**
**Noon** Agg: Cp; NS.
**Nose**, Discharge, with: Cp.
**Objects**, Seem to the right: Ns.
To turn in circle: Kp; Ks; **NM;** Np; NS; Sil.
**Occipital**: Km; Sil.
**Optical**, Defects, with: Mp.
**Pain**, During Agg: Sil.
**Passing** Over, or Seeing running water, Agg: Fp; Mp; Nm.
**Paroxysmal**: NM.
**Periodical**: NM.
**Perspiration** On forehead Amel: NS.
**Pregnancy**, During: NM.
**Rachitis**, With: Sil.
**Raising** up agg: NM.
Up arms, agg: Sil.
**Reading** Agg: Nm.
**Reeling**: Cp.
**Rising**, As if ground were: Sil.
**Rising**, On Agg: FP; Kp; Ks; **NM;** Ns; Sil.
Bed, from: FP; Ks; **NM;** NS; SIL.
Lying agg: Ks; Sil.
Seat, from: CP; Ks.
Sitting, while: Kp; NS.
Stooping, from: Nm; Sil.
Supine position, from: Sil.
**Rising**, On Amel: Nm.

**Room**, In Agg: Sil.
Warm Agg: Ks.
**Sea-sickness**, Nausea, without: Kp.
**Senses**, Vanishing with: Nm.
Suppression, of: NM.
**Side**, In right with: Nm.
Must walk to right: Nm.
**Sinking**, As if: Nm.
Down through or with bed as if: Cp.
**Sitting**, Agg: Nm; Np; SIL.
Up in bed Agg: Nm; Sil.
Amel: Sil.
**Sit** Up must: Sil.
**Sleep**, Before Agg: Nm.
During: Sil.
Half asleep, while: SIL.
On going, to: Nm.
**Sleepiness** with: SIL.
**Smoking** Agg: NM; Sil.
**Speech**, Mistakes of with: Nm; Sil.
**Spire**, Descending, from: SIL.
**Staggering** With: Cp; Fp; Kp; Ks; NM.
Old people, on getting up from sitting: Cp.
**Standing**, While Agg: Kp.
After sitting: KS; Sil.
Near, window: Nm.
**Stomach**, Empty feeling in, with: Kp.
**Stool**, After Agg: NM.
**Stooping**, Agg: CP; Cs; Kp; Ks; Nm; NS; SIL.

**Students**: Kp.

**Sun**, Facing the, Agg: Kp.

**Swaying**, Towards right as if: Nm; Sil.

**Swims** Everything, around, as if, could hardly move: Fp.

**Tea**, From: **NM.**

**Tobacco** or Snuff Agg: Sil.

**Trembling**, With: Nm.

**Turning** in Circle, as if: Nm; Ns.

On, Agg: Nm.

Bed in, to left agg: Cp.

Or moving the head, Agg: Kp; Nm.

**Unconsciousness** With: Nm.

Followed, by: Sil.

**Vision**, Dim: Nm.

Obscuration of, with: Fp.

**Vomiting** Amel: NS.

**Vomiting** of Bile, with: NS.

**Walking**, Gliding in air, feet do not touch ground as if: Nm.

**Walking** Agg: Cp; Cs; Kp; Ks; MP; **NM;** NS; Sil.

After long: Nm

Open air, in: CP; Kp; Sil.

**Walking**, While, Amel: Sil.

Open air, in: Mp.

**Warmth**, Amel: Sil.

**Weakness** And Oppression from the head, across the stomach, with: Cs.

**Whirling**, As if: **NM.**

**Wind**, Agg: Cp.

**Wind** blowing, as if through head: Nm.

**Window** near, Agg: Nm.

**Writing** Errors, with: Nm.

**VESICLES**: See Vesicles, under Eruptions.

**VEXATION**: See Anger.

**VIBRATIONS,** fluttering: Cs; KP; **NM; NS.**

**VICARIOUS:**

**VIGOUR,** Sense of: Np.

**VIOLENT** (Vehement): Cp; KP; NM.

**Trifles**, at: NM.

**VISE:** See Compression, and Squeezing under Pain.

**VISION: NM;** SIL.

**Accommodation.**

Defective: Nm.

Headache, during: MP.

Slow: Nm.

**Amaurosis** (Blindness): Fp; Kp; KS; **NM;** Np; **SIL.**

Coughing Agg: Km.

Day: SIL.

Eating, after: Sil.

Exertion, (sewing, etc.): NM.

Fainting, as from: Fp; NM.

Fixing, eyes: NM.

Headache, after: Sil.

Paralysis of optic nerve: Kp; NM; SIL.

Paroxysmal: Sil.

Periodic: NM; Sil.

Pregnancy, during: Sil.

Soup, while eating: Ns.

Stooping: Fp.
Sudden: NM.
Uterine affections, with: Sil.
Vanishing of sight: NM; Sil.
**Amblyopia** (Blurred, weak):
  Kp; Mp; **NM;** Ns; Sil.
Eyes, closing Amel: Cf.
Morning: Ns.
Pressure, Amel: Cf.
Writing, while: Cf.
**Asthenopia**: Fp; Nm; Ns.
**Black,** Sudden blind spells:
  NM; Sil.
**Blindness**: See Amaurosis.
**Confused: NM.**
**Coughing** Agg: Km.
**Dazzled**: SIL.
**Dim**, Blurred: CF; Cs; KP; Ks;
  NM; Np; NS; **SIL.**
Air, fresh amel: Ns.
Artificial light, in: Nm.
Chill, during: Nm.
Coition, after: KP; Np; SIL.
Diphtheria, after: SIL.
Distant object: Nm; Np.
Eating, while: Ns.
Exertion of eyes: Nm.
Firelight Agg: Nm.
Headache, after: Sil.
  before: NM.
  during: Fp; Nm.
Menses, before: Nm.
  during: Nm; Sil.
Reading, when: Nm; Sil.
Rising, from stooping: Nm.

Seminal emissions, after:
  Nm; Np.
Stooping, on: Nm.
Suppressed, foot sweat: **SIL.**
Walking: Nm.
Wiping eyes, amel: SIL.
Writing, when: Nm.
**Diplopia** (Double Vision): Kp;
  Mp; **NM.**
**Far sight**: See Hypermetropia.
**Flickering:** Cf; Cs; **NM.**
Headache, before: NM.
  during: **NM;** SIL.
**Flies:** See Muscae Volitantes.
**Foggy:** Cf; CP; Cs; Kp; Ks;
  NM; Np; SIL.
Reading: Nm.
Standing: Nm.
Writing: Cf.
**Headache,** Before Agg: NM.
After Agg: Sil.
**Hemiopia** (Half vision): Cs;
  **NM.**
Headache, then: Nm.
Vertical: Fp; NM.
**Hypermetropia** (Long
  sightedness): NM; **SIL.**
**Illusions** (optical): Cp; NM; Sil.
Circles: CP.
  objects turn in: Nm.
Colours, before: Kp; MP;
  NM; Np; Sil.
  black: NM.
    floating: SIL.
    letters change to points:
      CP.

spots: NM; Sil.

dark: Kp; Ks; Nm; Np; Sil.

objects: NM.

specks: Nm; **SIL.**

gray objects, seem: Sil.

spots: Cp.

green halo around light: Sil.

halo of colours, around light: Kp; Ks; Np.

objects change to gray spots: Cp.

rainbow: Sil.

striped: NM.

variegated: Ks; Mp.

Dazzling: Ks; **SIL.**

Distant, objects seem: Nm.

Fiery: NM.

circles: Cp.

points: NM.

pressure, amel: Cp.

shimmerings: CP.

zigzags: **NM.**

Glittering, objects: CP.

bodies, on blowing nose: Ns.

circles: CP.

Letters seem as if little birds were flying from left to right: Cp.

Lightnings: SIL.

Rain, seems looking through: Nm.

Run together, letters while writing: SIL.

objects: Sil.

Sparks: CF; Km; Ks; Mp; Np; Sil.

blowing nose on: Km.

coughing, on: Km.

headache, during: **MP.**

**Images,** Retained too long: NM.

**Leaf,** White, before, night: Ns.

**Letters,** Seem, as if birds were flying: Cp.

Change to a point: Cp.

Large: Nm.

Run together: **NM; SIL.**

writing, while: Sil.

**Lightnings:** SIL.

**Moving:** Cp.

**Muscae** volitantes: Nm; SIL.

Right: SIL.

**Myopia:** Nm; Np.

**Night,** eye, closing on: Sil.

**Nyctalopia:** Sil.

**Objects,** appear large: Nm.

Persons are, as if: Np.

Run together: Sil.

Turning in circles, as if: Nm.

**Pale:** SIL.

**Perceptive** Power, lost: Kp.

**Paralysis** of Optic nerve: Kp; Nm; SIL.

**Rain,** seems looking through: Nm.

**Rings:** Cp.

**Smoke,** Before: Km.

**Spots:** Nm; Sil.

**Stooping,** Agg: Fp.

**Swimming,** Object: NM.

**Veils,** Before: Cp; Nm; Np; Sil.
**Wavering**: NM.
**Weak**: Nm.
**Zigzag**: **NM.**
**VITAL Heat,** Lack of: Cf; **CP;** Cs; **KP; MP;** NM; NP; **SIL.**
Exercise during: SIL.
**VITREOUS Opacity**: Cf; Sil.
**VIVACITY**: See Cheerful.
**VOCAL CORDS**: See Larynx.
**VOICE Altered**: Nm.
  **Barking**: Km.
  **Colds,** Agg: Sil.
  **Control,** Lacks: Kp.
  **Croaking**: Nm.
  **Distant,** Seems: Nm.
  **Exertion,** Agg: Fp; Kp; NM.
  **Hoarseness**: Cf; CP; Cs; Fp; Km; Kp; KS; Mp; NM; Np; NS; SIL.
  Air open, amel: Cs.
  Chronic: Sil.
  Coryza, during: Fp; Km; Nm.
  Laughing, when: Cf.
  Leucorrhoea, with: NS.
  Morning, agg: **CP;** NM; SIL.
  Overuse of voice, from: Fp; Kp; NM.
  Painless: Cp.
  Paretic: Sil.
  Reading and reciting aloud: Cf.
  Room warm, agg: KS.
  Talking, from: NM.
  Walking, in open air agg: Cp.

  Weather, cold, damp agg: SIL.
**Hollow**: Sil.
**Husky,** Not clear: Nm; Ns; Sil.
  Morning: SIL.
**Lost**: FP; KP; Ks; NM; Np.
  Paralytic: Kp.
  Singers: Fp; NM.
**Nasal**: Nm.
**Rough**: Nm; Sil.
**Shrill,** sudden while speaking: Kp; MP.
**Weak**: CS; FP; **NM.**
**VOICE,** Hears (Delusions): Nm.
  **Dead** people, of: Nm.
  **Distant**: Nm.
**VOMITING**: CP; CS; Fp; Kp; Ks; NM; Np; SIL.
  **Agg**: Fp; Nm; SIL.
  **Acrid,** Sour: Cs; FP; Kp; Ks; NM; **NP;** NS.
  Eating, after: Ns.
  Fluid: NM; Np.
  Headache, during: Np.
  Scalding: Km; Sil.
  **Albuminous,** Glairy: Sil.
  **Bilious,** Bile: Cs; FP; Km; Kp; Ks; NM; Np; NS; Sil.
  **Bitter:** NS; Sil.
  **Blood:** Cs; FP; Km; Kp; Nm; Np; Ns; SIL.
  Bright: Fp.
  Clotted: Km.
  Dark: Km.
  Menses suppressed: Nm.

**Brain** Affections, with: KP

**Brownish**: NS.

**Cheesy**: Np.

**Chill**, Before, during, after: Nm

**Choking**, With: Kp.

**Coffee** Ground like: NM; Np.

**Coition**, After: Sil.

**Confusion**, With: Cp.

**Coughing**, From: Fp; KP; Ks; NM, Np; SIL.

**Curdled**: Nm; Np; Sil.

  Milk, in infants: Cp; Np.

**Drinking**, After: Fp; Nm; SIL.

  Any: Sil.

  Cold water, after: SIL

**Easy**: CP.

**Eating**, While, sudden: Sil.

**Expectoration**, On: SIL.

**Eyes**, Pain, with: Sil.

**Fever**, During: Nm.

**Food** of: Cp; Cs; FP; Km; Kp; Ks; NM; SIL.

  Bile, then: NM.

  Breakfast, after: SIL.

  Eating, while. Sil.

    immediately after: FP; Sil.

  Intermittents, in: FP; NM.

  Sour: Ns.

  Undigested: Cp; **FP**; Nm.

**Forenoon**: NS.

**Frothy**: Ks; Np; Sil.

**Glairy**, Albuminous: Sil.

**Green**: Fp; **NS.**

  Dark: Km.

  Fluid: Kp; NS.

  Pneumonia, in: Fp.

Yellowish: Np; NS.

**Hawking** up Mucous, when: SIL.

**Headache**, During: Cs; Fp; Cp; Ks; NM; Np; NS; Sil.

**Heat**, During: Fp; **NM.**

**Heated**, Becoming: Sil.

**Icecream**, After: CP.

**Incessant**: Km; Mp.

**Infantile**: Cf; Cp; Cs.

**Lifting**, Agg: Sil.

**Liquids**: **SIL.**

  Cold water only: Sil.

  Large quantity, in eating, after: Sil.

**Membranous**: Ns.

**Menses**, Before: Mp; Nm.

  During: Kp; Ks; Nm.

**Mental** Exertion: Nm.

**Milk**: Cp; Sil.

  After: **SIL.**

  Curdled: NM; Np; **SIL.**

  Mother's: **SIL.**

  Persistently: Cp.

**Morning**: **FP; NM;** Sil.

**Mucous**: Cs; Km; Kp; Ks; NM; Np; NS; SIL.

  Coughing: SIL.

  Greasly, white: Km.

  Thick white: Km.

**Mucous**, Amel: Nm.

**Night**: Fp; Nm; Ns; Sil.

**Nursing**, Immediately, after: Cp; Fp; **SIL.**

**Offensive**, Purulent: Ks.

**Pain**, During: Fp; Nm.

**Palpitation**, With: Kp.
**Periodic**: Ns.
**Persistent,** Immediately after eating: Mp.
**Pregnancy**: FP; KM; Kp; NM; Np; **NS;** Sil.
**Pressing** Upon epigastrium and stomach: Nm.
**Qualmishness**, With: Ns.
**Riding,** in Carriage: Fp; SIL.
**Salty**: NS; Sil.
**Sleep,** During: Fp.
  Then: Nm.
**Smoking,** From: Nm; NS; Sil.
**Sour**: Np.
**Stringy**: NM; SIL.
**Sudden**: Km; Sil.
**Ulcer,** With: Np.
**Urging,** To: Nm.
**Vertigo** During: Nm; Sil.
**Vexation,** After: NS.
**Violent**: Fp.
**Water**: NM; SIL.
  Food, then: Sil.
**White**: Km; Ks; Ns.
**Wine,** Taste of: Nm.
**Worms**: Nm; Sil.
**Yeast,** Like: Ns.
**VORACITY:** See Appetite, Increased.
**VULNERABLE:** See Healing, difficult.
**VULVA** (Labiae)
  **Abscess**: Kp; SIL.
  **Clitoris,** Erection, urination after, sexual desire with: Cp.

**Condylomata**: **NS.**
  Soft, red, fleshy: **NS.**
**Dry**: NM.
**Enlarged,** As if: Sil.
  Menses, before: Sil.
**Eruptions**: Nm; Ns; Sil.
  Herpetic: Nm; Ns.
  Itching: Sil.
  Painful: Sil.
  Pimples: Nm; Sil.
    painful: Sil.
  Pudendal: Nm.
  Vesicles: Ns.
**Excoriation**: Ks; Sil.
**Heat** (Burning): Cp.
**Inflammation**: Fp; Mp; NM; Ns; Sil.
  Follicular, herpetic: Nm.
**Irritation**: Nm; SIL.
**Itching**: Cs; KS; **NM;** Ns; **SIL.**
  Hair falling of, with: Nm.
  Leucorrhoea, from: Kp.
  Menses, after, during: Cs; NM; SIL.
  Pudendum, of: **NM;** SIL.
  Urination, during: Sil.
**Pain:** CP.
  Aching: Cp.
  Bearing down, during menses: Cs.
  Biting: Nm; SIL.
  Burning: Cp; Cs; Fp; Kp; Ks; Sil.
  Menses, during Agg: NM; Sil.
  Pressing: Cp.
  Pulsating: CP.

Sore, tender: Cp; Mp; SIL.

Stinging: Cp.

Stitching: CP; Ns.

   extends to chest: Cp.

Tearing: Sil.

Urinating, during: Sil.

**Swollen**: Cp; Ns.

**Tingling**, Voluptuous: CP.

**Tumours,** Encysted: SIL.

Erectile: Sil.

**Ulcers:** Cs; **SIL.**

**Varices** on Lábiae: Cf.

**Worms,** in: Sil.

**WAKING:** See Waking, under Sleep.

**WAKING,** on Agg: Cp; Cs; Fp; KS; NM; SIL.

**WALKING:** See under Legs.

**WALKING** Agg: **CS;** Km; Kp; MP; NM; NP; NS; SIL.

**Beginning,** of: Nm; SIL.

**Fast:** CS; Kp; NM; **SIL.**

**Open air in:** KP; **MP;** Nm; SIL.

**WALKING Amel:** Kp; KS; NM; Ns; Sil.

**Continued:** CF; Sil.

**Open Air, in:** Cs; **KS;** Nm.

**Slowly:** Cs; KP.

**WALKING Backward** Agg: Mp; Sil.

**Bare feet,** Amel:

**Bent,** Amel:

**Bridge** on narrow, or over water Agg: Fp; Mp; Nm.

**Cotton** on, as if:

**Dark,** in Agg: SIL.

**Eyes,** Closed with Agg:

**Hard,** Pavement on, Agg:

**Impulse** to: Cp; FP.

**WANDERING, Changing:** Erratic, complaints: KS; **NM;** Mp; Sil.

**WARMTH, Warm Agg:** KM; KS; NM; NS.

**Air** of: CS; **KS;** NM; NS.

**Becoming,** In open air: Nm; NS; SIL.

**Bed:** CS; Km; KS; NM.

**Room:** Cp; **CS; KS;** Nm; Np; NS.

**Stove:** Nm.

**Wraps:** Cs; **KS.**

**WARM Bed Amel:** CP; Kp; **SIL.**

**Stove:** Cf; **MP; SIL.**

**Wraps:** Kp; MP; SIL.

**WARTS**: See Warts, under Skin.

**WASH Impulse** to: Cs.

**WASHING, Aversion** to: MP; NS; Sil.

**Water** with, **Agg**: MP; NS; Sil.

**WATER Use** of, in any form Agg: Ns.

**Working** in: Cp; Mp.

**WATER Cannot** Bear touch of: Km; Np; Sil.

**Chokes,** Him:

**Dropping** or flowing on part: Sil.

**Sight** Of Agg:

**WATERBRASH**: CP; CS; Fp; Kp; Ks; NM; Ns; **SIL.**

**Afternoon**, Walking, while: Ns.
**Chilliness**, With: Sil.
**Eating**, After: Nm; Sil.
**Night**, At: Nm; NP.
**Pregnancy**, During: Nm.
**Sour** Things, after: Fp.
**Tongue**, Brown with: Sil.
**WATERY:** See Secretions, Watery, Thin.
**WAVERING:** See Fickle.
**WAVES, Ebullitions,** fluctuations, etc.: Sil.
**WAX** (Cerumen), in ear:
**Brown** and dark: Cs.
**Dark,** flowing: Cs.
**Increased**: Sil.
**Soft:** Sil.
**Thin:** Sil.
**WEAK, Feeble,** Enervated: CP; CS; Fp; KP; Ks; Mp; **NM; NS; SIL.**
**Coition**, After: KP; NM; SIL.
**Diarrhoea**, From: KM; **NS; SIL.**
**Diseases**, Acute, after: CS; Km; SIL.
**Dreams,** After: CS.
**Easy**: Kp; Nm; Sil.
**Emissions**, After: Kp; NM; Np; **SIL.**
**Evening:** NM; Sil.
**Exertion**, Slight: NM; Np.
**Heat**, from: Np.
Summer of: Nm.
**Influenza,** After: Kp.
**Intermittent** Fever, from: Ns.

**Lie** Down, unable to: Fp; Sil.
Stretch, and: Cs.
**Loss** of Vital fluids, from: Cp.
**Lying**, Agg: Nm.
**Menses**, After: Cp; Nm.
Before: NM.
During: Cp; CS; KS; Nm.
**Mental** Exertion, from: Nm; Sil.
**Morning**: CF; **NM;** Sil.
Awakening, after: **SIL.**
Rising, when: Sil.
**Moving**, Arms, on: Nm.
Difficult: FP.
**Nervous**: Cp; **KP;** NM; **NP; SIL.**
Females, in: Kp; Mp; Sil.
**Nursing,** Prolonged, from: Cp.
**Pain,** From: Kp; Mp.
**Paralytic:** KP; Np; Sil.
**Perspiration**, From: Fp; Nm; SIL.
**Rising,** On: NM.
**Sadness**, From: Cp.
**Scientific** Labour, from: Kp; Np.
**Sitting:** Nm.
Unable to sit: Mp.
**Sleep**, After: Sil.
**Stools**, After: Kp; Nm; **NS;** SIL.
**Storm,** Before and during: Sil.
**Talking,** From: KS; NM; Sil.
**Tremulous:** Nm.
**Trifles** Causes, from: Nm; Sil.
**Urination**, After: Cp.
**Vexation**, After: CP; NM.

**Waking,** On: Fp; Nm; Np.
**Walking,** From: Km; KP; NM; NS; SIL.
**Warm** Weather, from; Nm; Np.
**Writing,** from: Sil.
**WEALTHY** thinks, he is:
**WEANING,** Ill effects of: Cp; Kp.
**WEARINESS: CP;** Fp; **KP;** Ks; **NM;** NS.
   **Ascending,** Stairs: Cp.
   **Eating,** after: NM.
   **Evening:** NM; Sil.
   **Forenoon:** NM; Sil.
   **Menses,** Before: NM.
     During: Cp.
   **Talking,** After: Cp.
**WEATHER Autumn Agg:** Cp; Nm.
   **Bright,** Clear: Nm; NS.
   **Change** of: Cf; CP; SIL.
     Cold to warm: **KS;** NM; NS.
   **Cloudy:** Ns.
   **Cold wet: CP;** CS; Km; Kp; Nm; **NS; SIL.**
   **Damp:** Cf; **SIL.**
   **Dry:** Sil.
   **Summer:** Km; NM.
   **Warm** wet: **NS;** SIL.
   **Winter:** CP; Km; KP; Nm; SIL.
**WEATHER** Warm Wet, Amel: MP; Sil.
**WEDGE Plug,** sensation: Nm.
**WEEPING Agg:** NM.
**WEEPS** (Tearful mood): CP; **CS;** Fp; KP; Ks; Mp; **NM;** NP; NS; SIL.

**Admonitions,** From: Nm.
**Alone,** When, without knowing why: NM.
**Aloud:** NM.
**Alternating,** with Laughter: Nm.
**Bitterly:** Nm.
**Cause,** without: Nm.
**Convulsive:** MP.
**Crying,** and Continuous (religious): Kp.
**Delirium,** After: Ns.
**Dreams,** In: Cf.
**Involuntary:** NM.
**Looked** At, when: NM.
**Menses,** During: NM.
**Music,** From: Ns.
**Night:** NM; Sil.
**Noon,** Afternoon: Sil.
**Open** Air, Amel: NS.
**Past** Events, thinking of: NM.
**Piano,** Hearing on: NS.
**Pitied,** If he believes, he is: NM.
**Sleep,** in: NM; SIL.
**Spoken to,** when: NM; Sil.
**Stool,** During: Sil.
**Trifles,** At: Nm; Sil.
**Waking,** On: Sil.
**WEIGHT, As of a heavy:** See Heaviness.
**WELL Says he is,** when very sick.
**WENS** (Sebaceous Cysts): SIL.
**WET Applications Agg:** Sil.

**Getting**: Cp; Cs.
  Drenched: NM; **NS.**
  Feet: NM; **SIL.**
**Weather:** CP; CS; MP; **NS;**
  SIL.
**WET Warm** weather **Amel:** MP;
  Sil.
**WHEALS:** See Urticaria.
**WHEEZING**: See Respiration,
  Whistling.
**WHINING, Whimpering**: Ail-
  ments, little, with:
  **Attack** of sickness, before:
  Sleep, in:
**WHIRLING**: See Vertigo.
**WHISKERS**, Eruptions.
  Herpes: Nm; SIL.
  Pimples, burning: Cs.
  **Falling,** off: NM; Sil.
  **Itching**: Kp; Nm; Sil.
**WHISPERS:**
  **Ear,** in as if:
  **Herself,** to:
  **Sleep,** in:
**WHISTLES:** Ks; NM; SIL.
  **Fever,** during: Nm.
**WHITE, Whiteness**: KM; NM;
  **Chalky:**
  **Milky:** KM.
  **Spots: SIL.**
**WHITLOW** (Finger Felon): Cf;
  Cs; Ns; Sil.
**WHIZZING:** See Humming.
**WIFE is faithless:**
  **Run away,** from him:

**WHOOPING cough:** See cough,
  whooping.
**WILDNESS, At Unpleasant**
  news: Cp.
**WILFUL:** See Stubborn.
**WILL,** weak: Nm.
**WILY:**
**WIND** Air, draft Agg: CP; Mp;
  **SIL.**
  **Blowing** on part, as of a: Nm.
  **Cold Agg:** Cp; SIL.
  **North Agg: MP;** Sil.
**WIND PIPE:** See Trachea.
**WINDY,** stormy weather
  **Agg:** MP; Ns; SIL.
**WINE Agg:** Km; NM; SIL.
**WINKING:**
**WINTER Agg:** CP; Km; KP;
  Nm; SIL.
**WIPE must** (Eyes): Nm.
**WITHERED Shrivelled:** Kp; Nm;
  SIL.
**WITTY** (Jesting): Nm.
**WOMEN**: See Female affec-
  tions.
  **Aversion,** to: Nm.
  **Childless:** FP; **NM;** SIL.
  **Neurotic,** High stung: Kp.
  **Widows:** Cp; KP.
**WOODEN Feeling:** Fp; SIL.
**WOOLENS Agg:** Cs; Ks; NS.
**WORD Hunting:**
  **Swallows:**
**WORK Desires,** but on
  attemping the desire is
  gone: Cs.

**WORK, Mental,** aversion: Cp; Cs; Fp; Ks; Mp; NM; SIL.

**Complaints,** from: Nm.

**Impossible:** Ns.

**Seems** to drive him crazy owing to impotency of his mind: KP.

**WORKING in Clay, cold** water complaints, from: Mp.

**WORMS:** Np; SIL.

**Complaints:** Km; NM; NP; Ns; SIL.

**Fever:** Sil.

**Round** (Ascaris): **NM;** NP; SIL.

**Pin,** thread (Oxyuris): Km; Np; Sil.

**Tape** (Taenia): SIL.

**WORRY:** See Grief, Care.

**WOUNDS** (Injuries): Nm; Sil.

**Bleeding** Freely: Nm.

**Constitutional** Effects: Nm.

**Cuts:** Km; Sil.

**Granulations,** To promote healthy: Sil.

**Painful:** Nm.

**Penetrating:** Sil.

**Slow** To heal: Sil.

**Splinters,** from: Sil.

**WRAPPED,** body etc:

**WRAPPING Amel:** Kp; Mp; Nm; SIL.

**WRAPS up,** Summer, in:

**WRETCHED:**

**WRIGGLES:**

**WRINGLING:** See Twisting.

**WRINKLED:** Kp; Nm; SIL.

**WRISTS Right:** Cp; Np.

**Aching** Loss of power: FP.

**Caries:** SIL.

**Cold:** Cf.

**Compression:** Ns.

**Contraction:** Sil.

**Convulsion:** NM,

**Eruptions,** Pimples, back on: CP.

Vesicles: Cp; Nm.

itching: Cp; Nm.

radial side, on: Nm.

**Ganglion:** SIL.

Back of: Cf; SIL.

**Grasping,** Agg: FP; Nm.

**Itching:** Cp.

Inner side: Nm.

**Lameness:** Sil.

Bruised, as if: Cp.

**Menses,** During, after: Np.

**Motion,** On Agg: Cp; SIL.

**Pain:** Cp; Cs; Ns.

Aching: Cp; FP; NP; Sil.

Bed, warmth of, amel: Sil.

Boring: Cp.

Broken as if: SIL.

Burning: Cp.

scratching, after: Cp.

Cramps: Cp; Np.

motion, on: Cp.

Drawing: CP; Km; Nm; Np; Ns; Sil.

cramp like: Cp.

Extending, forearm, to: Fp.

writing, while: Fp.

Paralytic: Np.
Pinching: Nm.
Pressing: Cp; Ns.
Rheumatic: Fp; Np.
   outer side: Fp.
Right: Cp; Np.
Sore, bruised: Nm; Np.
Sprained, as if: Nm; Sil.
Stitching: NM; SIL.
Tearing: CP; Nm; **NS**; SIL.
   shoulder to: SIL.
   right: Cp.
Walking, while Agg: Ns.
Writing, while, Agg: MP; Sil.
**Paralysis,** Right and left ankle:
   Np.
   Sensation of (right): Np.
**Stiffness:** Ns.
**Tension:** Np.
**Weakness:** Nm; Np; SIL.
   Menses, after: Np.
   Right: Sil.
     and left ankle: Np.
**WRITING Agg:** Kp; **NM**; SIL.
**WRITING, Cramps: MP;** Sil.
**WRONG Cannot** tell, what is:
   CP.
   **Doing** something:
   **Everything** seems: Kp.
   **Had done** something: Sil.
**WRY NECK** (Torticollis): Sil.
**X-RAY BURNS:** Cf.
**YAWNING Agg:** NM; SIL.
   Amel:

**YAWNING:** CP; Kp; Mp; NM;
   Ns; SIL.
**Chill** During: NM; Ns; Sil.
**Eating,** Agg: Ns.
**Excessive:** Sil.
**Forenoon:** Cp.
**Frequent:** Nm; Ns; Sil.
   Riding in carriage, in
   evening: Nm.
**Hiccough,** With: Nm.
**Hysterical:** Kp.
**Lachrymation** With: Mp.
**Nausea** With: Nm.
**Sleepiness,** With: NM.
   Without: Nm.
**Spasmodic:** MP; NM.
   Violent as if dislocating jaw:
   Mp.
**Stretching** and Constant: Cp;
   Nm.
**Vehement:** Nm.
**Walking,** In open air, after:
   Nm.
**Wine,** Amel: Nm.
**YELLOW FEVER:** Fp; Kp; NS.
**YELLOWNESS:** See Skin, Jaun-
   dice.
   **Bright** or orange: KP.
   **Golden:** NP.
**ZEALOUS:**
**ZIGZAG:** NM.
**ZOSTER:** Km; NM; SIL.
**ZYGOMAE:** See Malar bones.
**ZYMOTIC FEVER:** KP; Ks.

■ ■ ■

# MATERIA MEDICA

## OF THE

# TWELVE TISSUE REMEDIES

*by*

## Dr. D.S. Phatak
*M.B.B.S.*

## B. Jain Publishers (P) Ltd.
### NEW DELHI

First edition - 1986
Second revised edition - 1997


© Copyright Dr. D.S. Phatak
            177 B Station Avenue Road
            Chembur, Bombay - 400 071




*Published by :*
**B. Jain Publishers Pvt. Ltd.**
1'2 , Street No. 10, Chuna Mandi,
P˙harganj, New Delhi - 110055 (INDIA)
Tele: 7770430, 7770572, 7536418

# PREFACE

Usually the Repertory is compiled from the knowledge of the Materia Medica.

In this book, Materia Medica is compiled from Dr. S.R. Phatak's Biochemic Repertory, as printed in 1937 and revised by him in late 1979. Ferrum Phos and Calcium salts were written when he was alive. He was satisfied with the writing but was skeptical about the length of the book. The source material from which Dr. S.R. Phatak compiled his repertory is given in the preface to that book.

Time only can decide whether such exhaustive materia medica of twelve tissue remedies is necessary. None the less the author is presenting it in its present form to the lovers of these remedies.

Introductory and other notes are the responsibility of the author. He believes that the key to better understanding of these remedies lies in the knowledge of their physiology. At present it is not easy to co-relate the actions of these remedies in terms of their physiology. The two are however placed in juxtaposition, so that the reader may correlate them in his own way. Late Dr. V.J. Patankar, Chief Surgeon of Mahatma Gandhi Memorial Hospital, has to be remembered in this context as he took keen interest in this project.

The real credit of getting this book written by me, goes to my nephew, Dr. Raghunath Phatak. He persistently reminded me to complete the book. His perseverance shook me from my inborn lethargy. If the reader finds this book useful, he should thank Dr. Raghunath Phatak, more than the author.

B. Jain Publishers deserve my thanks for publishing this book along with Dr. S.R. Phatak's Biochemic Repertory.

Bombay
July, 1986                                        **D.S. Phatak**

# INTRODUCTION

Materia Medica and Repertory are two sides of the same coin. Both are complementary to each other, and none is complete in itself. A good grasp of both is essential for a fairly good practice.

Mastery over Materia Medica is not that easy. There is no short cut or easy road to success. The symptoms given are just like a bony skeleton. You are to add flesh and life to it, by making them your friends. For that while reading every remedy, you must refer the repertory for every rubric or symptom, compare with other remedies given, learn their relative importance etc. This long drawn out effort is at times tedious, but does pay in the long run.

The best way to make friendship with them is to use them. (You can never learn swimming unless you jump into the water). You may succeed or fail. When you fail, review the case as to where you have gone wrong:

1. Taking the case

2. Interpreting the symptoms

3. Grasping the essentials of the symptoms.

Your failure if carefully analysed will teach you more than your success. Generalities, Modalities (worse and better), and mental symptoms are distinguishing features of the remedy. Peculiarities, which underlying pathology, cannot explain, are the identification marks of the remedy. Learn to recognise them by serious and repeated effort

When the cup is half full, it is half empty also. Please try to look at the same symptom from as many aspects as possible.

If you are conversant with homoeopathy, please use Dr. S.R. Phatak's "Concise Homoeopathic Repertory" along with biochemic Repertory. Both are now arranged on identical patterns. It is possible, that you may find better remedy in homoeopathy or vice a versa.

If you write freely to the author about the deficiencies of the book, it will help him to make this book more useful, in future editions.

Bombay:                                                    **D.S. Phatak**
July 1986

# How to use this book
## (Some Hints)

Materia Medica is written on the usual lines, Generalities, Modalities (Worse and Better), Mind and different regions. Signs for Agg. and Amel. are not used to avoid confusion. Instead of Agg. and Amel. Worse and Better are used.

Semi-colon is used with care. For instance, under Calcarea Phos under Generalities you will find "Convulsions; in children; clonic; epileptic; from suppressed menses: with falling; left sided or one sided". It means Convulsions: (1) In children, (2) clonic or epileptic in character, (3) suppressed menses is causation in certain cases, (4) with falling is concomitant, (5) one sided or on left side shows the location. These can be suitably combined.

At times the rubric is too lengthy. A separate paragraph is devoted to it. See pain under Generalities under Natrum Mur. It gives the character, location and modalities of pain, all put together. In the same paragraph you will find "pressing; externally; internally; load as from; muscles in; together". This has to be interpreted as shown above. A separate paragraph is not possible for every rubric. For example, in worse under Natrum Mur you will find Foods; of different types and at the end idleness. Here idleness has nothing to do with foods.

Three types Bold, Italics, and Ordinary are used to show gradation in that order.

Furthermore, what is given under Generalities can be applied to particulars. None-the-less Modalities are given under particulars. At times that can be applied to Generalities.

A person using twelve tissue remedies has limited choice. Hence he has to be very alert. Like a good detective he has to collect all the evidences, weigh the different symptoms carefully and select one or two most suitable remedies and combine them if necessary.

I hope, these few hints will enable the beginners to wade through the mass of details with little more ease.

# CALCAREA FLUOR

**GENERALITIES:** Calcarea Fluor is useful in most of the affections of the bone. Development of the bones is tardy. Slow repair of broken bones. Non-union; necrosis of bones. Suppuration; in bones, periosteum. Swelling of bones. In most of the bone conditions Silica competes with it. **Exostoses:** *Osteo-sarcoma.* It disperses bony growths specially after injury. Deficient enamel of *teeth.* Periosteitis of lower jaw, ribs etc. Sequestrum; removal of.

This tissue salt relaxes elastic fibres, specially of veins and glands. *Glands enlarge* and become **stony hard.** *Veins dilate* and become varicose. Removes tendency to adhesions after operations.

**Indurations;** stony hard; glands of; tonsils of; neck tumours; specially after injury. Induration of margins of ulcers. Induration, threatening suppuration.

Aneurysm. Arteriosclerosis. *Fistula. Cataract.* Nodes in breast. Hodgkin's disease. Useful for abscesses, specially chronic, with stinking pus. Sinuses. Sequestrum was extruded through a sinus, the patient merely pulled it, with subsequent repair of bone.

In these patients there is lack of vital heat. Reaction is poor. Weakness, morning. Feeling of fatigue, all day. Numbness in different parts. Sluggish, temperament.

Synovitis. Rice bodies in cartilage. Nails hypertrophied. X-ray burns. Congenital syphilis; ulceration of mouth and throat. General stiffness. Discharges turn grass green. Cephalhematoma.

**WORSE:** Change of weather. **Cold** in general. Cold drinks. Cold food. Damp weather. Lifting. Sprains. *Beginning of motion.* Lying on painful side.

**BETTER:** Hot applications. Warmth of stove. Rubbing. Lying on painless side. Menses. **Continued motion.** Pressure.

**MIND:** Anxiety about money matters. Thinks he is poor (delusion). Fear of poverty, misfortune. Indecision. Fickle.

**HEAD: Exostoses. Cephalhematoma** of new born infants. Headache worse in evening. Sensation of cracking noise in head, preventing sleep.

**EYES: Cataract.** Cornea; opacity; phlyctenular keratitis; *spots on; ulcer.* Pain in eyes, worse on writing; better by closing and pressure. Subcutaneous palpabral cysts. Amblyopia; while writing; better by pressure. Vision; dim; foggy. Sparks and flickering before eyes.

**EARS:** Noises; of bells' ringing. *Caries of ossicles; sclerosis of.* Calcareous deposits on tympanic membrane. Chronic discharge, from. Periosteitis of mastoid.

**NOSE:** Bones; caries; diseased; growth of. Periosteitis. Coldness and hardness of external nose. Catarrhal inflammation. Fluent discharge; greenish; offensive. *Ineffectual efforts at sneezing.*

**FACE:** Eruptions on. **Exostosis;** of lower jaw. Hard swelling on cheek with pain or tooth-ache. Small, hard, cold sores on lips.

**MOUTH:** Cold sores. Gum boils. Teeth; caries of; deficient enamel; loose; ache; worse; during pregnancy. Fistula dentalis. Tongue; cracked; indurated; chronic swelling. Ranula. Periosteitis; lower jaw.

**THROAT:** *Adenoids.* Diphtheria, involving trachea. Disposition to hawk. Chronic follicular pharyngitis. Pain worse by cold drinks; better by warm drinks. Relaxed.

Suffocative sensation, specially at night, better by warm drinks. Constant disposition to swallow, due to tickling in larynx. Pain and burning; amel. by warm drinks. **Tonsils enlarged.** Mucus plugs in crypts. Elongated uvula. *Goitre;* hard, lumpy. Induration of external glands.

**STOMACH:** Cancer. Cannot bear tight clothing. Vomiting of infants; of undigested food. Acute indigestion from fatigue and brain-fag; in overtaxed children.

**ABDOMEN:** Colic; while sitting; amel. by bending forward or double; walking, lying on painless side. Flatulence, of pregnancy; riding in carriage. Pendulous. Pain, right hypochondriac region, cutting; lancinating. Hernia; inguinal. Liver; cutting pain agg. by sitting and bending forward. Constipation. Fissures. Fistulae. Piles; blind, with backache. Prolapse of rectum. Gushing stools; first natural and then loose. Putrid odour.

**URINARY:** Pain in bladder. Cloudy urine. Dark or pale. Copious; agg. 8 A.M. to 3 p.m. Pungent odour. Scanty. Clear water. Stitching pain in kidney. Burning pain in urethra and meatus.

**MALE:** *Induration of testes.* Ulcers on penis; edges hard. Oedematous swelling of scrotum. Hydrocele. Varicocele.

**FEMALE:** Mammary glands; inflamed; spoiled milk in; nodules sensitive in. Uterus; flabby; indurated; displaced; **fibrous polypi** of. Varices on labia.

**HEART:** Atheroma. Aneurism. Distended arteries. Heart; general affections, dilatation; chronic inflammation (myocarditis). Veins; varicose; as if would burst. Varicose ulcerations. Vascular tumours of veins.

**RESPIRATORY:** Asthmatic breathing with difficult expectoration. Cough; from elongated uvula; from tickling or irritation in larynx. Cough; croupy; hacking; paroxysmal; spasmodic. Cough agg. by eating and bathing. Expectoration; globular; lumpy; yellow. *Larynx;* nearly closed (in diphtheria); spasmodic croup in; tickling in; scraping in; wants to clear, hence hawking. Hoarse voice, while reading aloud or laughing.

**NECK & BACK:** Aching. Lumbago; with restlessness. **Curvature of spine.** Backache agg. while sitting; amel. by gentle motion, walking, external warmth.

**EXTREMITIES: Arthritic nodosities. Exostoses.** Caries of bones. Joints; easy dislocation, fingers of; swelling of. Cold wrists. Ganglion, on back of wrists. Callosities on hands. Chapping on palms; desquamation. Varicose veins. Milk leg (phlegmasia alba dolens). Nodes on tibia.

**SLEEP:** Dreams; confused; cutting of a woman, for salting; of danger; of the dead; death of relations; events of previous day; frightful; journey, new places etc.; vivid; trying to get out of window. Sleep, unrefreshing.

**FEVER:** Long lasting fever.

**SKIN:** Cheloid. Cicatrices; affections of. Carbuncle. Gummata. Nodes. Occasional erysipelas. Ganglia. Naevus. Ulcer; **fistulus;** indolent; with hard edges. Whitlow.

# CALCAREA PHOS

**GENERALITIES:** Calcarea phos. affects nutrition and growth. If these twins are remembered, many of the symptoms can be easily understood, for instance, dwarfishness, leanness, marasmus (in children), rickets, anemia etc.

**Anemia;** from nutritional disturbances; with menstrual derangements. **Chlorosis.** Cancerous affections, epithelioma. Chronic disease to begin treatment. *Convalescence.*

Convulsions; in children; clonic; epileptic; from suppressed menses; with falling; left side or one-sided.

Affections of cartilages. Bones; crumbling; development tardy; abscess about; injuries; necrosis; **non-union;** pain in. Bones; *slow repair; softening;* suppuration; swelling. *Rickets.* Dropsy; from heart or kidney disease; from loss of blood. **Dwarfishness** (growth tardy). Emaciation; **in children** (marasmus). Exhaustion. Falling apart as if. Fistulae. Flabby feeling. Formication. **Heat;** *lack of vital.* **Loss of vital fluids.** *Leukemia.* **Lean people.**

Inflammation of serous membranes. Jerking; **muscles.**

Desire to be magnetised. Numbness externally; in single part from unpleasant news. *Nursing children.* Nutritional disturbances. *Old people.* Complaints from over-lifting; after operations for fistulae.

Pain; *in bones;* as if broken; burning, externally; cutting internally; growing; pressing externally; in *small spots; stitching* tearing; wandering; shifting.

**Polypi.** Disorders of pregnancy. Psora. *Puberty* and *youth.* *Pulsation* (throbbing); internally. *Rickets.* Scrawny. Scrofula. Separated as if. Sexual excitement indulged or suppressed; irregularities of. Shocks; electric like. Impulse to stretch. Symptoms, alternate.

**Tendency to take cold.** Tendons; injured; inflamed. Tobacco, abuse of. *Trembling;* during menses. Tumours cystic. *Weakness; weariness;* during menses; after talking.

**WORSE: Morning. Afternoon. Night. Air open cold**; *Ascending.* Autumn. **Change of weather.** *Change of temperature* **Cold;** in general; **air;** becoming; entering a cold place. **Wet weather.** Company. Consolation. Dentition. **Eating after. Emotions.** Exertion physical.

**Food;** coffee, cold drinks; frozen; fruits. Fright. **Uncovering head.** Lifting. Lying, on moist floor. **Menses; before; beginning of;** during. Motion. *Pregnancy.* Pressure. Sexual excess. Sleep; falling to; during. Snow; melting; air; or exposure to. Spring. Stooping. *Swallowing;* empty. *Talking;* **thinking;** of complaints. Touch. On waking.

**BETTER:** Eating. Eructations, sour. *Flatus passing.* Holding or being held. *Lying; on abdomen; on side.* Magnetism. Motion. Repose. Sneezing. Summer. Warm bed.

**MIND:** *Agitated. Ambition;* loss of. *Anger;* ailments after. **Anxiety;** in children; when lifted from cradle. Aversion for school; *for company.* Desire for company. Censorious. Cheerful. Learns with difficulty. *Confusion of mind;* agg. on putting hat; amel. cold bath, washing face and motion. Contradiction; does not tolerate. Delirium, with sleepiness. Delusion; away from home, must get there; as if bed is sinking. Illusions of fancy. Visions of fire. **Discontented;** wants this and that. **Dullness; in children.** Ailments from grief, and excitement. **Fear;** of hearing bad news; of dark. Fickle. Forgetful. Feeling as if she is frightened. Grasping or reaching at something, making gestures as if. Home, desires to go.

Ideas, abundant. Clearness of mind. *Idiocy.* Imbecility. *Indifference. Indignation;* at unpleasant dreams. *Indolence;* aversion to physical work. Industrious; desires activity; after coition. *Irritability; in children* during headache; during perspiration.

*Jealousy.* Ailments from disappointed love. Sick with one of her own sex. Reproaches himself and others. Memory, active. Weakness of memory. Mistakes; speaking; writing; repeating words; using wrong words. Prostration of mind; from talking. Quiet disposition, walking in open air. *Restlessness;* anxious; agg. lying on back; amel. lying on side. *Nymphomania.* Sadness; in girls; before puberty; on waking. Sensitive; oversensitive. Sentimental. *Shrieking;* in children; feels as if she must; grasping with hand and *during sleep.* Stupefaction. Stupidity. Suspicious. Talk; indisposed to; silent; taciturn. Talk; slow learning to. Thoughts wandering from one subject to another. Travel, desire to. Violent. Vehement. *Weeping,* tearful mind. Wildness at unpleasant news. Aversion to mental work.

**HEAD:** Brain; anemia; congestion; during menses. Brain fag. *Tubercular meningitis.* **Pain along sutures.** Sensation as if, brain pressed against skull. Head; caries of bones; chilliness; coldness icy. **Occiput. Vertex. Open fontanelles.** Eruptions; scurfy, black. *Formication, fungus.* Hair falling; in spots; painful. Headache; aching; distensive; full; pressing asunder; pulsating; *sore,* bruised; tearing around the head. **School girls in.** Headache is due to: constipation; tension; exertion; gastric; pressure of hat; from pressing at stool. Headache may be accompanied by cool feeling in head; flatulence; mental weakness; pain in neck; vomiting, transparent phlegm. Headache; agg. by exertion, mental; by *washing;* stepping hard, missteps; amel. by *cold applications;* tobacco smoking. Head; *unable to hold up. Hydrocephalus. Large head.* Head; *motions of,* during sleep, wobbling. Numbness, sensation of; *in occiput. Thin cranium. Ulcers.*

**VERTIGO: In general.** *Constipation from.* Old persons in; with aching in bones; falling forward; nausea; nose discharge; staggering, old people in getting up from sitting. Worse; *headache during;* menses during; *motion; rising from seat, on; stooping:* turning in bed, to left; windy weather.

**EYES:** Perspiration on eye-brows. *Cataract. Conjunctivitis.* Keratitis; herpetic; syphilitic origin; phlyctenular. Cornea; opacity; spots on; ulcers; ectasia. Eyeballs; *inflamed;* from cold; scrofulous. Lachrymation, when yawning. Pain due to artificial light; reading. Pain is; aching; drawing; *as from* foreign body; sore, bruised. *Photophobia.*

Protrusion of eyeball; stiffness. *Redness of eyes.* Sensations of; coldness; heat; swelling; *foreign* body as of. Strabismus, squint. Lids; heat in; spasm of. Paralysis of retina. *Vision;* foggy. Optical illusions; circles, fiery; spots; objects, glittering, change to gray spots; letters seem as if little birds were flying from left to right.

**EAR:** External; redness; eruptions; heat; erysipelatous inflammation; itching; soreness of; swelling, of glands; twitching; ulceration about. Itching with burning in external auditory canal; agg. in warm room, after riding. Pain. Polypus.

Noises in ear (tinnitus); after stool; like singing.

Pain; in front of ear; from left to right; in damp weather. Pain is; aching; burning; in spots jerking; soreness; *stinging, stitching;* tearing; agg. cold air, at night, touch, and warmth. Pulsations. Mastoiditis. Discharge from ear; excoriating; ichorous. Hearing; impaired; *deafness;* because of hypertrophied tonsils, adenoids.

**NOSE:** External; coldness of; eruptions; acne; itching; formication; swelling. Internal; **bleeding, (epistaxis);** in anemic persons; from blowing the nose. Dryness, in warm air. Foreign body as of, in. *Coryza;* with chilliness; laryngitis, with **salivation;** sore throat. Chronic fluent discharge, extending to sinuses. Obstructed. *Polypus. Sneezing.* Pain; sore, bruised; biting; as from foreign body. Tickling. Ulcers round septum.

**FACE: Pale. Yellow. Chlorotic.** Earthy. Bluish. Sallow. Waxy. Pimples, at puberty. Pustules. Heat; during chill; with *cold body or limbs.* Prosopalgia (pain); damp weather; extends to other part; rheumatic. *Perspiration on face.* Lips; cracked; indurated. Pain. Upper jaw, parotids.

**MOUTH:** Dryness. Pain inside cheek (right). *Salivation;* sour. Taste bad, (morning); bitter, bread and water; insipid; metallic; putrid; sweetish.

Teeth; *caries;* for prevention of; crumbling. **Dentition difficult;** slow; with diarrhoea. Pain in teeth; boring; drawing; extending to eyes; stitching; stinging; tearing; rheumatic; from warm drinks; from anything cold; when chewing.

Tongue; numb; cracked; blisters (on tip). Pain on swallowing.

Throat; *adenoids;* diphtheria; redness. Hawk; disposition to; after breakfast; during sleep; while talking. Clergyman's throat. *Inflamed.* Pain; burning; drawing; sore; agg. empty swallowing; yawning. Throat; *relaxation;* roughness. Scratching; weariness in; swelling. Spasm of glottis. Sensation; as if pharynx has disappeared; contracted; suffocation; amel. by warm drinks. Tonsils; enlarged; chronic tonsillitis. Pain, redness and swelling of uvula.

**STOMACH:** Appetite; **increased,** noon, 4 p.m. Constant desire to nurse, *with marasmus.* Appetite; diminished. Aversion, to smoking accustomed cigar. Cannot bear tight clothing.

Desires; bacon; coffee; *fat food;* ham; indigestible things; meat, salted, smoked; condiments; pork; potatoes; raw food. Distended; feeling of. Eructations; difficult; drinking after; forenoon; loud; sour; *waterbrash.* Gagging; after breakfast. Heartburn. Hyperacidity. Hiccough; amel. by hot applications.

*Nausea;* after breakfast; after coffee; during headache; riding in carriage; on stooping; *smoking after;* 4 p.m.

Pain; *burning; cramping; cutting; pressing;* sore; with diarrhoea; agg. cold drinks; amel. by **eating,** *eructations.* Retching. Sensation of; *anxiety;* distension; *emptiness, goneness;* not relieved by eating; *fullness; hanging down,* relaxed as if. Thirst; with dryness of mouth and tongue.

Vomiting; easy; of food; of milk, curdled; infantile; immediately after nursing; when hawking mucus; after icecream.

**ABDOMEN:** Colic; in children; extending to chest; downwards to thighs, to vagina; alternating with head; **menstrual.** Pain; as in stomach; followed by burning leucorrheal flow. Distended. *Flatulent;* rumbling, before menses.

Sensations; as of something alive in; emptiness; movements in; numbness; sense of weakness; sunken. Hard; in hypochondriac region (right). Hernia (inguinal).

**Liver;** gall bladder, to prevent re-formation of stones. Tabes mesenterica. Pancreas. Spleen; cutting pain. Umbilicus; discharge from; bloody (in newborn); retracted.

**RECTUM & ANUS:** Boils in anus. Constipation; in children; *in old people.* *Diarrhoea;* anger after; emotional, fright, grief etc.; in children; alternating with eruptions; chronic; after cider; during dentition; in emaciated people; fruits and icecream agg. Fissure. Fistula. Flatus, during diarrhoea; after drinking; difficult; offensive.

Haemorrhage; from anus. Haemorrhoids (piles): external; *protruding during stool.* Moisture. Mucus discharge. Pain; cutting; pulsating; after or during stool. Polypi in rectum.

Stools; balls (sheep like); bilious; bloody; copious; difficult; flaky flatulent; flocculent; hard; hot; knotty; lumpy; lienteric; mushy; offensive; purulent; shooting out; small; soft; spluttering, noisy; undigested; urging; white.

**URINARY:** Calculi; to prevent re-formation. *Urination;* frequent urging; difficult (dysuria); feeble, from retention, with violent pain in bladder; involuntary (enuresis). Addison's disease. Pain in kidney;' agg. blowing nose, digging when, from jar, lifting. Pain in prostate gland.

Urethra; agglutination of meatus; burning in with chordee; gleety discharge; **chronic gonorrhoeal discharge; white discharge,** in anemic subjects. Induration; chronic. Cutting in; during erections; agg. before, during, and after urination.

**Urine;** albuminous; burning; copious; strong odour. Sediment; flocculent; phosphates; sand; sugar (diabetes mellitus).

**MALE:** Erections; painful; while riding; without sexual desire. Ill effects of masturbation. Seminal emissions. Sexual desire increased; voluptuous feeling. Weakness; stool after.

Scrotum; pimples on; excoriation; itching; moisture; sore; perspiration; relaxed. Testes; hydrocele; inflamed; indurated.

**FEMALE:** Sexual desire; **increased;** insatiable; violent (nymphomania). Leucorrhoea; slimy; bland; milky, creamy; offensive; transparent white; before or after menses. Mammae; full; enlarged; indurated; milk spoiled, **child refuses;** sensitive nodules in; painful; tumours, specially left and in males.

Menses; black, bright red; **clotted; dark;** offensive; with flushed face and / or urinary symptoms. Menstruation; scanty; amenorrhea; before the proper age, delayed; dysmenorrhea; frequent; irregular; during lactation; copious (menorrhagia).

Uterus; contractions in; displacement; heavy; pain, extending to thighs; small, infantile; prolapse of.

**HEART:** Sluggish circulation. Non-closure of foramen ovale. Stitches; agg. deep inspiration, rising from sitting. Palpitation; in anemia; during cough. Varicose veins.

**RESPIRATORY:** Cracking sternum; **Pain;** aching; cutting; **stitching;** clavicular region, sternum, sides, ribs, etc; agg. during cough, touch. Trembling. Ulcers on sternum and clavicle. Chest; tightness; cracking in. Heat in. Pulsation. Quivering.

Cough, crawling in larynx; croupy; dry; hacking; suffocative; amel. lying on; copious; **yellow.**

Larynx; **catarrh;** tuberculous; mucus in; scraping, clearing; tickling sensation. Hoarseness; painless; from mucus in larynx; agg. **morning,** open air.

Lungs; emphysema; haemorrhage; **phthisis, incipient.**

Respiration, accelerated; deep, desire to; difficult; panting; **sighing; suffocative.**

**NECK & BACK:** Right to left. Spina bifida. Fistulae. **Pain;** aching; cutting; tearing; on walking; yawning; amel. when carried. Spasms, opisthotonus. Air draft unbearable on nape; emaciation; heaviness. Stiffness (neck). Tumours, malignant, on neck. Spine and cord; caries (Pott's disease); **curvature of;** weakness; tired feeling.

**EXTREMITIES:** Arthritic nodosities. Bursae. Caries of bones. Coldness. Curving and bending of bones. Eruptions on joints. Heaviness. Lameness. Numbness. Pain; in **joints; rheumatic;** wandering; shifting. Paralysis. Stiffness; during menses. Hands; cold; *trembling;* sucking the thumb.

Psoas abscess. **Late learning,** *to walk.* Flat foot. Cramp in calves. **Hip joint disease.**

SLEEP: Abdominal position. Deep; **morning.** Disturbed; by dreams. Dreams; amorous; anxious; cats; danger; of death; fire; frightful; vivid.

Sleepy; during day; **morning;** while sitting; waking difficult. Yawning.

CHILL & FEVER: Chill ascending, creeping. Fever; hectic; intermittent.

SKIN: Branny. Burning. Cicatrices; break open. **Coldness.** *Yellow, jaundice.* Dry. Boils, furuncles. Pimples. Formication. Freckles. Itching: biting; burning. Lupus. Sarcoma cutis.

# CALCAREA SULPH

It is Dr. Schussler's **connective tissue** remedy. Sulphate radical gives suppurative properties and thick yellow lumpy discharges.

GENERALITIES: *Abscess; glands of;* recurrent; running. Burns and scalds, when suppuration sets in. Suppuration. Pus; bloody; lumpy; scanty; thick. *Cancerous affections.* Cancerous ulcerations. Tumours. *Cystic; fibroid; polypi.* Convulsions; *consciousness without. Epilepsy.* Epileptiform, fever with. Granulations, exuberation. **Haemorrhage;** clotted. Heat; flushes of; eating while. Lack of vital heat. *Reaction poor; lack of.* Inflammation, surgical. Lumps, lumpy effects. Secretions; lumpy, thick. Mucus secretions altered. *Pulsation, throbbing. Sprains,* strains. *Stiffness.* **Motion, aversion to. Swelling of glands**. *Tendency to take cold. Twitching* hysterical; menses during.

Weak, enervated; after acute diseases; dreams after; unable to lie down and stretch; unable to sit up; *menses during;* females in; pain from.

WORSE: 10 to 12 noon. **Night.** 9 p.m. to 4 a.m. Air draft. **Bathing.** Cold in general. *Emotions.* **Exertion;** physical. **Milk.** Heat; room of. *Lifting. Motion.* Onanism. Reading. *Sexual excess. Standing.* Stooping. Swallowing. *Touch.* **Walking.** Warmth; *air of; bed; room. Weather, cold wet.* Getting wet. Wraps.

**BETTER:** Air open, desire for. Bathing *cold, face;* uncovering. Drawing up limbs. Eating after. Hot applications, warm.

**MIND:** Absent minded. Agitated (excitement). Amorous. Anger; ailments after. Answer, aversion to. **Anxiety;** fever during; health about; salvation about. Aversion; bathing; mental work; company.

**Bashful;** timidity. Brooding. Capriciousness. Confusion; morning; on waking. Death, desires. Discontended, displeased. **Dulness.** Delusions; sees images, phantoms; night, while trying to sleep; frightful; visions, spectres. *Excitement.* Fickle. Forgetful. Fear; of death; of dark; of insanity; of misfortune. Desire for green things. Hatred; persons who do not agree with him. Hurry. Hysteria. Imbecility. Indifference (apathy). Insanity. **Irritability.** Lamenting, because he is not appreciated. Mania-a-potu.

Memory; weakness of; for what was about to do; sudden and periodical. Mirth; evening; changing suddenly to melancholy. Mood; changeable, variable. Obstinate; offended easily. Mistakes; speaking. Prostration of mind. Restlessness.

Morose. **Sadness;** afternoon; morning, mirthful in evening; perspiration during. Sits quite stiff and meditates. Starting, startled; easily; from sleep, as if wanting air. Stupefaction. Suspicion. Talk; indisposed to; silent, taciturn. Thoughts; persistent; vanishing of. Sudden unconsciousness. **Weeping;** perspiration during. Work, desire to do, but on attempting to do it, desire is gone.

**HEAD:** Brain; anemia. Congestion of brain; alcoholic liquors from; coughing on; menses during; menses suppressed from; night; warm room in.

Cold; chilliness; vertex of. *Dandruff.* Eruptions, bleeding on scratching; crusta lactea; yellow crusts; suppurating; favus (scald head); pimples, under hair. Formication. **Itching.** *Perspiration. Heat of head;* forehead; warm room in.

Headache; *forehead;* occiput; supra-orbital; vertex. *Aching,* constrictive; distensive, full. Heaviness. Pulsating; beating; throbbing. Tearing, head around. Headache; concussion from; gastric; *injuries mechanical;* shaking head; sun, exposure to; spirituous liquors from; washing head; catarrhal; periodic, nausea with. Worse; forenoon;

looking upward; reading; rising, lying from; shaking head; talking. Better by pressure.

Vertigo; exertion of vision from; optical defects with. Fall; tendency to; *nausea;* floating as if; stooping on; walking.

**EYES:** Inner canthi; inflamed; burning; red. Pus in anterior chamber. Conjunctiva; **mucus discharge;** creamy, profuse; yellow. **Conjunctivitis,** neonatorum. Smoky cornea. Cornea; ulcers, deep; abscess.

Eyeballs; **inflamed;** gonorrhoea; *scrofulous;* itching; injury, after effects of. *Pain; sore, bruised;* aching; burning; foreign body as from; pressing. Looking down piece of paper agg. Photophobia. *Redness of eyes.* Lids; **inflamed;** agglutinated. Eyelashes, falling. Vision; foggy; flickering; dim. Hemiopia.

**EAR:** *Itching.* Erysipelatous inflammation **inside; abscess.** *Caries* of *ossicles. Pain* (Otalgia), stinging. *Pulsation.* Stopped as if. Eruptions and pain behind the ear.

*Acute otitis media.* **Chronic suppuration. Thick, purulent.** Offensive; **bloody,** discharge. Wax; brown and dark; flowing. Noises; buzzing; *ringing; roaring;* singing.

**NOSE:** Caries of bones. *Itching. Sore. Swelling.* Quivering at the root of nose, goes to cheek. **Epistaxis;** scrofula with; face washing after. *Dryness;* air open in *agg.* and *amel.* Coryza (inflammation); right; after bath; bloody in children, epistaxis with; indoors agg.; laryngitis with; washing cold water with, amel.

Discharge; **excoriating;** fluent; thick; **purulent; yellow. Crusts,** scabs. Watery; left at night; right during day.

Obstruction, *stuffiness.* Offensive, odour. Smell; diminished; **wanting; lost.** Sneezing; open air amel. Closure of posterior nares. Yellowish green discharge.

**FACE:** Pale; sickly. *Swollen;* cheeks; upper jaw; toothache *from.* Suppuration. *Eruptions; acne;* boils; eczema; herpes; *pimples* at puberty; pustules. Scurfy. Itching; stinging. Heat; flushes of. Nodes, on. Pain, cutting, from becoming cold; cold application amel. Perspiration. Pain, *upper jaw.*

Lips; pain and sore inside; *cracked;* vesicles, lower. Burning pimples, whiskers. Parotids; sore bruised pain. Submaxillary glands, *swollen.*

**MOUTH:** Breath offensive. Dryness; mouth, tongue; throat. *Inflammation* mouth; tongue; when suppuration threatens. Slimy mucus, in; morning. Slimy saliva. Taste; acrid; *bad;* bitter; metallic; soapy; sweetish. Vesicles, in. Swelling. Gums bleeding; cleansing when; boils, burn like fire; sore; *swelling,* decayed teeth around. Sore palate. Teeth; *caries.* Cold drinks agg. and then amel. Ulceration of roots of teeth.

Tongue; cracked; red, fiery, lines; yellow base; looks like half dried clay; flabby; burning pain; puckered at root.

Throat; *constriction.* Pharyngeal discolouration. *Inflamed. Mucus.* Mucus, drawn from posterior nares; yellow.

Throat pain; burning; left upper in; pressing; *rawness; sore;* stitching. Scraping. Hair or thread as if. Lump, plug, as if. Swallowing difficult. Itching. Swelling. **Ulcers.**

Tonsils; about to discharge, as if; suppuration; peritonsillar abscess. Swelling of cervical glands.

**STOMACH:** Appetite; **increased; ravenous;** wanting, diminished. Constriction. Aversion to coffee; *milk;* **meat,** but desires smoked meat. Desire; cold drinks; alcoholic drinks, claret; fruit, acid, green; green and sour vegetables; things, green, refreshing, salty; sour; acids; tea.

**Indigestion. Distension;** eating after. Eructations; *sour;* bitter; empty; tasteless; food of; foul; morning; night. Heartburn. Nausea; headache during; entering a warm room, after being in open air.

Pain; burning; cramping; cutting; gnawing; convulsive, stool before; digging; pressing; sore stitching. Afternoon agg. Stool before and after agg. Cold drinks amel. Emptiness; weak; sinking. Fullness. Heaviness, weight, in morning. Stone as if in. Pulsations. Feeling of weakness; seems to come from head. **Thirst; extreme;** forenoon. *Vomiting;* headache during; acrid, sour; bile; bitter; food of; infantile. *Waterbrash.*

**ABDOMEN:** *Colic;* burning; cramping; cutting; dragging; pressing, sore; stitching; cold things, drinks, amel. Distension. Fullness. Pulsations. Heaviness as from a load. **Flatulence;** eating after. Inflammation, typhoid fever in. Rumbling. Sensation of coldness in. Skin were too tight. Tension. *Appendicitis. Cramping* in hypochondriac region. *Hepatalgia;* pressing; sore; stitching. Stitching in left inguinal region. Tabes mesenterica.

**RECTUM & ANUS:** Peri-rectal abscess. Fistula-in-ano. Constipation; consumption during; hectic fever with; constriction; cramp. Diarrhea; excoriation; **children in;** bloody; eating after; change of weather; painless.

*Haemorrhage;* from anus. Piles, (haemorrhoids); external. Burning; stool after. Moisture at anus.

Pain; aching; burning; pressing; sore, bruised; stitching, shooting; stinging; stool during; stool hard after. Tenesmus. Rectum; prolapse of. **Formication in** anus.

Stool; *difficult;* dry; *hard; knotty;* nodular, lumpy; insufficient; unsatisfactory. Large. Lienteric. Involuntary. Scanty. Soft. *Purulent.* Ineffectual urging. White coated. Yellow.

**URINARY:** Catarrh of bladder. Retention of urine. Nephritis. Pyelitis. Discharges; **bloody;** gleety; **gonorrhoeal;** chronic; **purulent** yellow. Burning pain.

**MALE: Impotency;** seminal emissions with. Prostatic suppuration. Hydrocele (of boys). Testes, drawing pain, morning: sore, afternoon; suppuration.

**FEMALE:** Abortion, tendency to. **Leucorrhoea;** *excoriating; burning;* copious; menses after, *before;* white; purulent; yellow.

Mammae, inflamed. Amenorrhoea, delayed menses. Menses; frequent, too early, too soon. Irregular; late, delayed and prolonged; protracted copious (profuse); meno and metrorrhagia. Menses dark, pale; suppressed scanty flow.

Uterus; *fibroids;* cancer. Pain. Prolapse. Vagina; itching; menses during and after. Ulcers. Pain; burning; bearing down; during menses, in vulvae and labia.

**HEART:** Pericarditis.   Pain in heart, to thighs. Palpitation; ascending, agg.

**RESPIRATION:** Bronchitis. Chest, eruptions; eczema; rash; vesicles. Itching.

**Pain;** cutting; burning; rawness. stitching; sternum at, sides of chest. Inspiration; cough; stool before; agg.

Constriction; tightness; weakness. Fluttering. *Oppression.*

Cough; croupy, only after **walking; dry;** night; hacking; hoarse; loose; rattling; sharp; spasmodic. Worse; *bathing,* wet getting; lying; talking. Better by air cold, open.

Expectoration; clear white; bloody, mucus; **copious, profuse; lumpy;** thick, viscid; *purulent;* transparent; **yellow.** House in agg.

Larynx; laryngitis; **catarrh; croup; recurrent;** sore; *scraping;* clearing; crawling; dust as from. *Hoarse.* Sudden shriek while speaking. Rawness in trachea.

Pneumonia; results of. Hemoptysis. Hepatisation (lungs). Resolution. Phthisis. **Empyema.** Asthma, hectic fever with. Dyspnea; rattling. Worse on coughing; lying while; walking.

**BACK:** Coldness. Heat. Pain; drawing; stitching; coughing; menses during; motion on; *sitting from,* while. Stiffness; walking amel.

Stiff neck; sore, bruised; across the back; vertex to. Curvature of dorsal spine, **lumbo-sacral spine.** Pain and itching between scapulae. *Spina bifida.* **Weakness;** lumbo-sacral; used feeling, riding on.

**EXTREMITIES: Stiffness.** Awkwardness. Arthritic nodosities. Coldness. Pimples; inflamed, sensitive. Paralysis. Weakness.

Pain; joints in **gouty;** *rheumatic;* sore; bruised; chill during. Numbness.

Hands: cold; *cold perspiration; burning pain;* stitching. Trembling. Heavy, tired legs. Gouty joints. Dropsical swelling.

**Deep ulcers.** Paraplegia. Trembling. Weakness; *walking after. Lameness* (knees). Stiffness (thighs). Hip joint; *tuberculosis; pain;* suppuration.

**SLEEP:** Restless. Dreams; anxious; *frightful.* Sleepiness; hectic fever with; night sleeplessness; midnight before; thoughts from; activity of mind from. Waking, with dreams of convulsions. Startling up, as if wanting air, in sleep.

**CHILL & FEVER:** Chill; shaking. Covers; drinking; eating agg. Fever; **hectic;** intermittent; small-pox. Uncovering a.ne¹. Perspiration; profuse; on coughing.

**SKIN:** *Corns; burning; painful; pressing.* Cracks. Pale. Yellow (jaundice). **Dry. Crusty.** Boils; *furuncles.* **Eczema;** in infants. Discharges, yellow. *Pimples.* **Herpes.** Psoriasis. Whitlow.

Skin; *unhealthy; would not heal.* Pulsating. **Warts.** Tubercles. Rash, scaly. Ulcers; **deep;** offensive, *putrid;* crusty, cancerous; bleeding; burning; indolent; indurated. Urticaria; vesicular. Excoriation. Intertrigo.

# Note on Calcium

Calcium and phosphates are widely distributed throughout living tissues. The great majority is found in bone and the ability of the skeleton to turn over calcium and phosphate is essential for growth, the prevention and healing of fractures, and skeletal remodelling in response to physiological and pathological stress.

The extracellular fluid concentration of calcium is critical to maintain normal neuromuscular activity; and a fall in plasma concentration results in tetany and convulsions. Also a rise in extracellular fluid calcium has many adverse effects including delayed neuromuscular conduction and paralysis.

The total amount of calcium within soft tissues is similar to that found in the extracellular fluid. However, cytosol calcium concentrations are thought to be 100 to 1000 times lower than extracellular. Within cells, mitochondria are capable of accumulating large amounts of calcium against electrochemical gradient.

Hormonal activity, enzyme activity, membrane function, and cell division are all important roles for intracellular calcium. Calcium is also essential for neurotransmitter release as well as for the release of hormones and other secretory products. This is true for every endocrine that has been thus far studied.

Calcium has a role to play in coagulation of blood and milk.

There is a significant exchange of calcium between extracellular fluid and bone. Studies with radioisotopes in normal human adults show that between 1 and 2 per cent of total body calcium is exchanged over in few days.

# FERRUM PHOS.

**Introduction:** Ferrum phos is by far the best of the twelve tissue remedies for inflammation, specially in anemic subjects. This is not the place to go into details of inflammation. Inflammation is the tissue reaction to an irritant. The irritant may be injury, chemical; new growth or bacterial (more common). The cardinal signs of inflammation are: 1. heat, 2. redness, 3. swelling, 4. pain. The result is altered function.

Ferrum phos is useful in inflammation of all tissues of body except perhaps bone. Understanding of the symptomatology of Ferrum Phos will be easy if the main idea of inflammation is properly grasped. It all depends on:

1. The tissue.

2. The stage of inflammation.

3. Body defences.

For instance, in the nose if it is catarrhal stage, there is increased discharge from nose. Further, nose gets severely congested and bleeding i.e. epistaxis may ensue. Similarly, in lungs it may be pneumonitis, pneumonic consolidation, hemoptysis, etc. Pleuritis may be dry or with exudation.

If the inflammation is in inner organs, the body tries to **guard the organ by muscle contraction. That is the explanation** of guarding seen in appendicitis or localised peritonitis. In muscular nollow organs, the muscle in the wall may contract, thus producing constriction. In vagina, it leads to vaginismus. Prolonged contraction may lead to exhaustion of muscles leading to relaxation and prolapse.

In rectum, the stages may be proctitis, constriction, haemorrhoids, bleeding, prolapse.

If this general idea is assimilated, then the understanding of Ferrum phos is the application of it to different organs of the body.

Certain things are left out, which cannot be explained on the basis of pathology. These are the peculiarities of the drug. We know the drug by its peculiarities, which are its identification marks.

**GENERALITIES:** Useful in anemia, haemorrhages and diseases of veins. It affects the venous circulation of **lungs;** *ears;* nose (root); and eustachian tubes. Useful in inflammation, induration and enlargement of blood-vessels. Indisposed to physical exertion. Physical and mental lassitude. Neuralgic pains; orbit; right; agg. morning. **Full; soft, flowing, pulse.** Hyperaemia. *Passive congestion and weakness.* Bloody discharges. Bruised soreness; chest, shoulder, muscles. Inflammation of soft parts. Burning rawness.

Abscess. *Anemia. Anxiety;* general, physical. Congestion of blood. Dropsy external; heart disease from. Swelling; affected parts of, inflammatory. Haemorrhage; orifices from; passive oozing. *Hard bed sensation.* Heat, flushes of. Injuries. *Inflammation.* Lassitude. Lie down, inclination to. Orgasms of blood.

Pain; sore; bruised; stitching; tearing; downward. Paralysis (rheumatic). Complaints from suppressed perspiration. Plethora. Post-operative disorders. *Puberty* and *youth.* Pulsation (throbbing). Rickets. *Scurvy.* Secretions: blood-streaked; meat-water like. Sensitiveness. Symptoms; alternate; ascend; to right. Pain goes to side lain on.

Tendency to take cold. Trembling. Weak; unable to lie down; moving difficult; waking on. Weariness.

**WORSE:** Morning 4 a.m. to 9 a.m. Noon 12 to 6 p.m. Evening 6 to 9 p.m.; 6 p.m.; at the same hour. Midnight after. Air; open cool. Cold; air; becoming; while sweating or hot. Breathing deep. Coughing. Eating; before. Foods; cake; coffee; tea; herring; meat, sour. Heat of fire, sun; becoming overheated. Jarring. Lifting. Light. Lying. Motion. Noise. Right side. Standing. Stooping. Swallowing; empty. Talking, speaking. Thinking of complaint. Vomiting. Waking.

**BETTER:** Bleeding, haemorrhage. Cold applications. Company. Motion. Sleep after. Urination.

**MIND:** Agitation (excitement). Ambition, loss of. Anger; ailments after; trembling with; violent. Anxiety; conscience of (as guilty of crime); fear with; fever during; hypochondriacal. Aversion; motion of; mental work. Cheerful. Company; amel.; aversion to. Concentration difficult. Confusion; motion amel.; washing the face amel. Delirium; very talkative, being wide awake. Discontented. Excitement; evening; loquacity with; unnatural.

Fear; apoplexy; crowd in a; death of; evil of; misfortune of; people of. Forgetful; names, faces etc. Hysteria.

Ideas, abundant. Clearness of mind, Impetuous; evening, Indifference; pleasure to. Indolence. Irritability; own mental sluggishness, loquacity, Mania-a-potu. Memory, weakness of. Mirth. Mood, alternating. Morose. Obstinate. Restlessness; heat during; tossing about in bed; driving out of bed.

Sensitive, oversensitive. Silent; indisposed to talk. Thoughts; changing suddenly from pleasant to unpleasant. Unconsciousness; fever during. Weeping.

**HEAD:** Brain; anemia; *congestion, heat of face* with; *menses during.* Brain-fag. Sensitive to least jar. Sore, bruised.

Head, coldness. Hair falling, combing when. Hard scalp. Heat of head; menses *during;* vertex. Itching. Hydrocephalus, impending. Rolling motions of head, with moaning. Pushed forward as if. Tired feeling. Sensitive; to cold air; to touch. Shocks, blows.

Headache; concussion from; emotions *excited;* heat; menses, before, during; shaking head; sun exposure to; anemic; coryza with; earache with; fever with; vertigo with; vomiting undigested food.

Pain; *aching;* constrictive; distensive, full; heaviness. Pulsating, beating, throbbing. Sore, bruised. Stitching. Tearing.

Forehead. Sides, down sides. Supra-orbital. *Temples. Vertex,* down sides, menses agg.

Headache is worse, bending forward; chill during; on closing eyes; motion, shaking head; pregnancy, during 3rd month; stooping;

vomiting; wrapping head. Better by; cold application; air cold; nose-bleed; pressure; tea; profuse urination.

Vertigo; exhaustion from; menier's disease. Fall forward. Throbbing headache, with flushed face. Nausea, Staggering. Intoxicated as if. Swims, everything around, could hardly move. Obscuration of vision with. Vertigo agg. by: afternoon; chill during; on closing eyes; head moving; looking downward; lying down; passing over or seeing running water; riding in a carriage; *rising* on, from bed.

**EYES:** Pain; reading while. *Conjunctivitis,* discharge. Cornea, abscess. Eyeballs; burning; inflammation acute; dentition during. *Lachrymation.* Pain; aching, burning; sand as from; stitching, shooting; amel. profuse urination. *Photophobia,* headache during; menses during. Protrusion of eyeballs; exophthalmus. Foreign body as of. Sunken. Iritis. Eyelids; redness, styes, lower, right; swollen, cystic tumours. Amaurosis; fainting as from; stooping. Dim vision during headache.

**EARS: Erysipelatous inflammation,** external ear; inside. Pain and inflammation in external auditory canal. Hypersensitive to noise, sounds, etc. Pain, *otalgia;* **aching** drawing; hammering; stinging; tearing. Touch agg. Night agg. Open air amel.

Pulsation. Mastoiditis. Tympanic membrane; dark beef red; thickened; red, bulging. *Acute otitis* media; suppurative. Bloody discharge. *Hearing, acute;* deafness; hearing, difficult.

Noises in ear; lying while, *buzzing;* humming; ringing; singing; like running water.

**NOSE:** Epistaxis; anemic persons; bright; blowing the nose from; cough with; fever during; headache during; old people in; posteriorly; predisposition to; puberty at. Inflammation; catarrhal, ordinary cold in head.

**Coryza;** cough with; inflammation in larynx with; warm drinks agg. Discharge; crusts, scab; excoriating; purulent. Pain; rawness posterior nares; inspiration agg. *Sneezing.*

**FACE:** Bluish circles around the eyes. Chlorotic, earthy. Hippocratic. **Pale.** *Red,* alternate with paleness; circumscribed; during pain, headache, menses and dysmenorrhea. Sallow. Sunken, Swelled. Oedematous, *yellow.* Eruptions, forehead. Heat 6 p.m.; flashes of;

sitting while.  Pain (Prosopalgia); inflammatory, pressing; pulsating; stinging; stitching.  *Motion, stooping agg.* Cold application amel.

Perspiration.  Pulsation.  Hot cheeks, with toothache.  Eruptions on chin, jaws, dislocated as if, lips; bluish; pale; dryness; swelling red.

Parotid glands; pain, swelling, mumps.

**MOUTH:** Bleeding.  Dryness.  *Salivation.* Taste; insipid; putrid; sweetish.  Gums; bleeding; red; inflamed; swelling.  Toothache; with swelling of cheek; inflammatory; external warmth or warm things agg.; cold water or anything amel.

Tongue; clean and red; dark; white.  Burning pain.  Swelling under.  Ranula.

**THROAT:** Predisposition to abscess.  Blood oozing.  Redness. Hawks greenish lumps.  Acute *follicular inflammation.*

Pain; burning; rawness, sore; singing agg.  Lump, plug as of. Swallowing empty painful and agg.

*Tonsils,* red; enlarged; tuft like exudation.  Quinsy; acute inflammation.  Predisposition to suppuration.  Exophthalmic goitre.

**STOMACH:** Appetite; increased; relish without; wanting; diminished.

Aversion to; acids; coffee; meat; milk.  Cannot bear tight clothing. Desires; alcoholic drinks; ale, brandy; cold food; sour; stimulants. *Indigestion;* distension after eating.    Eructations; bitter; empty, tasteless; **food of;** greasy; sour; vexation after.

Heartburn; coffee after; meat after; sour things after.  Waterbrash. Hiccough; hot application amel.  Inflammation of stomach.  Flushes of heat.  Fullness of.

Nausea; anxious, deathly; *eating after;* morning, rising on; pregnancy; sleep during; wakes him at night; sudden attack of, in throat.

Pain; burning; cramping; pressing; sore, bruised.  Eating 2 to 3 hours after agg.  Pressure agg. Cold drinks amel.

*Thirst; large quantities for;* night.

Vomiting; coughing; drinking after; headache during; heat during; **morning;** night; pain during; *pregnancy; riding in carriage. Vomiting; acrid, sour; bile; blood, bright; food of, immediately after eating, intermittently,* **undigested.** Green mucus..

Relaxation of pylorus.

**ABDOMEN:** Sensitive to clothing. Colic; burning; cramping; *pressing;* sore, tenderness; agg. during menses and before stool. Distension. Flatulence. Gurgling. Rumbling. Fullness. Heaviness, as from load. Inflammation; peritonitis; enteritis.

Hard: In spots, layer of hard substance as. Tension. Weakness of. Inflammation in cecal region (Typhlitis) Strangulated hernia. Liver enlarged, *pain* (Hepatalgia). Spleen; enlarged; inflamed.

**RECTUM & ANUS:** Constipation; habitual. Constriction, closure; stool after. *Diarrhoea;* painless; eating after; afternoon, night agg.; hot weather. Dysentery. Haemorrhoids; bleeding; inflamed. Prolapse; children in; stool during. Tenesmus, night.

Stools; corrosive; excoriating; bloody; bloody green; brown; difficult; frequent; hard; involuntary; *lienteric;* mucus bloody, muddy dirty water; small; soft; odourless; thin, watery, liquid; undigested. Ineffectual urging.

**URINARY:** Bladder, haemorrhage; cystitis. Pain; neck in; standing agg.; urination amel. Paralysis. Retention of urine; children in; fever or acute illness from. Urging to urinate; constant; daytime only; frequent; night, painful, sudden, hasten must or urine will escape.

Urination; after every drink; *frequent; involuntary;* cough during; day-time only; lying down amel.; laughing; night; *sneezing when;* walking while. Kidney. Chronic nephritis. Pain. Discharges; gleety; *gonorrhoea;* mucus; haemorrhage.

Urine; albuminous; cloudy on standing; bloody, last part; dark colour; red; pale; copious, profuse; headache with; night. Ammoniacal. Scanty. Haemoglobin sediment. Mucus. Sp. gravity increased. Suppressed; heat from.

**MALE:** Erections; troublesome. Seminal emissions. Sexual passion; increased; with weak powers; wanting.

Prostate, inflamed. Testes, inflamed. Epididymitis. Seminal vesicles; *acute inflammation*. *Varicocele;* pain, aching.

**FEMALE:** Abortion; tenoency to. Coition aversion. Conception, difficult (sterility). Sexual desire diminished. Dryness. Leucorrhoea; excoriating; bland, menses before; milky, white; thin, watery. Inflamed mammary glands. *Amenorrhea.* Menses painful (dysmenorrhea); with frequent urging to urinate; preventive as a. Menses; frequent, too early, too soon; intermittent; irregular; late, delayed. Copious, profuse (Menorrhagia); puerperal. Metrorrhagia, protracted.

Menses; *scanty flow; suppressed;* bright red; pale; thin, watery; with flushed face. Inflamed ovaries.

Uterus; pain; after pains; ovarian pain with; bearing down with ovarian pain; coition during. Prolapse.

Vaginismus. Vagina; dry; burning; sensitive; digital examination agg.; pain, crampy, coition during.

Vulvae, labia; inflamed, burning.

**HEART:** Sluggish circulation. Congestion of blood. Arteritis. Dilatation. Distension of arteries. Aneurysm. Varicose veins; in young persons. Pulse; **flowing; frequent; fast;** *full;* **soft.**

Heart; dilatation. Goitre heart. Myocarditis. Endocarditis. Pericarditis. Angina. *Pain;* to left spine; external pressure agg.; stretching the body amel. Palpitation; *audible;* motion walking rapidly on; noise from; noise every strange agg.; sitting while agg. Anxiety in the region of. Constriction. Contraction.

**RESPIRATORY:** Asthma; soreness in chest with; spasmodic; night. Anxiety in *chest.* Tightness. Oppression. Congestion, fullness, heat. **Bronchitis,** *capillary.*

Chest; sensitive to clothes. Hard as if. Pain; rawness; soreness; stitching; intercostal region; sides; right. Pain agg. during cough; inspiration; deep breathing.

Cough; irritation in chest or air passages from; asthmatic; constant; dry; morning; evening; hacking; loose; nose bleed with; painful; paroxysmal; spasmodic; tickling; tormenting; whooping. Cough agg. by air, cold open; bending downwards; deep breathing;

eating; fever during; lying; sleep daytime; pregnancy during; rising on, morning; singing; talking.

Expectoration; **bloody,** blood-streaked, bright red; dark; after a fall; copious; daytime only; difficult; frothy; mucus, greenish; offensive; purulent; putrid taste; scanty; thick, viscid; yellow; watery.

Larynx. Dryness. Laryngitis; membranous; tuberculous; singer's. Voice hoarse; coryza during; *lost.*

*Lungs; congestion. Haemorrhage;* bright red; concussion of, fall after; cough with; tubercular. **Pneumonia;** *in aged* persons; secondary. Phthisis; **acute,** florida, sycotic, **pituitous.** Pleurisy. *Dyspnea.* Rattling, shallow respiration. Agg. cough with; lying while; *night;* motions.

**BACK & NECK:** Coldness. Crick in; cervical region. Pain between scapulae. Pain; stitching; tearing; *menses during;* agg. by sitting, standing, walking. Stiffness, cervical region. Pain lumbar or lumbo-sacral region. Weakness, sitting while.

**EXTREMITIES:** Coldness. Cracking in tendons. Heaviness, tired limbs. Awkwardness; drops things; stumbling etc. Inflammation of joints; synovitis; rheumatic; gouty. Pain; joints. in; gouty; rheumatic; stitching; motion on. Dropsical swelling of joints. Weakness of joints.

Drawing pain in deltoid (right); shoulder (right); extends to chest and wrist; motion agg. and amel.; night agg. Elbow; swelling, sprain from. Wrists; forearm; agg. while writing or grasping anything.

Hands; **coldness;** heat reading while; numbness, right. Dry heat in palms. Fingers; chilblains; contraction; nodes; numbness. Nails, blue, felon.

*Coldness of feet;* during fever; crampy pain. Jerking. Joints, gouty, rheumatic. *Sensitive.* Twitching. *Sciatica.* Cramps in thighs, legs; feet. Pain; hot *swelling of knees;* weakness of. Heaviness of legs; numbness. Restless (legs); weakness.

Pain in ankles; *extending upwards.*

**SLEEP:** Sleepiness; stools after. Sleeplessness, with sleepiness. Dreams; anxious; confused; falling of; insane becoming; quarrels; nightmare; vivid.

CHILL & FEVER: Periodicity regular and distinct. Shaking chill. Fever; **in general;** *chill without; dry heat;* internal heat; perspiration on hands with.

Fever; adynamic; catarrhal; chicken-pox; dentition during; inflammatory; influenza; measles, haemorrhagic, bronchial symptoms with; puerperal; scarlet; yellow.

Perspiration; *in general,* **clammy;** cold; exhausting; profuse; night at, of phthisis.

SKIN: Burning. *Chilblains.* Coldness. Pale. Red. Dry. Desquamating. Warts. Erysipelas, red, shining recurrent, chronically inflamed.

# KALI MUR

(Kali mur shares the weakness and other properties of potassium. It resembles Nat mur in certain respects because of its chloride ion.)

GENERALITIES: Abscess. Anemia with skin affections. Ball, globus (feeling). Bathing, dread of. Burns; blisters from burns. Cancerous affections. Hodgkin's disease. Hypertrophy. Contraction; general sense of.

Convulsions; **nervous children** in; with dyspepsia and urticaria. Clonic. Epileptic. Epileptiform. Eyeballs bulging. During sleep. Suppression of skin eruptions, from.

Dropsy; external; internal; heart disease from; liver or kidney disease from. Exudation; effusion; hard. Fibrous tissue. *Induration; stony. Swelling of glands.*

Formication. Full feeling internally. Haemorrhage; blood clots quickly (contrast with Kali phos). Heaviness; externally; internally. Infiltration. Inflammation; to favour absorption. Injuries. Glands. Itching in bones. Reaction; poor; lack of.

Lassitude. Lie down inclination to. **Loose, torn as if.** Mottled. Patchy. Muscles; relaxed. Numbness; externally.

Pain; *cutting* externally; in bones. Extort cries. Shooting. *Stitching. Wandering.* Paralysis; one sided; organs of. Pulsations; throbbing. **Scurvy.** Discharges; bland; milky; slimy; *sticky; thick; white.*

Sensitiveness. Sluggishness. Sprains and strains. Symptoms; crosswise; outward. **Syphilis.** Tendons; crating in. Tension; muscles. Twitching. *Vaccination, ill effects of.*

Weak; diarrhoea after; acute diseases after; walking from. *Whiteness.* Wounds; cuts; shrinking.

**WORSE:** 5 p.m. Night. 9 p.m. to 4 a.m. **Midnight.** *Midnight after. Air open, cool* (aversion to). Bathing; sea. Clothing; tight. Cold; in general; air; becoming; wet weather. Damp dwellings; being in. Eating after. Exertion. Food; alcoholic, beer; cold drinks; cold food; fat; pastry; *rich.* Heat; body of. *Warmth;* bed of. Summer. Lifting. Lying; bed in; painful side; right side. Menses before, during and after. Motion. Walking. Sitting while. Periodically. Suppressions. Touch. Wet *getting.* Winter.

**BETTER:** Bleeding with (mental symptoms). Cold applications in general. Drinks, cold. Hair, letting down. Sun light desire for. Sun exposure to. Hot, dry applications. Rubbing. *Scratching.*

**MIND:** *Anger;* at trifles. Desires death. Delusions; he must starve. Discontented. Fear; evil of. Fickle. Imbecility. Indifference; to pleasure. Indolence. Insanity; with moaning. Mirth; alternating with sadness; amel. by nose-bleed. Sadness; evening; with chilliness. Obstinate.

Sit; inclination to; in complete silence or moody silence. Quiet meditation.

Startled. Taciturn. Talks in sleep. Unconsciousness; in advanced stage of brain and meningeal disease.

**HEAD:** Loose as if. Dandruff; white. Eruptions; crusta lactea; favus (scald head).

Headache; constipation from; fatty food; hawking up white mucus, vomiting white mucus. Headache is; bursting; cutting, darting; heaviness; weight as from; sore, bruised; *stitching;* extending to teeth.

Occiput. Vertex across (ear to ear). Binding up the hair; pressure; urine; stooping and 2 to 3 a.m. agg. Wrapping amel.

Shocks, blows, jerks; occiput.

Vertigo; alcoholic liquors from; after violent exertion; with headache. Menier's disease. Occipital. Periodical. Peculiar feeling in cervical muscles. Worse on lying down.

**EYES:** Burning. Twitching; inner canthi. Cataract. Clear discharge. Trachoma. Redness.

Cornea; keratitis, syphilitic; spots on; ulcers, flat; vesicles, pustules; abscess. Pus in anterior chamber. Iritis.

Eyeballs; eruptions about; itching; inflammation. Lachrymation with cold in head. Pain in; as from sand; pressing forward; suddenly in right; stitching; shooting. Protrusion of eyeballs; forced out of head with cough as f; in goitre.

Eyelids; scabs; crusts; granulations. Suppurating points on the edge of. Retina; exudation; irritable.

Smoke before eyes; sparks; on blowing nose, coughing or sne ezing.

**EARS:** Eczema; behind the ear. Inflammation, erysipelatous. Swelling of glands, about ear. Soreness. Ulceration of ring hole. Mastoiditis. Pain behind the ear, stitching.

Granulations; inflammation; polypus; external auditory canal. Eustachian tubes; catarrh; itching; obstruction; soreness. Tympanic membrane; granular proliferous inflammation; retracted. Middle ear; catarrhal inflammation; acute and chronic suppuration. Discharge; milk white. Pain (otalgia); cold air agg. Stopped as from plug. Stuffy. Tingling.

Deafness; from eustachian catarrh; exposure to cold; from swollen glands about the ear; old age; thickened drum; from throat affection.

Noises in the ear (tinnitus aurium). Chirping. Snapping. Blowing nose; sneezing; swallowing when; turning head on.

**NOSE:** Acute catarrhal inflammation. Copious discharge; excoiating; fluent; purulent; thick; viscid; white; cough with; abuse of mercury from. Coryza; dryness. Crusts. Itching. Obstruction (stuffiness); *Diphtheria* in; evening; with mucus. Sneezing; desire to; tension n cheeks with. Sinus in general. Thick; tough; viscid; yellowish green discharge from posterior nares.

**FACE:** Bloated; bluish; dirty looking; sickly, suffering expression. Sunken. Painful swelling. Cancer; lupus. Acne. Flashes of heat. tching; right. Parotid gland; swollen; enlarged; inflamed; metastasis, o testes. Submaxillary glands; inflammatory swelling.

Pain; right; paralysis with; lancinating; becoming more frequent gradually; stitching; chewing when agg.; touch agg. Tension. Twitching; coughing, eating, or speaking when. Swelling of cheeks. Pain in jaw; extending to other parts.

Lips; ulcers; dry, peeling; swelling; eruptions mouth around. Excoriation, angles of mouth. Epithelioma.

**MOUTH:** *Aphthae;* in children; mucus membrane red. Saliva; ough, stingy. Taste; bad; bitter; breakfast, dinner after; metallic; putrid; saltish; sour.

Ulcers; nursing mother in; syphilitic. Vesicles. Bleeding. Red. Gums, scorbutic. Teeth: on edge and loose; aching; stitching; with swelling of cheek; with swollen gums; evening agg.

Tongue; aphthae; eating cold amel.; grayish; violet; white at base; dirty yellow; dryness; tumour growing on, as if. Swelling. Ulcers.

**THROAT:** Chronic constriction. Diphtheria; croup with. Grayish; white; tenacious mucus. Redness. Dry; cough with. Hawks; cheesy, etid lumps. Heat. Acute follicular inflammation.

Pain; extending to ear; chronic; sore; cold amel. Scraping. Sensation of; coldness; crawling. Stiffness. Swallowing difficult; must wist his neck to get it down. Swelling. Ulcers; soreness from. Uneasy feeling in oesophagus.

Tonsils; inflamed; acute (quinsy); enlarged, swollen; caseous deposits on; gray; ulcers gray.

**STOMACH:** Appetite increased; attack of; between regular periods of eating; wants to eat every hour; drinking water amel. Appetite; diminished; after drinking water; habitual.

Aversion; fats; rich food; meat. Desires; cold drinks.

Stomach; disordered; indigestion; fat food after; pastry. Constriction. Inflamed from hot drinks.

Eructations; bitter; alternating with pain in chest and abdomen; food of (regurgitation); hot drinks from; incomplete; ineffectual; morning; night.

Emptiness; not relieved by eating. Heaviness; night. Thirst; chill during; extreme. Gagging; gulping of white mucus with.

Vomiting; scalding; bile; blood, clotted, dark; food of; green dark. Incessant. Sudden. Mucus. Waterbrash.

**ABDOMEN:** Pain; cramping. Menses appear, as if would. Stool before, during agg. Distension; whooping cough in. Flatulence; night; preventing sleep. Inflammation (peritonitis); exudation with.

Rumbling; stool before. Emptiness. *Fullness; eating after.* Tension. Swelling. Appendicitis. Typhlitis. Pressing pain, right hypochondriac region; tension; griping pain, hypogastric region. Inguinal bubo.

Liver; atony of; fullness (congestion). Jaundice. Spleen; enlarged; pressing pain. Cutting pain, umbilical region.

**RECTUM & ANUS:** Condylomata. Constipation. Diarrhoea; day time only; fats from; pastry after; vaccination agg. Dysentery; blood only. Haemorrhage from anus. Haemorrhoids (Piles); bleeding; dark venous blood; external; large; walking agg. Itching; stool after. Pain; sore; stinging; stool after, during; walking while.

Paralysis. Coldness in anus. Crawling; stool after. Formication. Worms complaints; thread worms. Perineum, bald sensation.

Stools; corrosive; oily; gray coloured; copious; flocculent; green; dry; hard; involuntary, on passing flatus; large; mucus; slimy; bloody; white; offensive; pale; pale ochre-coloured. Constant urging.

**URINARY:** Bladder catarrh; cystitis, acute and chronic. Retention of urine. Ineffectual urging to urinate.

Nephritis; chronic; pain in kidneys. Urethra; gleety discharge, with eczema; itching; pain cutting.

Urination; *dribbling;* feeble; frequent at night; involuntary. Urine; albuminous, pregnancy during; cloudy; black; greenish black; pale; red; white. *Copious.* Scanty. Gelatinous. Sediment; mealy; sugar (diabetes mellitus), with derangement of liver. Urine; suppressed.

**MALE:** Erections; painful; troublesome. Sexual passion; chilliness and apathy with. Stinging pain in scrotum. Hydrocele (boys of).

Balanitis. Ulcers, chancres. Soft chancres. Testes; induration of; inflammation, from suppressed gonorrhoea, drawing pain.

**FEMALE:** Leucorrhoea; acrid, excoriating albuminous, slimy; bland; **milky;** thick; viscid; stringy; white.

Mammae; inflammation, before pus formation; soft nodules. Pain, soreness; **menses before.**

Menses; black; bright red; clotted; dark; tarry; viscid; thick. Menses; painful; scanty; suppressed; amenorrhoea. Delayed menses. Frequent menses, too soon. *Menorrhagia* (copious). Metrorrhagia. Vagina; acute and chronic inflammation.

**HEART:** Pulse; full; hard; intermittent; irregular; slow; soft; small.

Pericarditis. Cutting in region of. Sore, stitching. Deep inspiration agg.

Palpitation; dropsy with; excessive flow of blood to heart, from, morning; hungry when. Coldness of heart.

Lymphatic vessels; inflammation with acute glandular infiltration and swelling.

**RESPIRATORY:** Bronchitis. Chest pain; pressing; stitching; agg. respiration. Tightness, as from vapours of sulphur. Heat. Oppression, palpitation with. Rawness.

Cough; stomach from; as from sulphur vapours; barking; with coryza; croupy; racking; short; spasmodic; violent; whooping; evening lying down on; loose, morning. Worse; day only; lying; evening; night; **3 A. M.;** winter.

Expectoration; albuminous; grayish white; milky; gray; mucus; thick; transparent; viscid; white; bloody; flies from mouth; **evening** agg.

Larynx; dryness; irritation; inflammation, membranous, tuberculous. Hoarseness, coryza during.

Lungs; constriction; hepatisation. Inflammation; stage of consolidation. Pleurisy. Tuberculosis.

Respiration; deep; difficult; impeded; rapid; rattling; snoring. Asthma; with gastric derangement; at 3 A.M.

**NECK & BACK:** Coldness.  Pain; shooting; breathing when; sitting while; waking on.  Lying while amel.

Peculiar feeling in neck.  Stiffness; dancing after; exposure to drought of air, when overheated.  Morning.  Swelling of neck glands.

Lumbo-sacral pain; rising from bed; drawing; extending to feet; morning.  Wasting of spinal cord.

Scapulae; buzzing under left; pain between scapulae.

**EXTREMITIES:** Upper with lower (alternating or concomitant). Cracking in tendons. Cramps. Numbness. Pain; rheumatic, warmth of bed agg. Restlessness; evening. Weakness; morning. Shoulders; heaviness; right. Pain; left shoulder; pressing. Weakness (elbow). drawing pain in wrists.

 Coldness of hands and feet; evening.  Cracking of tendons on back of hand.  Heat.  Chilblains.  Lameness of fingers.  Twitching (thighs). **Crampy** pain in legs.  Bunions, foot.  Perspiration; cold, foot. Ingrowing toe nail.

**SLEEP:** Dreams; amorous; anxious; death of; previous events; frightful; misfortune of; pleasant; robbers; vivid; vexation; restless.

Sleepiness.  Sleeplessness; after midnight; 1 a.m. to 2. a.m.

Waking early; hunger with; 2 a.m. to 3 a.m.; cough with, sticking in chest.

**CHIL & FEVER:** Chill worse 6 P.M. Warm stove amel.

Fever; catarrhal chicken pox; typhoid; gastric measles; puerperal; scarlet; small pox.  Worse 2 P.M. to 3 P.M., 9 A.M. to 12 noon, 5 P.M.

Perspiration; **night; daytime only; midnight after.** Evening and through entire night.

**SKIN:** Barber's itch (Sycosis barbae). Chilblains. Coldness. Eruptions alternate with stomach and menstrual complaints. Carbuncle. **Crusty.** *Desquamating.* Dry. Eczema. Herpes zoster. Pimples. Scaly, brown like. Rosy erythema. Vesicles herpes. Erysipelas. Ganglia. Ulcers, bleeding night, suppurating. Warts.

# KALI PHOS

(Kali phos shares weakness of potassium ion as well as that of phosphate ion. It is very useful in weakness, physical or mental.)

**GENERALITIES:** Abscess. **Anemia.** Atrophy of glands. *Ball, globus.* Cancerous affections; encephaloma; noma; to remove pain; to remove deposits. **Leukemia.** Tumours; malignancy suspected.

*Chlorosis.* Chorea. Collapse; after stools. Convalescence. Convulsions; *in children;* hysterical. Degeneration; fatty, of muscles. Muscles; *progressive atrophy* of. Dropsy; external; internal. Emaciation. Exhaustion; early. Faintness; fainting. Fidgety. Flabby feeling. Haemorrhage; blood does not coagulate (contrast with Kali mur).

**Heat; vital lack of.** *Loss of vital fluids.* Inflammation; glands, (adenoids); gangrenous. Injuries. Irregular, incoordinate effects. *Lassitude.*

Motion; aversion to. Nervous patients. Numbness; externally; in single parts. Offensiveness; fetor; body of; smell like onions. Orgasm of blood; emotions after. Pain; paralytic, **stitching; tearing;** downwards. Paralysis; one sided; post diphtheritic. Prickling. Pulsations.

Scurvy. Secretions; milky; golden yellow, gray. Sea sickness; nausea without. Sensitiveness. *Sepsis. Septicemia.* Sexual excitement; indulged or suppressed. Side lain on; pain goes to. Symptoms, on *one side.* Sluggishness. Stiffness; paralysis from.

**Tendency to take cold.** Twitching. **Weak;** *coition after;* easy; emission after; influenza after; **nervous,** pain from; stools after; walking from. **Weariness.** *Yellow, orange or bright yellow.*

**WORSE:** Morning, 4 a.m. to 9 a.m. Afternoon, 12 to 6 p.m. Midnight after. *Air, open cool.* Alone when. Ascending. Cause, slight. **Coition. Cold** in general; air; becoming; entering a cold place; wet weather. Consolation. Coughing.

**Eating after;** while. **Emotions.** *Exertion.* Food; cold drinks; onions. **Fright.** *Heat of fire;* sun; overheated. Jarring. Light. *Lying on back;* side painful (Comp. Kali carb). *Menses during.* Mental labour. Motion; at the beginning. *Noise. Onanism.* Every tenth to fourteenth day. Rising; morning after. Scratching.

**Sexual excess.** Sitting while. Sleep, during; *falling asleep on* Sneezing. Standing. Stooping. Swallowing. Touch. Uncovering Walking; fast; *open air in. Winter.* Writing.

**BETTER:** *Bending double.* Company, pleasant. *Eating,* after Eructations; sour. Excitement; pleasurable. Hair, letting down. *Leaning. Lying.* Mind, being diverted. Motion; slow gentle. Pressure. Sleep after. Sitting or standing erect. Walking slowly. Warm bed. Wrapping

**MIND:** *Absent minded. Agitation.* Ambition; loss of. Anger ailments after; flies into passion; can hardly articulate. Answer aversion to. **Anxiety;** *with fear;* about future; about health; hypochondriacal, about money matters; about salvation  Aversion; husband to members of family; husband and baby, hatred of. (Comp. Sepia).

Bad news; ailments from. Bashful; undue sensitiveness. Brooding. Carried wants to be. Company; aversion to; desire for; alone while agg. Concentration difficult. Confusion. Cowardice. Death desires. Delirium tremens. *Delusions;* sees dead persons; fancy illusions of; sees figures, images, phantoms; frightful; familiar thing seem strange. Despair; *religious salvation.* Discontented. Dullness

*Excitement emotional;* ailments from; mental work from. *Fear of being alone;* in a crowd; death of; evil of; something will happen men of; people of; places; buildings of; work of. Fickle. *Forgetful* of words, while speaking. *Frightened easily.* Grief; ailments from

Making gestures; grasping or reaching something; imaginar objects; ridiculous or foolish; wringing of hands.

Hatred, husband and baby of. Held, wants to be. **Homesickness.** Hurry. **Hysteria.**

Imbecility. Impatience. Impetuous. *Indifference.* Indolence. *Insanity;* mental labour from. **Irritability;** headache during; menses during. *Spoken to when;* waking on.

Lamenting. Laughing; alternating with weeping. Love; *ailments from disappointed love.* Mania. Mania-a-potu.

Mildness. Mirth (hilarity). Memory active. **Memory weakness of.** Mistakes; in speaking; misplacing words; *in writing.* Mood; changing; variable. *Morose.* Move; dislike to; after being seated. *Obstinate. Out of humour;* discontent with everything.

**Prostration of mind.** *Religious affections. Restlessness.* Sadness; tired of life, but fears death; morning on waking. Senses; dullness of. Sensitive; children; light to; menses during; noise to. Sexual excess; mental symptoms from. Shrieking. Speech confused. Starting, startled; **easily;** *touched when.* Stupefaction. Suspicion

Talk, indisposed to. Silent, taciturn. *Tears things.* Thoughts; persistent; vanishing of. *Violent. Weeping;* crying; continuous (religious). Work; aversion to; seems to drive him crazy; owing to impotence of mind.

**HEAD:** Anemia and softening of brain. Concussion. Congestion; on coughing. Brain fag. Sensitiveness; jar, to the least.

Coldness; chilliness. Dandruff. Eruptions. Falling forward of head. Fontanelles open (tardy closure). Hair falling; margins of. Hair letting down amel.

Headache; emotions, excitement from; menses before and during; *nervous;* students; paroxysmal; violent; wakes from sleep, frequently; alternating with pain in teeth; coryza with; empty feeling in stomach; hungry when; noises in head; yawning, stretching with.

Headache is aching; boring; digging; burning; bursting; constrictive, as if in a net; distensive, full; drawing; heaviness; jerking; pulsating; sore; **stitching;** stunning, stupefying.

*Forehead;* extending to eyes or temples. **Sides.** Supraorbital; occiput to temples.

Worse; binding up the hair; lying on occiput; pressure; uncovering.

Better; air open; cheerful excitement; eating after; lying on back; menses appearing; motion gentle; rising after; rubbing; wrapping.

Heat of forehead. Hydrocephalus. Itching. Movements in head Perspiration; cold on mental exertion. Pins, stitching under. Pulled as if from occiput. Rocket had passed through. Shaking. Sensitive to cold air. Shocks, blows.

Vertigo; objects seem to turn in circle. Anemia of the brain from concussion of brain; sea-sickness, without nausea; students; fainting with; tendency to fall forward; nausea with; staggering; empty feeling in stomach with. Worse; in noon; eating after; headache during looking up; lying down; rising on; sitting or standing while; stooping facing the sun; turning or moving the head; walking, in open air. Better in open air, walking gently.

**EYES:** Conjunctivitis; injected; full of dark vessels. Discharge evening. Eyeballs; burning; dryness; dullness. Pain in eyeballs aching; biting; drawing; extending to occiput; pressing; as from sand sore, bruised; stitching, shooting, to temple; tearing. Waking; motion of eyes, reading, sunlight agg. Pressure amel.

Perceptive power lost. Photophobia; coition after; headache during.

Restless; crying hard as if. Staring. Strabismus, squint; diphtheria after. Sunken. Swollen. Twitching. Weak, after coition.

Eyelids; agglutinated; margins burning; falling, drooping of paralysis left. Styes; swollen. Pupils; dilated during disease. Retina inflammation; paralysis of.

Vision. Amaurosis (blindness). Amblyopia (blurred). Dim coition after. Diplopia. Foggy. Illusions; colours before; muscae volitantes; dark colours; halo of colours, around light. Paralysis of optic nerve; post-diphtheritic.

**EARS:** Eruptions. Heat. Swelling. Twitching. Ulceration, about of low form. Boils. Pimples. Itching. Swelling in external auditor canal. Pain behind the ear; stitching, shooting.

Pain (otalgia); cramp in; drawing; stinging, shooting, left; tearing noises agg. Pulsations. Stopped. Surging. Ulceration of tympani membrane. Chronic catarrh of middle ear; blood, offensive, purulent discharge.

Hearing; acute, to noises; voices; talking to. Hearing lost. Deafness; noises in ear with; paralysis of auditory nerve from; to human voice. Noises in (tinnitus aurium); vertigo with; fluttering; humming; reverberating; ringing; roaring; rushing; whizzing

**NOSE:** Itching (formication). Swelling. Pain, root of nose. Epistaxis; predisposition to; blowing the nose from; typhoid fever during. Coryza; dryness. Acute catarrhal inflammation; hay fever; hay fever annual; nervous. Discharge; bloody; crusts; excoriating; fluent; greenish; offensive; *purulent; thick;* watery; white; *yellow* or yellow orange.

*Obstruction* (stuffed); night. *Ozena.* Burning pain; sore, bruised. Smell acute; wanting or lost. Sneezing; frequent; violent; 2 a.m. Ulcers. Discharge from posterior nares; at night; must sit up to clear the throat. Itching in posterior nares.

**FACE:** Bluish, yellow at the edge of hair. Forehead (chloasmae). Careworn; chlorotic; dirty looking; distorted; earthy; greasy; pale; red, circumscribed. Expression; haggard; sad; sunken. Heat, flushes of. Eruptions; pustules on forehead.

Pain; right; drawing; stitching, tearing. Worse; *air open, cold.* Better; eating after; excitement; motion; talking, walking; touch; warmth. Paralysis; one sided; right.

Perspiration. Bluish spots. Tension. Cheeks; burning; glowing. Jaws; pain; necrosis of lower jaw. Lips; cracked; dryness; crusts scabs; pimples; vesicles. Lips; excoriated; peeling; swelling, as if, ulcers. Itching, lower lip.

Parotids; inflamed (mumps). Submaxillary glands swollen.

**MOUTH:** Breath (fetor oris); cheesy; putrid; *offensive.* Dryness. Inflamed. Mucus, slime in. Pain; burning; sore. Saliva; saltish; thick, salivation; eating after. Speech; slow; wanting. Swelling. Taste; bad; bitter; morning; fatty; greasy; insipid; putrid; sour; sweetish. Ulcers; ashen gray. Gums; bleed easily; detached from teeth; **scorbutic; spongy;** swollen. Palate; greasy.

Teeth; caries; chattering; grinding; during sleep. Looseness; brown mucus on. Pain; jerking; neuralgic; pulsating; sore, bruised; tearing; alternating with headache; as from cold; with bleeding gums. Agg. by anything cold, drinks; forenoon; masticating; after sleep. Brown sordes on teeth.

Tongue; brown; dirty, mustard; white; yellow, golden; greenish; dryness; morning; thick as if; sticks to palate. Swollen.

**THROAT:** Chronic constriction. Diphtheria; extending to tonsils. Dry; evening. Gangrene. Hawk; disposition to; cheesy lump. Inflamed. Mucus, saltish. Pain; burning, extending to ear; pressing; rawness; sore; swallowing agg. Paralysis; post-diphtheritic.

Scraping. Awns of barley, as if in. Fullness of; eructation amel. Lump as of; rising up. Swelling.

Tonsils; diphtheritic membrane on; pain; swollen; left.

**STOMACH:** Appetite; constant; increased; soon after eating, headache with; menses during; stool after. Appetite; diminished or vanishes at the sight of food. Aversion; to bread; food; sweets.

Desires; cold drinks, ice; sour acids; sweets; vinegar. Disordered digestion, atonic. Distension.

Eructations; bitter, eating after; empty, tasteless; food of (regurgitation); incomplete; ineffectual; sour. Heartburn. *Nausea;* cough during eating, after; eructations amel. during headache, menses, pregnancy.

Pain; burning; cramping; cutting; gnawing, 5 a.m. Pressing, menses during; night agg. eating after amel. Retching.

Sensations; Coldness. Emptiness; eating after, menses during, nausea during. Fullness of. Heaviness; eating after. Stone as if in.

*Thirst,* extreme; unquenchable.

Thirstless. Ulcers. Vomiting; choking with; coughing; headache during; menses during; palpitation with; pregnancy during. Vomiting; acrid; food of; fluid; mucus. Waterbrash.

**ABDOMEN:** Colic; left to right. Pain; burning, cramping; cutting; *dragging,* extending backwards; bruised; stitching. Pain is worse during diarrhea; coughing; menses before and during; sitting while; stool before. Pain; paroxysmal. Better by eating; lying on abdomen; menses, when flow becomes free.

Colitis; mucus. Distension; menses during; tympanitic. Dropsy (ascites). Flatulence; hysterical; obstructed; menses during. Hard. Heat. Peritonitis.

Rumbling; drinking after; menses during. Coldness (sensation). Emptiness. Heaviness. Tension. Swelling. Symptoms amel. when mind is employed.

Constant pain in epigastrium. Pressing in pelvis, downwards and backwards. Pain; stitching; sticking; across hypogastrium. Inguinal pain, during menses.

Liver; inflammation. Pain, sore; stitching. Pain; in sides of; on breathing. Spleen; aching pain; stitching; walking while or walking agg.

**RECTUM & ANUS:** Constipation; urging absent. Diarrhoea; after breakfast; with cramps in calves; eating after, while; excitement from; fright, emotions agg.; menses during; morning; nervous; night; painless; mental exertion amel. Dysentery; bloody only; blood with. Flatus discharge of; offensive; loud. Haemorrhage from anus, night.

Haemorrhoids (Piles); external. *Inactivity of rectum. Itching.* Orange coloured fluid from. Pain; pressing; stinging; stool after, during; stitching, shooting. Paralysis; after removal of piles. Relaxed. Dragging heaviness.

Stool; corrosive; blood; brown; gray colour; clay coloured; yellow, bright, greenish; of several colours; copious difficult; hard; knotty; involuntary; lumpy; large; lienteric *light coloured;* mucus slimy. *Odour,* **cadaveric;** *offensive;* **putrid;** *purulent.* Ineffectual urging after stool; watery.

**URINARY:** Bladder; catarrh; pressing pain, stitching, stinging. Paralysis; old people in. Urging to urinate; *ineffectual.*

Urination; dribbling, urination after; dysuria (difficult); feeble; frequent, day and night; interrupted, intermittent. Involuntary, from nervous prostration; night, in old people, with enlarged prostate; in typhoid fever. Urination; unsatisfactory.

Nephritis. Stitching pain in kidneys. Bloody discharge from urethra. Itching. Stitching pain in.

Urine: albuminous; burning; cloudy; dark; yellow saffron. Copious; **night.** Milky. Offensive. Scanty. Sediment; mucus; phosphate; red; sand (gravel). Specific gravity increased. Sugar (diabetes mellitus). Watery, clean water.

**MALE:** Coition, followed by prostration. Erections; painful; sexual desire without; violent, morning; wanting (impotency). **Seminal emissions;** erections without; frequent. Sexual passion; diminished; increased; wanting. Balanitis. Ulcers; phagedenic. Enlarged prostrate.

**FEMALE:** Abortion; tendency to; threatened. Coition, aversion to. Sexual desire; increased; insatiable, after menses. Labour pains; false; weak.

Leucorrhoea; excoriating, causing blisters; burning; copious; greenish; menses after; **offensive odour; putrid;** orange coloured; purulent; yellow, yellow green. Lochia, offensive.

Mammae; gangrenous offensive pus; milk spoiled; cutting pain under right nipple; stitching.

Menses; absent (amenorrhea); mental shock, from; delayed first, in girls; painful (dysmenorrhoea); irregular; late, delayed; too late and too scanty. *Menorrhagia,* copious menses. Metrorrhagia; during pregnancy. Protracted, menses. Scanty. Short duration. Suppressed, anemia from. Black. Not coagulating. **Offensive.** Pale, watery; thin. Headache, congestive symptoms, preceding and attending the flow.

Ovaries left, pain; bending double amel. lying on back or left side amel. Night. Pregnancy during. Sharp. Sleep on going to agg.; stitching.

Uterus; cancer; chronic metritis. Pain; after pains; labour like; menses during; night; pregnancy during; stitching. Prolapse of.

Vagina, burning. Vulvae, abscess; itching from leucorrhea. Burning pain in vulvae and labia.

**HEART:** Pulse; imperceptible; intermittent; irregular. Angina Pectoris. Fatty degeneration of heart. Palpitation, tumultous, violent;

ascending agg. flatulence, motion agg.; nervous irritability from. Constriction.

**RESPIRATORY:** Asthma, hay asthma; night; eating least food agg. Bronchitis. Chest, itching. Chest pain; burning; **stitching;** sides; left lower; agg. during cough, inspiration and motion. Spasms of chest.

Anxiety, felt in. Tightness; spasmodic. Fluttering. Oppression. Pulsation. Weakness.

Cough; irritation in larynx from; tickling in larynx; asthmatic; croupy; night; hacking; loose; paroxysmal; racking; rattling; short, spasmodic; sudden; tickling; whistling; whooping. Cough agg. by air cold; breathing deep; chill or 'fever during; dinner after; eating.

Expectoration; bloody; greenish; mucus, offensive; fetid; purulent; like soap suds; salty; sweetish; thick; viscid; white; yellow.

Larynx; croup; irritation; mucus in. Paralysis of vocal cords. Tickling. Hoarseness; from overuse of voice. Voice lost; suddenly; shrill while speaking.

Lungs; abscess. Haemorrhage. Inflammation. Oedema. Tuberculosis; *incipient;* purulent and ulcerative. Pleurisy.

Respiration; difficult; stitches in back with; suffocation threatened. Worse, eating after; **night.** Irritation in trachea; tickling; pain on coughing.

**NECK & BACK:** Right to left. Coldness; extending up. Eruptions. Heaviness. Itching, night. Pain burning; drawing; lameness; paralytic; pressing; sore; stitching, shooting; tearing. Agg. breathing when; exertion from; lying on back; leaning back; menses during; rest during.

Pain; rising bed from, sitting from, sitting while; standing while; touched when; must sit up to turn over. Better; leaning on something; gentle motion; walking while. Stiffness.

Pain in neck; aching; bruised. Stiffness; enlarged glands from. Swelling of neck glands. Pain, dorsal region; shooting.

Heaviness, lumbar region. Pain; aching; burning; drawing; stitching, shooting; tearing. Sacral pain.

Scapula; pain; pain between; under left in morning; right then left.

Pain, spine and cord; relieving headache; **sore, bruised;** ulcerative. Softening of spinal cord. Weakness, tired feeling, in spine.

**EXTREMITIES:** Coldness. Cramps. Emaciation; of paralysed limbs. Itching. Numbness, right. Pain; drawing in joints; gouty; stitching; tearing; on beginning to move; raising arm agg.; gentle motion, warmth amel.

Paralysis, post-diphtheritic. Paraplegia.

Restlessness. Swelling; dropsical. Trembling, twitching. Swelling of axillary glands. Perspiration, axillae in; garlic like.

Pain in shoulders; pressing, stitching; tearing; upper arms motion backwards and forwards amel.

**Coldness;** *of hands;* feet. Warts. Chilblains. Numbness (right); fingertips. Trembling.

Pain; up and downwards (lower extremities); sore, bruised. Agg. by motion; beginning to move; rising from seat. Stumbles easily, while walking. Weakness.

Hip joint tuberculosis. Pain in knees, drawing, downwards; sore bruised. Calf: blue spots. Crampy pain in calves; in cholera. Fidgety. Restless. Frost-bitten as if (foot). Stiffness, swelling (foot). Cracked heel. Itching, lameness, pain, crampy pain in soles.

**SLEEP:** Deep. Dreams; amorous; falling of; pleasant; of being naked; vivid. Position; back on. Restless. Sleepiness. Sleeplessness; excitement from; mental exertion after; with sleepiness. Vexation after. Unrefreshing sleep; from anger. Waking early; as from fright. Yawning; hysterical.

**CHILL & FEVER:** Chill; external; internal; one sided; shaking; worse, by open air; bed in; eating after; pains during.

*Fever;* alternating with chills. Dry heat; internal; perspiration absent; typhoid; hectic; scarlet; small-pox; yellow; zymotic; subnormal. Weakness after.

**PERSPIRATION:** Cold; offensive odour; onions or garlic like; profuse, eating while; **slight exertion** agg.; sleep during.

**SKIN:** Burning. Chilblains, Coldness; one sided. Yellow (jaundice). Dry. *Eruptions;* crusty; Discharges; moist, Herpetic, pimples. Psoriasis, Pustules, malignant, Urticaria, Erysipelas, Gangrene, **Inactivity.** Itching, crawling, stinging. *Sensitive;* sticking. *Ulcers; ichorous, yellow;* phagedenic; glands of. Vesicles. Wrinkled skin.

# KALI SULPH

(Kali sulph has the weakness of potassium. Sulphur radical makes it useful in suppuration or thick yellow discharges. It is known as Pulsatilla of twelve tissue remedies).

**GENERALITIES:** *Cancerous affections. Epithelioma.* Lupus. Chlorosis. Convulsions, epileptic; uremic. Fatty degeneration. Dropsy; external and internal. Emaciation. Faintness; before menses; from pain. Flabby feeling. Heat; flushes of. **Heat; sensation of.** Heaviness, externally, inflammation, specially of respiratory membranes, jerking; in muscles. *Latent disease.* Lie down; inclination to. Nodes. Orgasms of blood.

Pain; bones in; burning externally, internally; cutting externally, internally; glands in; gnawing; **stitching** internally; **tearing** in gland, in muscles; **ulcerative; wandering.**

Polypi. Post-operative disorders. **Pulsation;** throbbing. *Reaction; poor; lack of.* Sensitiveness. Suppuration; thick; yellow green yellow. **Sycosis. Syphilis.** Tendency to take cold. *Trembling.* Twitching. *Wandering; changing. Weak; during menses;* talking from. Weariness; talking after.

**WORSE:** 5 p.m. Evening 6 to 9 p.m. Bathing. Change of weather; **cold to warm.** Cold; becoming; while sweating or hot. Consolation. Coughing. Eating after. Emotions. Exertion. Fright. **Heat of fire;** sun; overheated. Warmth; **air of;** bed; **room;wraps.** *Jarring.* Lying in bed. Noise. Room in. Scratching. Sitting while. Sneezing. *Sleep during;* falling to. Spring. Stooping. Swallowing. Sympathy. Touch. Waking on.

**BETTER:** Air open; desire for. Cold in general; feels too hot. After eating. *Eructations.* Fasting (before eating). Flatus passing.

**Motion.** Uncovering. **Walking; open air in.**

**MIND:** Absent minded. Agitated. Loss of ambition. **Anger.** **Anxiety,** with fear. Business, averse to. Company, aversion to. Concentration difficult. Want of self-confidence. Confusion. Discontented. *Dulness. Excitement;* emotional. Fear; death of; falling of; people of; work of. Fickle. Frightened easily; at trifles.

Hurry. Hysteria. Ideas abundant; clearness of mind. Impatience. Indifference. Indolence. **Irritability;** before menses. Memory weak. Mistakes; misplacing words; in writing. Mood; changeable; variable. Obstinate. *Restlessness.* Sadness. Symptoms from sexual excess. Sensitive. Startled, easily. Shrieking; from undue sensitiveness. Sit; inclination to. Silent, taciturn. Weeping. Work; mental aversion to.

**HEAD:** Congestion of brain; on coughing. Warm room in. Loose, as if. Coldness; **chilliness;** vertex. *Dandruff;* copious; yellow. *Eruptions;* yellow; crusts; moist yellow; ring worm. Baldness in spots. Hair falling in spots.

Headache; eye strain from fasting; from shaking head; taking cold; catarrhal, rheumatic; violent coryza with.

Pain is **aching;** *boring; digging, bursting; cramping, squeezing;* distensive, full; drawing; jerking; *pulsating; stitching;* stunning; stupefying; tearing; headache; in forehead; sides; supra-orbital. Worse by bending head backward, to one side; chills, during; forenoon; shaking head. Better by cold air.

Heat of forehead; warm room in, itching. Movements in head; by moving head. Perspiration. Sensation; band; hoop; skull cap. Shocks, blows.

Vertigo; after violent exertion; from exhaustion; headache during or with; nausea; fainting with; staggering; tendency to fall backward. Worse; eating after; looking up; rising on; in warm room; standing while, after sitting; stooping. Better in open air.

**EYES:** Cataract. Conjunctivitis; yellow discharge; in new born. Cornea; abscess; opacity of; spots or specks on; ulcers. Eye balls; distorted; dryness eruptions about; inflammation; gonorrhoea; lachrymation.

Photophobia; daylight. **Redness.** Eyelids swollen; inflamed; redness; agglutinated; eruption on; scaly herpes at margins.

Vision: Amaurosis (blindness); dim. Foggy. Illusion of dark colours; halo of colours around light; variegated yellcw colours. Dazzling. Sparks.

**EARS:** Eczema. Pimples. Itching. Polypus. Eustachian tubes; **catarrh; inflammation.** Pulsations. Eruptions behind the ear. Pain (otalgia); aching; boring; cutting; stitching; shooting; evening agg.

Chronic catarrhal inflammation of middle ear; discharge from; brownish; yellow; yellow green; offensive; purulent; thin, watery.

Hearing, acute. Deafness; right; from **eustachian catarrh;** swelling of external ear; warm room agg.

Noises in ear; chirping; cracking; crackling; fluttering; humming; ringing; roaring; rushing; whizzing; **chewing when** agg.

**NOSE: Cancer, epithelioma.** Eruption. Itching (formication). Swelling. Epistaxis; blowing the nose agg. Coryza; *dryness.* Acute catarrhal inflammation, hay fever; left; discharge, bland, bloody, brownish, burning, excoriating (open air in). Fluent, greenish; offensive; **purulent, viscid, yellow** discharge; salty, thin.

Obstruction (stuffiness); after removal of adenoids; breathes through mouth. Ozaena. Pain. Smell; acute; wanting; lost. Sneezing. Septum; sore, bruised.

**FACE:** Chlorotic; distorted; drawn; pale; red; red circumscribed; sickly; suffering expression; swollen in scarlet fever; yellow.

**Cancer, epithelioma.** Eruptions; herpes. Flushes of heat. Itching; stinging.

Pain; tearing; **warm room** agg.; warm moist south wind agg.; air open amel. **Perspiration.** Twitching. Maxillary sinus, affections of. Caries of bones; upper jaw. Lips; cracked; peeling; eruptions; vesicles; swelling, lower; cancer.

Submaxillary glands; inflamed; swollen.

**MOUTH:** Offensive breath. Dryness. Heat. Mucus slime in. Saliva bitter. Salivation. Taste; sour; putrid; loss of. Painful teeth; warmth agg.; cold amel.; walking in open air amel.

Tongue, **aphthae;** yellow base, white edges; yellow; slimy.

Disposition to hawk. Heat. Inflamed. **Mucus,** morning. Pain; burning; rawness; sore; stitching.

**STOMACH:** Appetite; easy satiety; increased; relish without. Aversion to bread; hot drinks; eggs; food. Desires cold drinks.

Digestion, disordered; indigestion. Distension. Eructations; bitter; food or (regurgitation); *sour;* eating after. Heartburn. Waterbrash. Hiccough. Stomach inflamed. *Nausea;* cough during; headache during; eating after. Retching, cough with. Pain; cutting; cramping; drinking on; stepping on; while walking in open air agg.

Anxiety, coldness, emptiness, fullness, heaviness felt in stomach.

*Thirst;* burning. Thirstless. Vomiting; coughing; headache during, menses during. Acrid; **frothy.** white mucus.

**ABDOMEN:** Cold to touch. Pain; burning; *griping;* **cutting;** pressing; bruised; *stitching;* diarrhoea during agg. Flatulence, jarring, motion, menses before and during; agg. the pain.

*Distension;* tympanitic. Fullness. Heaviness, before and during menses. Dropsy (ascitis). Hard. Heat. Inflammation (peritonitis). Rumbling; stool before. Sensation of diarrhoea, after a normal stool. Pulsations. Trembling. Pressure (epigastrium). Pain above iliac crest. Aching, stitching in inguinal region.

Liver; enlarged. Jaundice, catarrhal. Pain; sore; stitching.

**RECTUM & ANUS:** Constipation; alternating with diarrhoea; habitual; menses during; obstinate. Inactivity of rectum. **Itching;** violent.

Diarrhea; then asthma; menses during. Flatus; discharge of.

Piles; blind; with constipation; external; large.

Pain, **burning;** diarrhea during; cutting; pressing; stinging, stool after, during; **stitching.**

Stools; corrosive; black; bloody; **difficult,** although soft; recedes; *dry hard;* incomplete, unsatisfactory; involuntary; knotty; lumpy; **large;** light coloured; *mucus;* **slimy; yellow;** offensive; purulent. Scanty;

sheep dung like; small; soft; thin, water; yellow black; ineffectual urging.

**URINARY:** Catarrh of bladder. Pain; pressing; stitching; stinging; urination before. Ineffectual urging to urinate.

Urination; dribbling; difficult (dysuria); frequent. Urine albuminous, after scarlet fever; burning; cloudy; red, copious; offensive, scanty; purulent.

Acute nephritis;--pyelitis;'stitching pain in kidneys.

*Urethra;* gonorrhoeal discharge; chronic; greenish; greenish yellow; mucus; purulent: yellow. Haemorrhage. Cutting pain in meatus.

**MALE:** Impotency; erections feeble. Sexual passion diminished. Itching, scrotum. Balanitis. **Empyocele.** Testes; swelling; inflammation; induration; from suppressed gonorrhoea; drawing pain in.

**FEMALE:** Abortion, tendency to. Leucorrhoea; acrid; albuminous; greenish; offensive odour; *purulent;* thick; yellow.

Menses; scanty; suppressed; late or delayed. Amenorrhea. Dysmenorrhea; fainting with. Bright red. Weight in abdomen; preceding and attending the flow. Menses; frequent; too early, too soon; every three weeks. *Menorrhagia. Protracted menses.*

Uterus; cancer. Pain; bearing down; menses during. Prolapse of.

Vulvae; excoriation; itching; burning pain.

**HEART:** Pain in the region of heart. Palpitation; tumultous; violent. Fatty degeneration of.

**RESPIRATORY:** Chest external; eruption; eczema; pustule; itching. Pain; burning; rawness; soreness; stitching.

Anxiety; tightness; oppression; weakness felt in chest.

Cough; croupy; dry; hacking; loose, without *expectoration;* Paroxysmal: racking; **rattling;** retching; suffocative; tickling; **whooping.** Worse; air hot; eating; fever during; lying, in bed; *warm room.* Better; air cold; cold drinks.

Expectoration; bloody; difficult; easy raising; greenish; mucus, gray, greenish; purulent; slips back; *must swallow, what has been loosened;* viscid; yellow.

Larynx; catarrh; dryness; irritation; mucus in; rawness; soreness; stitching. Rattling. Scraping, clearing.

Hoarseness; mucus in larynx from. Warm room agg. Lost voice.

Lungs; inflammation; hepatisation; haemorrhage. Stage of resc- lution; delayed resolution. **Tuberculosis.** *Pleurisy.* **Empyema.** Bron- chitis; chronic; winter catarrh. Mucus in trachea.

Respiration; **difficult;** asthmatic, with difficult expectoration, warm room agg.; **rattling** without expectoration; wheezing; whistling. Worse, cough with; lying while; *warm room;* walking. Air open amel.

**BACK:** Pain; aching; burning; drawing; evening; periodical; shooting; wandering. Breathing when agg. Menses during and beginning of agg. Warm room, sitting while agg. Better, walking while.

Stiffness, neck and back.

Neck; pain; head inclined to right, shoulder raised. Swelling of neck glands. Pain stitching. In dorsal region. Pain, between scapulae. Weakness lumbar region. Pain, sacrum.

**EXTREMITIES:** Coldness. Cramps. Eruptions, hot water amel. *Psoriasis, Scabs. Ulcers, varicose.* jerking. *Numbness.* Trembling. Twitching. Weakness.

Joints; cracking in; inflamed (fungoid); swelling, white; stiffness of, stitching pain; chill during; air open amel.; *motion, walking* amel. *Wandering pains.*

Coldness of hands and feet. Psoriasis, near elbow, palms. Perspiration palms of. Eruptions; moist vesicles; on back of hand; fingers. Growth of nails, interrupted. Burning. Itching. Cracked skin.

**Hip joint tuberculosis.** Pain; thighs; sitting while agg. Twitching (thighs). Sore, bruised tibia. Restless. **Ulcers.** Cold perspiration; swelling and stiffness of foot.

**SLEEP:** Dreams; anxious; death of; disease; frightful. Sleepi- ness. *Sleeplessness;* midnight before. Somnambulism. Waking early; frequent.

CHILL & FEVER: Chill; quotidian; shaking; worse on exertion. Fever; chill with. Dry heat, perspiration absent. Fever; typhoid; gastric; hectic; intermittent (malaria); measles; scarlet; night agg.

Perspiration; easy; profuse; exertion even slight agg.

SKIN: *Burning;* dry: inability to perspire. Coldness. Cracks. Red spots. Eruptions; burning; moist; crusts; scabs; discharges moist; desquamating; eczema; herpetic. Hot water amel. Painful. Papular. Psoriasis. *Pustules.* Scaly **yellow.** *Smarting.* Suppressed (eruptions). *Suppurating.* Tubercles. Urticaria, nodular. Vesicles.

Formication. Itching; burning; crawling. Seborrhoea. Inactivity. Hairs fall out. *Sensitive.* Stickling. Swelling. Dropsical ulcerative pain. **Ulcers;** bleeding, burning; crusty; flowing; thin, watery; indolent. Pulsating.

# NOTE ON POTASSIUM

(98 per cent of total body potassium is intracellular. The ratio of intracellular to extracellular potassium is a critical determinant of the membrane potential of excitable tissue).

**Effects of Hypokalaemia:** Marked potassium wasting impairs muscle function with weakness sometimes progressing to paralysis, absent reflexes and on occasion acute rhabdomyolysis, particularly after exercise. The smooth muscle of the gut is also affected with reduced motility or frank ileus complicating hypokalaemia. The force of myocardial contraction is increased in *vitro,* when the bath fluid potassium concentration is low but *in vivo* hypokalaemia is associated with cardiac failure. Myocardial excitability is increased and digitalis intoxicity is enhanced. Arrhythmias associated with hypokalaemia include atrial tachycardia with block, atrio-ventricular dissociation, ventricular tachycardia or fibrillation.

The effects on kidney include nephrogenic diabetes insipidus, a fall in glomerular filtration rate, and a tendency towards sodium retention. Hypokalaemia may be associated with hypophosphatemia with evidence of renal tubular phosphate leak.

There may be no symptoms attributable to hypokalaemia. Muscle weakness or paralysis may affect respiratory muscles. Paralytic ileus is seen most commonly in surgical wards. Failure of renal water conservation results in thirst and polyuria. Symptoms of paraesthesia may occur and in rare cases tetany has been described.

Hyperkalaemia is less common than hypokalaemia, but more dangerous. Very rarely hyperkalaemic patients may complain of muscle weakness, but cardiac arrest is the only clinical manifestation.

# MAGNESIA PHOS.

(*Note:* Magnesium is mainly an intracellular ion. Its functions are similar to that of potassium. Its extracellular concentration is very little 2 to 3 m/eq per litre. Increased extracellular concentration depresses activity in the nervous system, and also depresses skeletal muscle contraction. This latter effect can be blocked by administration of calcium. Low magnesium concentration causes greatly increased irritability of the nervous system, peripheral vaso-dilatation and cardiac arrhythmias).

**GENERALITIES:** Suitable to tall, slender, dark and neurotic persons or tired languid exhausted subjects. It is a remedy for *cramps. Convulsions, neuralgic pains* and spasmodic effects; showing its influence on **nerves** and muscles.

Pain is crampy, *neuralgic; paroxysmal; radiating, shooting, lightning;* **night only.** Pain extort cries; is *wandering,* changes places suddenly. Appears gradually and disappears suddenly. Jerking externally. In small spots. Prolonged exertion agg.

Ball, lump, globus internally. *Band, hoop* as of a. Relieves pain in cancerous affections. Constriction, externally; *internally,* convulsive movement. Convulsions; in children; during dentition; after diarrhoea; puerperal. *Epilepsy.* Tetanic rigidity; tonic.

Adenitis. **Nervous patients.** *Occupational disorders.* Here and there. *Paralysis agitans.* **Repeated paroxysms.** Relapses, recurrences. Sensitiveness or want of; to pain. Scrawny. Pain goes to side lain on or right side. Symptoms; here and there; erratic; radiating to distant parts. Tension. Tightness. Trembling; nervous. Twitching.

Weak, enervated. *Washing aversion to;* complaints from working in clay; cold water.

**WORSE:** 11 a.m. *night.* 9 p.m. to 4 a.m. Air draft. **Cold in general;** becoming; feet. *Bathing.* **cold.** Washing with water. Working in water. *Cold drinks. walking;* open air in; wind north; *windy stormy weather.* **Uncovering.** Touch. Grasping objects, when. Writing. Piano playing. Lying on back, right side.

**BETTER: Hot applications;** bathing hot, poultices. *Warm stove.* Weather, *warm* wet. Wrapping. Day during (pain). Pressure hard.

Lying *doubled up or bent;* bending or turning affected part. Menses.

**MIND:** Always *talking of her pains.* Talks to herself constantly or sits still, in moody silence. Sits quite stiff; meditates. Aversion to mental work. Indisposition to study; to mental work. Learns with difficulty. Carries things from one place to another and back again. Cheerful; afternoon.

Delusions; movement, loss of, as if. Fear; motion; of touch; contact. Frightened, on waking. Shrieking; pain with. Weeping; convulsive. Lamenting.

**HEAD:** Dandruff. Brain, large and heavy as if. Contents of head, as if liquid. Swashing of water, as if in. Hat, as if on. Skull cap. Scalp adherent to cranium, as if. Shocks as if from electric sparks. Trembling.

Headache, *infra-orbital;* supra-orbital; extends to face. Nervous. Student's. With nausea and chilliness. Nail as from pressing. Optical defects with. Sudden increase and decrease. Shooting. Wandering. Mental exertion, uncovering agg. Darkness; **hard pressure; external warmth;** wrapping amel. Walking in open air amel.

Vertigo; fall forward, backward. Optical defects, with. Exertion of vision agg. Passing over or seeing running water; closing eyes on. Walking agg. Walking in open air amel.

**EYES:** Eye-balls; movement, convulsive, involuntary. Strabismus, squint; convergent. Nystagmus (trembling). Photophobia. Pain goes backward. Right side agg. Pressure amel. Pupils, contracted.

Eyelids; falling drooping of, sensation. Drawn together sensation. Paralysis; right upper. Spasms. Twitching.

Vision; **during headache,** sparks. Accommodation defective. Amblyopia. Diplopia. Illusions; colours before eyes.

**EARS:** Proliferative inflammation of tympanic membrane. Deafness.

Pain goes to side of neck. Cold air, and turning head agg. Warmth of bed and wrapping amel.

**NOSE:** Albuminous discharge. Lumpy, obstructive plugs. Smell; wanting, lost.

**FACE:** Distorted; colic and pain from. Bluish or red during cough. Red, during headache. Swollen; as from bees' sting.

**Prosopalgia** (pain). Right. Alternating with pain in shoulder. Repeated attacks. Infraorbital. Exposure to cold from. *Periodical. Wandering. Cramp like.* **Lancinating.** *Stitching.* **Tearing.** Pain is relieved by motion; **pressure;** sleep; **warmth.**

Pain is worse at noon, 11 a.m. to 2 p.m., by air cold, dry open; *bed in; chewing when;* **cold applications;** *draft,* eating while; motion of lower law. Pain is worse at *night,* in bed, **driving him out of bed;** during rest; touch. **Dry cold wind** agg.

**MOUTH:** Lockjaw. Corners of mouth, cracked. Vesicles, upper lip. Twitching; around mouth; corners. Mumps. Inflamed submaxillary glands. Balls of mucus in mouth. Saliva sticky. Scalded as if.

Speech difficult; chorea from; thick; *stammering; heaviness of tongue from;* begins to speak with closed teeth.

*Bitter taste.* Twitching (tongue). Tooth ache; **neuralgic;** *rheumatic; stitching;* in a whole row; inflammatory; in nervous patients. Toothache is worse by *anything cold;* during eating or drinking; filling teeth, after; touch, tongue of; *night;* in bed. Pressure; *warm drinks* **external warmth** amel. Tender, sensitive teeth.

Tongue, brown; clear and dry; swollen.

**THROAT:** *Constriction; convulsive; swallowing liquids.* Pink, salmon colour. Tenacious mucus. Rawness. Soreness; aching in body and chilliness with. Pain goes to ear. Corn husk, lodged in upper part as if. White of egg dried up and causing tension as if. Spasms of glottis. Stiffness. Swallowing difficult; with pain in back of head. Can swallow only liquids. Constant disposition to swallow. Scraped as if. Oedematous swelling. Goitre.

**STOMACH:** Aversion to coffee. Desires sweets. Cancer. Eructations; food of; eating *immediately* after; while eating. *Heartburn, Hiccough;* convulsive; day and night; *fever during;* with meteorism; with retching; spasmodic; violent; obstinate. Hot drinks or applications amel.

**Cramping pain:** Worse from cold drinks. Bending double, eating after; and pressure amel. *Hot drinks or food* and **warm applications,** give relief.

Retching; with cough, vomiting, menses before; incessant; persistent; immediately after eating.

Band, tightly drawn across the body. Thirst for *cold drinks.*

**ABDOMEN:** *Colic;* **cramping;** cutting. **Spasmodic** pinching. Extends backwards. With eructations, without relief (comp. Carbo veg.) Tossing about in anxiety; no relief from flatus; worse in children.

Drawing up legs; bending body forward; pressure; walking; rubbing and *warmth* amel.

*Contraction.* Flatulent, painful distension. Must loosen clothes. Prevents sleep at night.

Hard. Knotted feeling in. Tension; spread into thighs. Cramping, griping in hypogastric region before and *during* menses. Gall bladder stone colic.

**RECTUM & ANUS:** Constipation; in children; from hard feces. Diarrhea; at night; cramps in calves with; painful dysentery. Diarrhea ceases; spasms or other brain trouble set in.

Copious flatus. Prolapse; with feeling, as if torn.

Stools; forcible; sudden; gushing; hard first then soft; ribbon shaped, flat.

**URINARY:** Bladder pain crampy, cutting. *Retention* of urine; catheter from. Spasms of neck. Spasmodic constriction neck, as of.

Urination, involuntary, in children; from catheterisation; *frequent;* menses during. Urine alkaline; colourless; phosphates.

Kidneys; pain, pressing outward.

**MALE:** Flaccidity. Seminal discharge. Neuralgic pain in testes.

**FEMALE:** Threatened abortion. Labour pains; spasmodic; excessive cramps in legs with. Membranous **dysmenorrhoea.**

Menses; too early; interrupted and reappearing; tarry; stringy; viscid; with urinary symptoms.

Ovaries; inflamed; right; stitching, shooting pain; relief bending double.

Uterus; after pains. Pain; crampy; cutting; menses before and during. Pressure and *music amel.* Cancer.

Acute and chronic inflammation of vagina. Sore vulvae, labia. Vaginismus.

**HEART:** Intermittent; irritable pulse. Angina pectoris. Pain squeezed in vise as if. Expiration, inspiration agg., sensation of constriction, contraction.

Palpitation; nervous irritation; paroxysmal; apex beat visible through clothing. Lying amel.

**RESPIRATORY:** Asthma; spasmodic; chest pain with; *flatulence* from.

Chest pain; intercostal region; tearing; *tightness;* during cough. Oppression, with desire to take deep breath.

Cough. *Dry,* paroxysmal; retching; spasmodic; suffocative; violent; whooping, with stiff body; with cynosis. Cannot speak because of cough. Lying; talking; warm room agg. Air; cold; open; amel.

*Shallow; sobbing;* paroxysmal; tremulous respiration. Desire to take deep breath.

**BACK:** Pain cutting; stitching. Sensitive. Episthotonus. Coccyx bent back as if. Lumbago. Vertebra absent as if.

**EXTREMITIES:** Cramps; exertion after. Pain; neuralgic; paroxysmal; rheumatic; *wandering;* **writing while;** playing piano and violin. Motion agg. Pressure amel. water in agg. Trembling on slight motion.

Fingers; clenching; *during convulsion.* Contraction; spasmodic; during epilepsy. Thumb drawn inwards. Numbness and stiffness of finger tips.

Lower extremities, alternating with upper. Neuralgic pain extending downwards. **Sciatica.** Crampy pain in hollow of knee; legs. Painful calves; during pregnancy; in tailors.

*Cold* feet. *Perspiration;* cold; *offensive. Ingrowing nails.* Sensitive. Hip joint pain; to feet. Walking; ambulatory; tottering and stumble easily.

**SLEEP:** Sleepiness, during day; study during. Sleeplessness; indigestion from. Yawning; spasmodic; lachrymation with. Wakes with impression, as if someone is in the room.

**CHILL:** *Waves in; along spine. Coldness;* worse in evening and night; worse after stools. Fever; *with shivering.* Bilious. Intermittent.

**SKIN:** Barber's itch.

# NATRUM MUR

### Introduction

Natrum mur is one of the most versatile amongst the twelve tissue remedies. Silicea is another remedy which competes with it.

The human body cells are bathed and surrounded by interstitial fluid and plasma (internal environment of Claude Bernard). The most important constituent of this tissue fluid is Sodium Chloride. The fluid inside the cell is called intracellular fluid as against the extra-cellular or interstitial fluid.

The extracellular fluid is kept more or less constant with respect to acid-base equilibrium, osmotic pressure, concentration of individual solutes (Sugar+, Na+, K+, Ca++) and temperature. This constancy is preserved not by inactivity but by ceaseless activity.

Sodium and Chloride ions are very important ions of extracellular fluid. The proper concentration of these two ions is necessary to maintain the requisite osmotic pressure. It is necessary to maintain the excitability of nerves, skeletal muscle and heart muscle.

Natrum mur is thus useful in wide variety of symptoms with (at times) opposite modalities.

**GENERALITIES:** This salt profoundly affects nutrition. The patient is thin, *thirsty,* poorly nourished on account of digestive disturbances. **Anemia** may be from grief; after haemorrhages or with menstrual derangements. Lassitude. Lie down, inclination to, specially after eating. Muscles under-developed. Children talk late. Emaciation; in parts; with good appetite. Emaciation; in **children;** descending; of neck or abdomen. Faintness. Fainting; crowded room in; exertion on; fever during; hysterical. Sense of fainting, specially in warm room. Convulsions; clonic; consciousness with. Epilepsy, mental premonitions as aura; general nervous feeling before; grief after; hysterical; left; left sided; menses during; periodical; puerperal. Irritability. Irregular, inco-ordinate effects. Jerking; internally; convulsions as in; muscles, during sleep. Chorea; attacks few minutes to several days; facial; fright from; jumps high. Clumsiness. Motion; aversion to; sensation of.

Hodgkin's disease. Leukemia. Cancerous affections. Fungus hematodes. Lupus.

Heat; flushes of; sleep during; warm water dashed over as if. **Heat,** *sensation of.* Heaviness internally.

Inflammation; cartilages, internally, nerves. Injury; pains returning. Constitutional effects of injury. Abscess; bone about.

Coldness; in joints. Constriction; external, *internal;* orifices. Orifices; affections of. Contraction; muscles of, congenital. Contraction, stricture; post-inflammatory. Convalescence. Cyanosis.

Contradictory; alternating states.

Formication; all over body; bones in. Fullness, internally. Numbness; parts lain on; single parts. Overlifting; complaints from.

*Pain;* periodical; with the Sun; one sided. Beaten as if; benumbing; boring; compressing; squeezing. Cutting. Digging, extort cries F.e. Glands in. Jerking externally; in bones; in glands; internally Neuralgia. Load as if. Paralytic. Pinching. Pressing; externally; internally; load as from; muscles in; together. Pain, in small spots. Sore, bruised. Stitching in joints. Pain; tearing; ulcerative. Pain goes to side lain on.

Paralysis; feeling externally and internally. From emotions. After intermittent fever. One sided; right. Of organs. Painless or from pain. Pollution or coition after. Post-diphtheritic.

Complaints, from suppressed perspiration.

**Plethora.** Plug sensation; internally Pregnancy. Sense of pressure. Prickling. Psora. Puberty and youth. Pulsation and throbbing; internally; during sleep; better by motion.

**Quinine,** abuse of. Quivering.

Reaction; poor; lack of. Relapses, recurrences. Roughness. Salt, abuse of (halophagia). Scurvy.

Secretions; hair destroying; slimy; sticky; thick; urinous odour. Mucous secretions, altered; increased. Loss of vital fluids, agg.

Senses; special dulled. Sensitiveness. Shocks; electric like; on going to sleep; during sleep. Sinking sensation. Sluggishness.

Short as if; tendons. Shuddering, nervous. Sit; inclination to. Stretching, impulse to. Sourness. Hyperacidity. Strained.

Sprains; old; as if. Suppuration, profuse. Swelling; of affected parts; inflammatory; of bones; glands.

Sycosis. Symptoms; ascend; go backward; left upper, right lower i.e. diagonal; to side lain on.

**Tendency to take cold.** Tension; tightness; internally, muscles. Torpidity. *Trembling;* before breakfast; after emotions; exertion agg.; internally; morning; noon, after sleep; weakness from.

*Twitching;* here and there; hysterical; before menses.

**Wandering;** changing; erratic complaints. Uneasy feeling.

**Weak;** coition after, emissions after, evening, slight exertion agg.; heat of summer, from; lying agg.; menses, before, during and

1 F.A.

after; *morning;* moving arms on; nervous; perspiration from; rising on; sitting; vexation after; walking from; warm weather from.

**Weariness;** eating after; evening; forenoon.

Whiteness. Wounds; bleed freely; painful; constitutional effects.

**SENSATIONS:** Alive internally. Ball, lump, globus internally. Bead like. Band hoop as of a. Coat of skin, was on, as if. Egg dried on, as if. Floating or flying, as if. Flowing like water, as if. Fullness, internally. Formication, all over body. Falling, forward. Fine or hair. **Heat.** Loose, torn as if; flesh from body. Swashing, splashing as of water. Touch, illusions of. Trickling.

**WORSE:** *Morning.* Forenoon. Noon. Periodically. Alternate days. Air; open; cool; aversion to. Draft. Seashore. Alone when but company agg. Ascending. Autumn. Bathing; in sea. Bending or turning affected part. Bending; backwards; sideways. **Biting.** *Chewing.* Bleeding. *Blowing nose.* Breakfast after. Breathing when.

Change of weather. Weather; bright, clear; cold wet. Chill during. Closing eyes. Clothing tight. Cold; air; becoming; and heat. Company. Consolation. Conversation. Darkness. Drawing up limbs. Drinking; after rapidly. Driving in carriages. Riding in car.

*Eating after;* fatigue; long after; over eating; while.

**Emotions. Exertion physical.** Foggy weather.

*Foods;* alcoholic drinks; beans and peas; bread; butter; cabbage; coffee, odour of; farinaceous; fat; flatulent. Idleness.

Jerking. Kindness, sympathy. Lain on pain. Light; artificial; candle. Lying; on bed; in side on; left; painful.

Menses; before and after, beginning; during and after.

Mental labour. **Vexation.** Chagrin. Mortification.

Moon phases; first quarter. Sun, exposure to.

Motion; affected parts of. Raising; affected parts. Reading. Rising. Sitting while. *Standing.* Sneezing. Stooping. Talking, speaking; by others; hearing others. Touching; cold things. Turning around; over in bed. Scratching. Sewing. Working. Yawning. Swallowing.

11 F.B

Narcotics. Noise. Periodically. Perspiration; except headacl·e. Pressure; clothes of. Onanism. *Sexual excess.* Room in; full of people. Rudeness of others.

Sea-shore. Smoke. Summer. Storm; approach; during. Winter.

Sleep; at beginning; after; during; before; falling to; loss of from.

Stools; before, during and after. Sympathy.

Thinking of complaint. Uncoverings; single part; throat.

Vomiting. Waking on. Walking; beginning of; fast; open air.

Warmth; air of; becoming in open air; bed, room; stove of. Weeping. Wet; getting, drenched.

**BETTER:** Air, open, desire for. Alone when. Bathing cold. Coffee, cold. Breakfast, after. Breathing deep. **Cold in general,** feels too hot. Company. Constipation. Dancing. Drawing up limbs. Driving. Eating, after. Eructations. Flatus passing. Exertion. Fasting; before eating. Hanging down, limbs.

Leaning. **Lying;** *on back; in bed;* hard surface on; side on; **right.**

Occupation. **Perspiration,** except headache. Pressure. Raising. Rest. Rising. Rubbing. Running. Salt. Sea-shore. Sitting. erect; down on first. Standing. **Stool after.** Support. Touch. Walking fast; open air in. Wrapping.

**MIND:** *Abrupt.* **Absent-minded.** *Absorbed;* as to what would become of him. Abstraction. Affectionate. **Agitation.** Alone, like to be. **Ambition loss of.** Amorous. Anticipation; complaints from. Anguish; empty feeling in head. **Anger;** ailments after when obliged to answer; with silent grief; with indignation; violent.

**Anxiety;** alternating with indifference; conscience of; fear with; fever during; forenoon; future about; hypochondriacal; menses before and after; sleep on going to, during; uneasiness; and must uncover.

*Aversion;* to answer; motion; spoken to; reading; school; tobacco; women; work; mental work.

Bad news; **ailments** from. Bashful. *Besides himself.*

Careless. Censorious. Cheerful; alternating with ill humour, sadness. Cheerful; coition after; evening, forenoon. Cold; frigid.

Company and aversion to strangers, during urination. Confidence; want of. Concentration; difficult; learns with difficulty. Consolation agg. Contempt; ailments from. Cowardice. Cursing.

**Confusion;** calculating when; on attempting to concentrate mind. Does not know, what he ought to say.

Dancing. *Dark side of things;* looks on. Death *desires;* presentiment of. *Delirium;* maniacal; muttering; raging; very talkative, being wide awake. *Delusions;* sees dead persons; did not touch the bed when lying; every one pities him; faces when stooping; head belongs to another; house full of people; insane he will become; objects appear different; sees people; rocked was being specially on lying down and closing eyes; sick, imagines himself; **spectres;** Ghosts; stepping on air; talking as if with dead people; sees thieves in house, will not believe the truth, till search is made; voices hears, distant; dead people of.

**Despair;** salvation (religious) of. *Disappointment.* **Discontented** with everything. *Dream,* as if in. *Duality;* sense of. *Dulness.* Dwells on past disagreeable things.

*Estranged,* from her family. **Excitement; ailments** from; sleep before.

*Fancies,* vivid; falling asleep when. **Fickle,** ideas in. **Fright;** complaints from. *Forgetful;* eating after; mental exertion from; words of, while speaking.

**Fear;** anxious; restless; crowd in; death of; disease of impending; evil of; falling of, when walking; happen, something will; insanity; men of; misfortune of; palpitation with; people of; pursued being; reason, loss of; robbers; recurrent; sleep, to go to; trifles of; walking of; work of.

**Grasping,** hand, involuntary motions of. Picks at bedclothes. **Grief;** ailments from; boisterous; cannot cry, from; about his future; silent. Guilt, sense of crime.

*Hatred* of persons, who had offended. Homesickness. Hurry. *Hypochondriasis. Hysteria;* fainting hysterical.

*Ideas;* abundant; clearness of mind; deficient; fixed. Illness; sense of sick feeling, *imbecility.* Impetuous; perspiration with.

Impudence. *Inconsolable.* **Indifferent;** alternating with anxiety; mental exertion after; pleasure to; when in society. *Indignation,* pregnant while. *Indiscretion.* **Indolence;** aversion to physical work. *Insanity;* neuralgia, with disappearance of; paralytic debility with. **Irritability;** alternating with cheerfulness; business about; chill during; coition after; headache during; menses agg. perspiration during; questioned when; waking on; spoken to when.

*Jesting,* averse to. Lamenting. Life; unworthy, weary of. Learn poorly.

*Laughing;* immoderately; involuntarily, serious matters over; spasmodic, convulsive; hysterical. Looked at, cannot bear to be. Lose her senses, she would. Ludicrous, things seem.

Mania; puberty of. **Mania-a-potu.** **Memories;** disagreeable, recur. Memory; involuntary recollection. **Memory;** weakness of; in expressing one self; sudden and periodical; for mental labour. **Memory** weakness of; for what has happened, said, read, thought; words, about to say or write. **Mildness.** Mirth; alternating with irritability; evening. Misanthropy. *Mistakes,* localities; **speaking,** what he intends, misplaces words; writing. Mood, changeable. *Nymphomania.* Offended easily.

Passionate, hasty temper. Prostration of mind. Rage, fury, with headache. Reproaches, himself, others. Reserved. *Revenge and* **hatred. Restlessness;** anxious; tossing in bed; driving out of bed; internal; midnight at.

**Sadness;** alone when; cause without; heat during; labour during; masturbation from; menses before; **night;** perspiration during; **weep cannot.**

Searching, for thieves, at night, after having dreamt of them. Sensitive. Senses, dullness of. Sighing. Singing. Sit, inclination to. Speech; confused; intoxicated as if; mistakes of. *Starting. Startled;* easily; sleep during; as if coming from feet, waking her. *Stranger, sensation as if one were a.* **Stupefaction.** *Stupidity. Sympathetic.*

Talk; indisposed to; silent, taciturn; forenoon. Talk; sleep in; slow learning to; takes pleasure in his own. Talks, dead people with; laconically.

Thinking; affected; aversion to; difficult; slow; inability of. *Thoughts;* disease of; persistent; evening; haunted by unpleasant subject; slow; tormenting; vanishing of, mental exertion on; wandering; what would become of him. Torpor, Trifles; **vexed over;** seen important.

*Unconsciousness;* on moving head, sitting while; transient vertigo during; automatic acts during. Unsympathetic.

Verses make, after falling asleep. Violent; trifles at.

Weeping; admonitions from; alone when; aloud, *involuntary;* laughter, alternating with; looked at when; menses during; past events, thinking of; pitied, if he believes he is; sleep in; spoken to, when.

Will weak. Work; complaints from.

**HEAD:** In general. One sided. Alternating. Begins on one, agg. on other side. Loss of vital fluids from. Chronic; continuous; constant.

Distensive, full. Disturbances of vision with. Emotions excited from. Eye strain from. Fatty food from. Grief from. Head injuries, after mechanical. Jerking; fright from. Head getting cold on. *Heaviness;* loss of sleep as from. Heat; cold bath amel. hands cold with; occiput; vertex; menses during. Numbness as if. Numbness; tingling of lips, tongue, and nose with. Stiffness; rheumatic; sensitive to cold air, touch.

*Sensations* are: Air, wind through. Asleep. Band, hoop. Blow, shock, through as of. Brittle. Crushed; as if shattered to pieces. Burning. Displaced as if. Dragging in. Drawing. Empty, hollow. Enlarged expanded as if. Swollen or distended feeling. Looseness; feeling of; in forehead; on shaking the head. Motions in; ascending stairs while; by moving the head. Rope, tight drawn around. Separated from body; as if. Shaking as if; scalp of. Thick as if. Step; every felt in. Waving. Weakness as if. Tired feeling.

Pain, may be constant, continuous, chronic; dull; extending backwards; boring, digging; burning; lancinating, vertigo with, laughing agg.; bruised, sore; **bursting;** constrictive; cutting, hammering, *maddening;* nail as from; periodic; shooting; stitching, extending to chest; tearing; ulcerative; violent; school girls in; gnawing; prickling, needles like; pulsating, to chest and neck; hammers as from little; nausea and vomiting with; before 10 a.m.; throbbing in; pressing, stone as from; vise as if in.

Drinking quickly from. Drowsiness with. Face pale with, Gums painful with. Hawking up watery mucous. *Nausea* with. **Nervous.** Toothache with. **Unconsciousness** with. Vomiting with, transparent mucus.

*Pain, worse;* **anger.** Ascending; into, right. Bending downwards or forwards. Stooping. Looking downward, fixedly at anything. Breakfast after. Fasting during, but eating amel. Chill; before, during and after. Coition. Constipation from. Cough. Increases and decreases with Sun; decreasing gradually. Forenoon. Heat during. Sun exposure to. Summer. Frowning. Leaning against something, while. Lying on occiput. Midnight, after. Motion. eyes of; quick from. Exertion mental. Head; shaking; supporting. Sneezing; during; after. Talking. Turning body. Twisting. Uncovering. Walking in Sun. Wrinkling forehead. Stool from pressing at.

*Pain, better:* Air, open, cool. Cold application. Evening. Eyes closing on; pressure on. Lying; with head high; side on. Morning. Rising on. Sitting. Sleep. Walking, in open air. Wrapping. Yawning after. Perspiration; musty; forehead. Perspiration, amel.

**VERTIGO:** Afternoon agg. Alcoholic liquors from; as from. Blindness, blackness before eyes. Chronic, one sided headache with. Closing eyes on. Coffee. With dulled mind and senses. Epileptic. **Eructations** during. Fainting with. Tendency to fall forward. Flickering before the eyes. Headache during. Head moving agg. Haemorrhoids; flow suppressed from. High places. Intoxicated as if. Memory, thinking, affected with. Nausea with. *Nausea periodic.* Objects seem to turn in circle. Pain; paroxysmal. Pregnancy during. Senses; vanishing with; suppression agg. Side, in right. Sinking, as if. Speech, mistakes of, with. Staggering. Swaying towards right, as if. Trembling with. Turning in circle as if, whirling as if. Unconsciousness with. Vision dim. Wind blowing through head, as if. Writing errors, with.

**WORSE:** Afternoon. Ascending. Bathing. Bed going to. Chill, before and during. After dinner. Eructations, during. Exertion; mental and physical. Looking; moving objects at; window out of; *steadily at.* Passing over or seeing running water. Lying; head low with. Menses, after. Moving; moving head. Raising up. Reaching up. Reading. **Rising on;** after; **bed from;** stooping from. Sitting up in bed. Sleep; before; on falling to. Smoking. Standing near window. Stool after.

Stooping. Tea. Turning; on; or moving the head. Walking; after, long. Window near.

*Better:* Cold application. Lying while; head high with.

**EYES:** Eruptions about eye brows; itching. Canthi; burning; crack; discharge eye gum; itching. Pain in canthi; inner, outer left; stitching; styes, inner, towards inner. *Cataract.* Ciliary neuralgia; paralysis, spasm of muscles. conjunctiva; granular inflammation; bloody discharge; **injected;** swollen dermoid. Cornea; spots or specks on, white. Cornea; ulcers, deep; vesicles.

Eyeballs; burning; smarting. Dryness; reading. Eruptions about; itching; spongy. Inflammation. Itching; morning; rising after. *Lachrymation;* affected side; cough with; laughing when; morning; open air; pain during. Tears; acrid; biting; smarting; burning; leave varnish mark; whooping cough with; wind with. Eyeballs; half open; during headache.

Pain; aching; begins morning, worse; then ceases in the evening. Boring. Burning. Smarting. Sand in, as if. Foreign body as from. Crampy. Drawing; together; stiff sensation in muscles. Pressing; extending to head; 11 a.m. Sore, extending to canthi. Stitching; shooting; right. Worse; after coition; fine work; during heat; light, artificial. Worse, by looking down; *sharply; steadily;* white objects at. Worse; morning, on waking; vision, exertion on; reading; writing; motion of eyes. Periodical. Raising lids. *Sunlight* to sunset. Twilight. Better; evening; walking in open air.

*Paralysis* of muscles; internal recti. Photophobia; artificial light. Protrusion; exophthalmus. Redness; reading; sewing. Scrofulous affections.

Sensation are: contractive; crossed as if; drawn together; enlarged, distended as of; fullness; heaviness, before and during menses. Sand in as of. Left smaller as if. Smarting as from smoke. Swelling of. Stiffness. Strabismus; sense of derangement. Suffused; swollen. Tension, (glaucoma); decreased. Twitching; menses before. Weak; emission after; reading, writing on. Wipe must frequently; and pull at the lashes.

Iris; discolouration; inflammation.

Fistula lachrymalis. Inflammation and swelling of lachrymal gland; of lachrymal canal.

Eyelids; agglutinated, night. Bleeding. Close; desire to; with headache. **Spasmodic closure.** Eruptions on; pimples. Eversion, after use of silver nitrate. Excoriation. Heaviness. Inflammation; redness, margins. Narrowing of interval between (eyelids). Opening difficult, night. Paralysis; right. Quivering; right upper. Stiff. Suppurating points on the edges of. Thickening. Tumour. Twitching; menses before; right.

Orbits; itching; osteoscopic pains. Pricking, left. Twitching. Pupils contracted. Retina; hyperaesthesia; retains image too long.

Vision: Accommodation; defective; slow. **Amaurosis;** exertion, sewing, etc; fainting as from; *periodic;* vanishing of sight. *Asthenopia; confused.* Vision; dim, artificial light in, chill during, distant object. Dim; exertion of eyes from; headache, before and during; menses before, during; reading and writing when; rising from stooping; seminal emissions after; stooping on; walking. Diplopia (double vision). Foggy; reading, standing. Hemiopia; headache then; vertical. Hypermetropia (long sightedness). Myopia (short sight). Paralysis of optic nerve.

Illusion. Objects seem distant; turn in circle. Colours; bright; black; floating, muscae volitantes. Spots; dark; objects. Fiery; points; zigzags. Flickerings; headache before and during. Glittering objects. Letters; seem large; run together. Rains; seems looking through. Swimming, objects. Veils, before. Wavering **zigzags.**

**EARS:** External; redness; concha of; one sided. Boils on lobes; itching. Pimples. Formication. Hot; afternoon; coffee after. Inflammation, concha of. Swelling. Twitching.

Eustachian tubes; catarrh; inflammation.

External auditory canal; boils; pimples; inflammation; pain; swelling.

Internal ear; cancer of ossicles.

Noises in; bubbling; chiming; fluttering; humming, ringing; roaring; rushing; singing; trickling. Chewing when; eating while; lying while; vertigo with; walking while.

Pain; left; to neck outward; shoulder to, left; aching; blow as from; boring; **burning,** right; cramp in; digging; drawing; *stinging; perioaic;* swallowing agg.

*Pulsations.* Sensations: *Air bubble in;* stopped, yawning *amel.* tingling; torn out, as if; twitched out of ear, with hook something were; wind blowing as if.

Eruptions, behind the ear. **Itching,** behind, followed by burning. Pain; aching, pressing, stitching.

Hearing; acute. **Deafness;** from eustachian catarrh. *Paralysis* of *auditory nerve.* **Difficult.** Lost.

**NOSE:** Burning pain in bones, soreness. Constriction, contraction, deadness, desquamation; redness, left side of external nose.

Eruptions; burning; *crusty; eczema;* nodular; *pimples*; scurly; *vesicles; inflammation;* left. *Lupus,* of. Numbness, one side. Perspiration, on. Sore, when compressing wings. *Swelling* left. Twitching.

Pain; boring; bruised, sore; smarting inside; drawing; *pressing;* stitching; *tearing; to forehead.* Vesicles. Squirming in, as from small worm; blowing nose, stooping, touching. agg.

Bleeding; blowing the nose from; chill, in place of; cough with; at night; puberty at; stooping.

Boring into nose, itching, until it bleeds. Redness. Dryness. Foreign body, as if. Formication, crawling. **Scraping.**

**Inflammation. Coryza;** with aching in limbs; chronic; cough with hay fever, annual; laryngitis with; suppressed; uncovering the head from; perspiration, amel.

Discharge; **Albuminous; white;** like white of an egg; thick, like *boiled starch; crusts;* burning; excoriating; *bloody;* **fluent,** dripping; sudden gushing; watery; **copious; purulent, yellow.**

Itching, numbness. Obstruction, alternates with discharges; cough agg.; night. *Ozaena. Sneezing:* frequent; ineffectual efforts; violent; uncovering from. Discharge from posterior nares. Sinus catarrh.

**FACE:** Anemic. **Pale.** Menses after. Bloated, **swelled,** oedematous. intermittents in; wrinkled in headache; *bluish,* circles

around eyes; brown yellow at the edge of hair; *yellow.* **Chlorotic.**
**Cyanotic.** *Earthy.* Emaciated. *Greasy,* shiny, spots oily, as of. Hairy.
Lead coloured. *Red;* circumscribed, headache during, heat of fire
from, one sided.

Expression; confused, *haggard;* **old looking,** suffering; **sallow;**
wretched; looks in glass to see; sickly.

*Eruptions: Acne,* comedones; boils burning, **eczema; forehead;**
**herpes;** *circinatus. Itching.* Forehead, pimples; pustules; vesicles;
*urticaria;* burning.

Growth of hair, on child's face. Heat, itching, *stinging,* on cheek,
chin etc.

Pain, in jaw, cheeks, malar bones, parotid glands, etc.

**Pain; paralysis** with; **periodical; quinine abuse of;** *with the*
**Sun; suppressed ague from.** Pain; burning, drawing, pressing,
sore, stitching. Worse, **chewing when;** *menses during;* toothache
after, touch. Better, open air. Paralysis. *Perspiration;* cold; eating
while. Red cheeks, chin etc. Tension. Twitching. Ulcer. White of
an egg dried on, as if.

*Lips:* **Chapped. Cracked.** Bluish, **during chill.** *Dryness, Erup-*
*tions;* **mouth around; vesicles.** Peeling of. Pouting. Rough, upper,
Salty. Sensitive. **Swelling.**

*Ulcer;* corners of mouth; **upper;** *tingling.*

*Parotid gland. Induration; inflammation;* pain, pinching, tearing
when drinking.

Whiskers; herpes; *falling of;* itching.

**MOUTH:** *Aphthae; burning.* Breath; *hot;* fetorous; **offensive;**
**putrid;** sense of.

Cold sores; pale; **dry; thrush with.** Foam, from. Heat. Pale,
mucous membrane. **Mucus in;** viscid. *Ranula.*

Saliva, bloody; menses before; diminished; expectoration of;
**frothy;** green; *saltish;* sour; watery.

Salivation; cough with; evening, in bed; mercury from; pain with
sleep during; **gushes,** sudden attacks of, scalded as if.

*Speech; difficult; thick;* weakness; of organs of speech. Spitting constant; *sticky. Stomacae.*

Taste; altered, eating after; astringent; bad, morning, water tastes bad, **bitter;** food tastes, eating during and after, intermittents in, tobacco taste; clammy. Inky. Insipid. Metallic. *Putrid,* water tastes, sour, morning, eating before and after. **Loss of, in coryza. Tastelessness of food.**

*Ulcers;* corners of, burning, painful to touch. Vesicles; biting; burning, blood.

*Gums: Aphthae.* **Bleeding,** scurvy. *Boils, Epulis, fistulae,* Inflamed, sore, eating when, *swelling. Ulcers, putrid.*

Palate; dry sore, stiff; ulcers.

Teeth: Caries, Deadened. Chattering. Bluish. Fistulae dentalis. *Looseness. Pain,* boring; broken as if; cutting; drawing; radiating to ear, eyes, throat etc; *pulled out as if; pulsating; stitching,* tearing; with involuntary flow of lachrymation or saliva. Pain; agg. by, chewing; air draft; **cold drinks; eating after; masticating;** menses; pressure; touch; warm things.    Amel. by pressure. Teeth; edge as if on; *elongated as if;* foreign substance, in as if. Sensitive; to air; brushing cold air; touch; *warmth.*

*Tongue: Aphthae.* Bleeding. *Blisters on tip. Cold.* Clean, moist, red, smooth. *White;* base at; patches; red insular with; yellow. Tongue; *dry, thirst without; foam beads,* edge; flabby; heaviness; *herpes; inflammation; mapped;* **mucous collection** on as if; *numbness;* one side; obtrusion. Pain; *burning on tip;* smarting. Ringworm, right side. Sensations; asleep as if; *biting;* **broad, seems too; dryness;** enlarged; **hair on,** as if. Swelling; stings of insects after; tip of; under the (Ranula), with stinging pain. Trembling. Ulcers. **Vesicles; tip.**

*Throat:* **Catarrh.** *Choking;* **drinking when;** *swallowing on;* water from, *Diphtheria.* **Dryness;** eating after. *Food lodges in. Glazed appearance.* **Hawk,** disposition to. Hawks; gluey, viscid mucus; difficult to raise up. *Inflammation;* **acute follicular;** chronic, tobacco from; pharynx of. *Liquids taken* are forced into nose. **Mucus; albuminous;** *from posterior nares; morning; saltish;* thick; **white.**

Pain; **burning;** drawing ear to; oesophagus, on swallowing; *pressing;* raw; sore; spots; smokers; *splinter as from; stitching* like a hot needle. Pain, agg. by coughing; laughing; night; smoking; swallowing.

Throat: *Paralysis,* post-aiphtheritic. Sensation; warm drinks seem cold; *hair or thread of;* **lump,** *rising up, swallowing on, not amel. by swallowing;* when not swallowing; narrow; tension, *Glottis, spasm of;* constant disposition to swallow; swallowing, difficult; can swallow only liquids; food goes wrong way; must drink to swallow; paralysis from. *Swelling.* Ulcers.

Oesophagus; burning; itching; dryness *sore spot;* **strict re.**

Tonsils; *enlargement of;* chronicity. Uvula; adheres to right tonsil; *elongated;* hangs to one side; stitching; shooting.

**STOMACH:** Appetite; better after beginning to eat; changeable; constant; *easy satiety;* **increased, ravenous;** alternating with loss of; **relish without; emaciation or marasmus** with. Appetite; **wanting, diminished; hunger with;** vexation after.

Aversions: **Bread;** beer; *butter; coffee; fats* and *rich food;* fish; food, **hunger with;** *salt food; tobacco, smoking; water, cold;* wine.

Cannot bear tight clothing. Constriction, convulsive.

Desires. Cravings: *Beer; bitter food;* coffee; bread; cold drink, *icy;* farinaceous food; fat food; *fish;* **salty things,** during pregnancy; *milk;* piquant things; pickles; sweets; *sour; acids; warm,* soup; wine.

**Indigestion;** bread after; **farinaceous food** from; pregnancy during. Distension. **Eructations;** afternoon 4 p.m. air, in open; bitter, eating after at night; burning; *drinking after; water after.* **empty; food of;** foul; rich food or milk after; **ineffectual** (incomplete), *menses before, milk after; ingesta tasting of; menses* before; morning; nervous; night; repulsive; **sour, eating after;** *sweetish* before menses, pregnancy during; *water-brash; pregnancy during.*

Heartburn, eating after, pregnancy during. *Hiccough; quinine after;* **violent.** *Hyperacidity.*

Nausea: *Breakfast during.* Chill, before, during. Coffee after. Cold drinks after. Cough during. Eating and drinking after. Epigastrium in, evening, in bed. Eye symptoms with. Faint like. Fish after. *Headache* during. Lying down on, but right side or side amel. Menses agg. Morning. Pain during. Periodic. Pregnancy during. *Salt thinking of.* Sea-sickness. Shuddering with. Smoking while. *Stools after.* Vexation after. Waking after. *Yawning* when.

   **Pain:** Burning, some hours after eating; *clawing;* **cramping; pressing;** scraping; *sore;* stitching; *ulcerative; nausea with;* weakness with; *paroxysmal; night in bed.* Agg. *by tight clothing, drinking,* heat during, deep inspiration, sour or fat food, **touch.** Amel. by, bandaging, clothes tightening, yawning.

   *Retching; cough with;* warm drinks from.

   Sensation: Anxiety, rises to head. Burrowing. Bursting. *Coldness,* burning with, diarrhoea during. *Emptiness;* aversion to food with; *hunger without;* not relieved by eating; *headache during; fatigue* agg.; 11 a.m.; morning, anxiety with. Foreign body or stone as if in. *Fullness.* Hanging down, relaxed as if. *Heat flushes of, heaviness.* Lump, eating after.

   Sensations: Movements in. Pulsation, cough with, *eating, after, eating* while. Tenderness, to contact, pressing. Tension. Tickling. Tingling. Turning. **Twisting.**

   **Thirst:** Burning, **Chill during,** *after,* before. Dread of liquids with. **Extreme,** *unquenchable; headache with;* **heat during; large quantities** and often. Walking after. Small quantities. Without desire to drink. Thirstless. *Ulcer.*

   *Vomiting:* Chill after. Cough with. Drinking after. Headache during. **Heat during.** Menses agg. Morning. Night. Pain during. *Pregnancy. Vomiting: acrid. Bile. Bitter.* Blood, coffee *ground like.* Curdled milk. Food of, then bile, undigested food. Mucus. *Stringy. Urging. Taste of urine.*

   *Waterbrash;* eating after;' pregnancy during. Weak, *relaxed* stomach.

   **Abdomen:** *Colic; abdominal ring;* extends to testes.

   Pain: *Burning. Cramping.* **Cutting.** *Dragging.* Drawing; extends downwards, to anus, rectum, testes, thigh, urethra. *Pinching. Pressing.* Sore. Stitching. Tearing. With, pain in arm, heat of body, leucorrhoea, nausea. Worse: Bending to one side. Breathing deep. Coffee after. Constipation. *Coughing.* Drinking after. Exertion. Laughing. Lying; with legs extended; *left side; painful side;* right side. Malaria after. *Menses after, during.* Motion. Night. Periodical. Riding. Rising seat from. *Sitting, while.* Stool, before, during, after. Stretching on. Urination during *Walking.* Better: Bandaging. Bending, body to the side, forward. Dinner. *Flatus passing.* Leucorrhoeal discharge. Pressure, clothes of. Rubbing. Yawning.

Contraction; muscles of; desire for; stools during; urina tion after; walking agg. Discolouration; inflamed spots.

**Distension:** *Beer after.* Breakfast after. Flatus passii g amel. Hemicrania during, painful. Stool after. Stool, amel. Sudcen.

*Flatulence;* here and there; noisy; *obstructed;* offensive; stool during. Fermentation. Gurgling; motion amel.

Eruptions; pimples; ringworm. Hard. Jerks. Retraction. *Rumbling;* breakfast during; coffee; after; eating after; stool, before, after; diarrhoea before.

Sensation: Bubbling. Constriction, band, hoop; stool during; desire for; walking when. Disagreeable feeling. Distension or falling out as of. Fullness, urination after. *Heaviness;* as from load; motion during. Movements in morning, after. Relaxed feeling; walking while. Rough substance as of a. Stone as of a. Squeezing. Swashing. Tension. Sunken. Weakness. Worms were griping in.

Epigastrium: Anxiety felt in. **Bruised. Suppurative festering pain. Swollen.** Foreign body or lump above, as if. *Pulsation.*

Pain, distension, tender to touch in hypogastric and hypochondrium.

Clicking sound, as if two bones slipped over each other, in inguinal region. Hernia, internal ring, cough agg. Swelling of gland. **Hair falling from,** pubic region. **Distension,** *pressing,* **pushing sensation,** at sides of abdomen. Swelling of inguinal glands.

Umbilicus: Constriction. Contraction. Discharge. Distension. Pain; crampy, cutting, sore, to rectum. Protrusion, as if hernia would. Tension.

Liver: *Atrophy.* Fullness. Inflammation, chronic. Lump in. *Pain; pressing, stitching,* extends to *back* and right. Worse, eating after. Better, bending forward.

*Spleen: Enlarged. Inflamed.* Sensitive. Stretched, sensation. Swelling, heat during. Pain; *aching;* lancinating; *pressing,* stitching, *walking while;* thrusting; worse heat during and pressure of clothing.

**RECTUM & ANUS:** Congestion. **Constipation, alternate day agg.**

Constipation: Alternating with diarrhoea. **Hard feces from.** *Habitual.* Haemorrhoidal. Heart symptoms with. Menses, before, **during.** Must remove stools mechanically. Painful. *Urging with. Women.*

*Constriction:* Spasmodic. Stool; *before,* **during,** *preventing.* Urinating on.

**Diarrhoea:** Breakfast after. Children in. *Cholera, infantum.* Chronic. Coffee after. **Day time only.** Emaciated people in. **Farinaceous food.** Gushing. *Hot weather,* Indiscretion, slightest, in eating, Menses after. Midnight after. 3 A.M. to 11 A.M. Morning, rising after. *Opium* or quinine after. **Painless.** Night, children in. School girls, in. *Vegetables* agg. *Motion,* walking agg. Urination during.

**Eruptions** about *anus: herpetic, Excoriation, nates between. Fissure. Flatus discharge of:* Afraid to pass, lest feces escape. *Copious.* Drinking after. **Offensive.** Stool before.

**Haemorrhage** from anus; stool, after, **during, from hard.**

*Haemorrhoids* (Piles): Bleeding, stool during. External. Large. *Motion,* agg. **Night. Painful.** *Pregnancy during.*

*Heat* (Burning); *stool after. Itching; walking while; stool after.* **Inactivity of rectum.** Moisture at. *Narrowing of.*

Pain: **Burning,** constant. *Constrictive.* Forenoon. Griping. Lancinating, even after soft stool. Pinching. Pressing. **Pulsating, throbbing.** *Sore, Stitching. Stinging.* Tenesmus, coffee after.

Paralysis. *Prolapse, stool after.* Redness. *Stricture.* Swelling.

Sensations: Bubbles. Escaping. Coldness. Insects were crawling. **Feces retained** as if. Lump, foreign body as if. *Pulsation.* Tickling. Rough substance as if.

Pimples on, worms, round.

**STOOLS: Acrid, Albuminous.** *Balls, sheep dung like. Black.* *Bloody.* Brown. Consistence, changeable. Copious. **Crumbling.** Covered with blood. Curdled. **Difficult;** although soft; recedes. **Dry.** **Hard;** first then fluid; heavy and tearing anus; must strain at. Gray; whitish in part. **Gushing. Frequent, frothy. Incomplete,** *unsatisfactory.* Scanty. **Involuntary;** sleep during; urination and stool during; on passing flatus. Irregular; now hard, now soft. Knotty. Large. Misshapen, triangular. Coated with mucus. Transparent. **White.** Oily. Offensive odour. Pasty. Looking as if, pepper in. Rough, as if. Urging; coffee after, constant; frequent; **ineffectual. Watery;** black; green; rice water, white; yellow, yellow orange.

**URINARY:** Bladder; catarrh. pain; *pressing;* stitching, *stool before*; *urination during;* walking while. **Unable to pass urine,** in presence of others. *Constriction.* Heaviness, compels him to bend forward.

Urging to urinate: **Morbid desire. Frequent,** with suppressed menses. Ineffectual. Night. Painful, with urging to stool. Sudden, violent.

*Urination:* Dribbling, stools after, urination after. Difficult, (Dysuria). *Frequent;* day and night; stool during. Involuntary, **enuresis; cough during;** *night; pregnancy during; sitting, standing,* walking while. *Irresistible,* hurried.

Kidneys: Heat in the region, while sitting. *Pain;* burning; burrowing; crampy, griping; *drawing in ureters; extending to ureters.* Pecking. Pulsation. Tension.

Urethra: *Agglutination* of meatus. *Burning,* 10 a.m. **night;** *contraction, with urging to urinate.* Discharges; *acrid;* clear and colourless; *gleety, itching with;* **painless; chronic gonorrhoea; milky; white;** yellow, chronic. Haemorrhage. Inflammation, moisture at meatus. Pain; burning biting, fossa navicularis, meatus; **morning; night;** coition after; *cutting;* erections during and after, morning agg.; pinching; during discharge of semen. Urination; agg. **after,** *at close of,* before, *during, when not.* Sensitive. Stricture.

Urine: *Acrid. Albuminous,* pregnancy during. *Alkaline. Bloody.* Burning. *Cloudy, muddy.* Colour; black; brown; menses during; clay; *coffee like; dark;* greenish dark; **pale;** *red;* white. **Colourless.** Frothy.

*Copious, amenorrhoea with, night. Offensive. Scanty, fever during. Sediment; adherent; bright; chalk; mealy,* **mucus, red; brick colour;** sand gravel. Specific gravity decreased. **Sugar.**

**MALE:** Coition; aversion, extreme to; *enjoyment absent;* followed by pollution and increased desire. Erections; *continued,* excessive, *frequent; incomplete;* night; painful; *sexual desire without;* stools after; *troublesome;* violent. Erections, wanting, impotency. **Hair falling from pubes. Irritability,** excited. Masturbation; disposition to; ill effects of. Stinky odour. Seminal discharge; absent during coition; cold; copious; feeble; scanty; every night. Seminal emissions (nightly); **coition after;** *erections* without; frequent; morning; stool after; night every. Sexual passion; diminished; **increased,** emissions after, erections without, excessive, **priapism with.** Sexual passion, wanting. Emission of prostatic fluid.

Penis and Glans: Excoriation. Blenorrhoea. *Formication. Balanitis. Itching.* Moisture. Pain. Perspiration. Pulsation. Redness. Paraphimosis. Cutting in prepuce, after urination. Scrotum relaxed, sensitive; swollen; moist eruptions; hydrocele; inflammation from suppressed gonorrhoea. Testes; pain; swelling; turbercles. Eruptions; eczema; herpes; pimples etc.

**FEMALE:** Abortion, from suppressed grief. Coition; aversion to, menses after; painful; *enjoyment absent.* **Conception difficult** (sterility); copious menses from. Conception easy. Sexual desire; *diminished;* increased; violent, involuntary orgasm with. **Dragging.** Dryness. **Hair falling** from **pubes.** Labour pains; ceasing; **weak.** Lochia; **protracted.**

**Leucorrhoea:** *Acrid.* **Albuminous.** Backache, preceding and alternating. Bland. Burning. *Copious.* Debilitating, replacing menses. **Greenish.** Headache with. Menses after, before, instead of. Milky. Morning. **Like boiled starch.** Thin. Watery. **Transparent. White.**

Mammae: *Atrophy.* Eruptions on. Itching. Milk, salty, thin, Nodules. Pain; sore; *stitching.* Sensitive to slightest touch.

*Menstruation:* Amenorrhoea, anemia from. Anger brings on the flow. Appear as if would. Dysmenorrhoea; convulsions with; forenoon only; irregular; from getting wet feet. **Frequent.** Late, **delayed. Menorrhagia.** Metrorrhagia. Night only. **Protracted.** Return, having ceased. **Scanty;** *short duration suppressed;* anemia from; getting feet wet; disappointed love from. Menses; *clotted;* dark, membranous; **pale;** *watery; thin; headache,* congestive symptoms with; ovarian pain with; during urination.

Uterus: *Cancer. Contraction in.* **Displacement.** Chronic inflammation. **Bearing down in the region of.** Pain, *after pains;* sleep during and after agg.; back on amel. *Prolapse; lying down* amel.; **morning agg.** String were pulling between sacrum and uterus.

Vagina: Aphthous. Coldness. Burning, sore. Pain; coition during. Vaginismus. Vulva and Labia: *Dryness.* Eruptions, herpetic. Inflammation, follicular. **Itching;** menses agg.; **pudendum of.** Pain, menses during.

**HEART:** Circulation sluggish. Arteries distended. Varicose veins. Pulse; *abnormal.* **Frequent** (fast), **motion** agg.; *vexation after.* Full. *Intermittent.* **Irregular. Quick.** *Slow, than heart beat.* Small. Soft. **Weak.** Tremulous. Tumultous.

Heart; beats felt all over body; *dilatation;* goitre heart; endocarditis, pericarditis. Pain; in region of; **aching;** crushed or bruised. Pressing; sore; worse by, ascending, *coughing.* Eating and drinking after, *lying on left side,* exertion, *mental,* deep inspiration, reading or talking aloud, on stooping, **touch;** better, in open air, *pressure of hand,* urinating after.

Palpitation: Alternating with beats in head. Anemia, vital drains from. **Ascending** agg. Audible. Chill during. Cough with. **Exertion** agg. Excitement, *fright,* after. Fainting with. *Hysteria in.* **Unrequitted affection** from. *Pregnancy,* during. Shaking the body from. *Throat to.* **Tumultous.** Visible. Noise from strange.

Waking, on or waking the patient. Lying, **on left side** agg. on right side amel.

Sensations: Broken were. Coldness; **icy,** chill during; in *region* of; **mental exertion** agg. **Constriction.** Jerks. Movements in as of. Tension. Tightness. Trembling, fluttering.

**RESPIRATORY:** Chest: Anxiety in. *Asthma;* cough with; evening agg. Chilliness, left side. Clucking sound. Coated sensation, inside. Cracking on motion. Congestion, *pregnancy* during. Dropsy. Foreign body sticking behind sternum. Itching. **Constriction;** band as from; exertion agg. lying while; spasmodic. *Fluttering; air open* amel. **lying while on left side,** faintness after. Fullness. Gurgling, rumbling on right side. Narrow as if, too. Oppression; erect after rising or sitting bent.

Chest pain: Aching. Burning. **Rawness. Cutting.** Gnawing. *Pressing.* Extends to arms, back, left, scapula, shoulder. Spots in. Tearing. **Stitching.** Thrusting. Clavicles. Intercostal. Sides *left. Sternum.* Worse; bending forward; *chronic;* respiration; *pressure;* standing; while *talking* or walking; touch. Better; air open; placing hand on  head; pressure; walking. Twitching in muscles.

Cough; from abdomen, constriction of trachea, dryness of throat or larynx. Irritation in *larynx;* stomach; elongated uvula from. Asthmatic; breathing obstructed, choking. Constant day and night. **Dry.** Cutting in chest with. Pain in cervical glands with. **Evening. Hacking.** Racking. Hollow. **With thrusts in hypogastrium.** Pain in inguinal region. Lachrymation with. *Morning. Painful.* Paroxysmal. Rattling. Retching. Saliva accumulation with. *Short. Spasmodic. Whooping,* flow of tears with. Suffocative. *Reflex sympathetic.* **Tickling** *tormenting.* Worse; evening 8 to 11 p.m.; exertion, mental labour from, **motion of arm;** drinking; **fever during;** lying back on, bed in, on becoming warm. Night. *Room,* entering in, from open air. Sour food. Standing erect while.

Expectoration: Acrid. **Albuminous. Glairy. Mucous.** *Bloody,* streaked, menses during, after violent erection. Frothy. Grayish. Greenish. Hawked up mucus. Lumpy. Purulent. Taste; bitter, copper like; metallic; flat; repulsive; *salty;* sour. **Transparent.** Viscid. *White.* Yellow. Walking while agg.

Larynx: *Catarrh. Constriction. Croup. Dryness, inflamed. Chronic catarrh.* **Irritation.** *Swallowing empty* agg. **Mucus in;** *copious; after each paroxysm of cough; ejected with difficulty.*

Rattling in. *Scraping in.* Pain; *rawness;* tearing; soreness; stitching to ear; cough and inspiration agg. Sensations; *crawling; dust as from; foreign substance; lump;* **tickling,** day and night, ulcerative.

Voice: **Hoarseness;** overuse of voice from; singing, talking; morning agg. Husky. *Lost.* Rough. Weak.

Lungs: Emphysema. Expand, have no room to. *Inflammation.* Pleurisy. *Oedema. Phthisis,* purulent, ulcerative.

Respiration: *Acclerated, rapid.* Arrested; cough during; evening; with griping pain in inguinal region. Deep. *Difficult,* suffocative attacks; wheezing; whistling on expiration. *Hot breath.* Impeded, obstructed. *Loud.* **Snoring.** Worse; **ascending;** *chill during;* **exertion,** walking **rapidly,** etc. Drinking when. eating after. Heat with. *Pain during.* Lying on back. better; air open; motion arms of.

Trachea: Dryness. Inflammation. Irritation. Pain, rawness. Tickling, also in throat pit.

**BACK: Coldness.** Eruptions; crusts; impetigo; moist; pimples; pustules. Heat. *Heaviness.* Itching.

**Pain: Aching.** *As if would break. Broken as if.* **Bruised, sore. Cutting.** *Drawing.* Extends to head, heart, *hips.* **Lameness.** Paralytic. Pressing. **Pulsating.** Stitching. Worse: Bed in. Breathing when. *Chill during. Fever during.* Coition. Coughing. Lying, *while, on back.* Night. Menses before. Pressure. Movements; raising arm up; straightening up; supporting; turning, in bed, frequently; walking while; work during. Better; bending backwards; *leaning on* something; lying, **on back, on hard surface;** *pressure;* turning, in bed, frequently; walking while.

Shivering. Spasms (Opisthotonos). Stiffness. **Tension.** Twitching.

Cervical Region: **Emaciation.** Eruptions. **Itching;** scratching agg. Pain; fatigued as if; extends to arms, down the back, clavicles, ear, eyes, head, occiput, shoulders; *pressing;* pulsating; **sore, bruised;** sprained, dislocated as if; stitching. Goitre, anteriorly.

Dorsal region: Formication. Pain.

Lumbar region: *Chill starts in.* Coldness. *Heat. Itching,* burning, to abdomen and thighs. *Numbness,* in morning or on rising. Pain (Lumbago); extends to thighs and uterus; lameness, with every breath; penetrating; **morning, rising from bed.** *Stitching. Paralysis; sensation of.* **Weakness.**

Stiffness of lumbo-sacral region. Scapulae; coldness, drawing, tension, between.

**Spine & Cord:** Myelitis. Spinal meningitis. Tabes dorsalis. Necrosis of vertebrae. Pain; **sore bruised;** tearing, downward. Sensitive. **Weakness, tired feeling.** Eating agg. **Manual labour.** Agg; **Sexual excess.** After.

**EXTREMITIES:** *Alternating between* (lower). Arthritic nodosities. **Awkwardness;** drops things; knocks against things; stumbling when walking. Band around bones as if. *Bandaged as if* (knees). Bubbling sensation. **Bursae in joints.** *Chilliness. Coldness;* standing while; of foot, to knees, headache during; of fingers, during chill; joints of. Cold, sensitive to. **Constriction of joints.** *Contraction;* muscles and tendons; knees, while walking. Cramps; hands, grasping a cold stone on; like pain, in foot. Discolouration, mottled. **Dislocation of joints,** easy, in lower. Drawn upwards (u). Emaciation of diseased limbs. *Eruptions;* boils; blotchy; gritty; in groups; *herpes; bends of joints;* itching; moist; red areola; *pustules;* rash; *urticaria; vesicle,* bloody serum; white. White spots on soles. Varicose ulcers. Varices. Formication. Hair on, as if. Heaviness; *tired limbs;* menses during, suppressed; motion amel. Heat. *Inflammation of joints. Itching; rubbing* agg; touch agg. violent, between toes; *cracked skin* with; palms and soles; water in agg. hands of. Lightness, sensation of. *Jerking; sleep during; on going to sleep.* Lameness (1). Loose sensation, bones (1). Motion; convulsive; involuntary. Nodes (1). *Numbness; left; lying on it;* hand into pocket, on; siesta *during.*

*Pain; aching;* bones; chill during. Boring. Broken as if. Burning. *Drawing;* downward. Joints in; *gouty; rheumatic.* Paralytic. Paroxysmal. Rheumatic. *Sciatica;* vertebral origin; with chronic tonic contraction. Sore, bruised. Sprained as if. Stitching. Tearing. Worse: Bending or turning the limb, backwards. Ascending steps and breathing (1). *Chill,* during. **Emotions.** *Exertion after;* motion on; backwards and forwards (arms). *Night. Lying. Periodically.* Pressure of clothes. Letting arm hang down. Raising arm up, riding after. *Rising from seat. Stepping* (1). *Uncovering.* Better; motion. Rest. Stretching limbs. **Continued walking** (1). Warmth.

Paralysis: *Anger* after. Suppressed intermittent fever from. Pain from. Post-diphtheritic. Painless. Emotions from, grief etc. Flexor muscles of. *Sexual excess from.* Stiffness with. Pulsation. Raise impossible to. *Restlessness;* sitting while; sleep before. Shocks. Sinking down. Sprains, tendency to. Short as if (1) *Stiffness;* joints of; paralytic. Suppleness, lack of (u). Swelling; *joints of; dropsical.* *Tension;* joints in; tendons short, as if, walking while (1). *Trembling;* exertion after; writing while. *Trembling; ascending stairs;* exertion after; *menses before,* during; *rising, after sitting,* on; *walking while* amel.

*Twitching;* as from electric shocks; joints of (u); sleep during or *falling to.* Warts. **Walk, late learning to.** Walking; *anxious;* falls easily, while; stepping high; stooped; *stumbles easily; tottering.* *weakness;* anger after (u); joints of; rising from bed, amel. rising from seat, agg. stiffness with; taking hold of something (u); vexation after; walking amel.

Axillae: Abscess; **crusts;** *scabs; glands; swelling; perspiration.* Shoulders; cracking in. Elbow; stitching in olecranon; tension bend of. Forearm; pain, hanging down agg.; downwards to radius. Hands: *Drops things;* callosities; desquamation; *dryness;* red and brownish spots; skin, cracked hard and rough; **trembling,** emotions from, unpleasant news, *writing while; warts.* Fingers; vesicles between; *chapped,* **nails about;** *formication, tips;* numbness; *sucking the thumb;* **tingling;** drops things, grasping when. Nails; cracks on, around; blue, *chill during; fellon, cold* application amel.; **hang nails;** *ulcerative pain; sensitive.*

Hips; tuberculous disease of joints, *tension.* Thighs; redness, between, **contraction of hamstrings;** tension, ascending steps, *downwards,* **hamstrings.** Knees; **contraction, hollow of;** compression; pain, nail driven as if in; *drawing; hollow of;* shuddering, walking amel, **tension, hollow of; weakness,** morning. Bandaged sensation. **Tension;** trembling. *Calf* in. Ankles; *weakness,* turn easily; **dislocation easy.** Foot; heaviness, menses during, *standing, while,* walking amel.; perspiration, offensive, sour, suppressed. *Restlessness,* uneasy, must move constantly. *Swelling, ascending steps* while, *oedematous,* sensation of. Soles; itching; perspiration; blisters on heels. Excoriation between toes; *ingrowing nails; numbness;* toes; *tingling, prickling tips.*

l=Lower u = Upper.

**SLEEP:** Comatose. Disturbed, dream by. Interrupted, thirst by limbs drawn up, position. Restless. **Unrefreshing;** with abdominal pain; blood ebullitions from. **Somnambulism.**

*Sleepiness;* **day during;** night wakefulness with; afternoon 3 p.m. unconquerable, but cannot sleep; eating after; **heat during;** musing (when unoccupied); overpowering; while *reading* or *sitting;* rising after; walking in open air, after.

Sleeplessness; *insomnia;* from anxiety, coldness; **grief, *palpitation, shocks;*** during heat, menses; **eating after;** *midnight before;* *morning;* frightened easily; late after midnight; sleepiness with; from activity of mind, (thoughts); from twitching in limbs, **vertigo; waking after.**

Dreams: Anger, quarrels, riots. **Anxious;** menses during; on falling asleep. Business. Carousing. Continued after waking. True, seem on waking. Cruelty. Disgusting. Death of. Exciting. Exertion of body. **Heavy, laborious day work. Fantastic.** *Fire.* **Frightful.** Ghosts. Nightmare. Lascivious. Love of. Many. Menses during. *Mental exertion.* Mind, affecting. *Pleasant.* Poisoned of being. Prisoner, of being taken a. Repeating. **Robbers; cannot sleep,** till the house is searched; menses during. Sad. Teeth pulled out. Thirsty. *Unimportant. Unpleasant. Unremembered. Vexation,* disgusting. **Vivid.**

Concomitant: Erections. Expectorating. *Saliva runs from mouth.* Screaming and shrieking. *Weeping.* Sobbing. Sinking in bed. Starting up as in fright. *Talking.* Throbbing in blood vessels. Tossing about. Twitching.

Waking; difficult. Dreams from. Early, 1 a.m., 3 a.m., 4 a.m. *Frequent. Fright as from.* Gastric symptoms with. From heat, palpitation. Late. Restlessness with.

Yawning: **Chill during.** Frequent, riding in carriage in evening. With hiccough, nausea. *Sleepiness with,* without. Spasmodic, and constant stretching. Vehement, walking in open air, after. Wine, amel.

**CHILL:** *Annual.* **Anticipating;** every other day, hour. Apyrexia, during. As if cold water dashed over him. **Autumnal.** Begins; *back in;* body right side; **feet; fingers** and **toes; hands** and **feet;** head, *creeping.* Coition, after. Exposure after; *living on water courses from; malarial influence; tropical countries; sea shore; soil freshly turned up.* Heated, over-heated during. *Internal.* One sided, right. Quartan. **Quotidian. Shaking.** *Tertian.*

Violent with delirium. Unconsciousness with. Warmth desire for, which does not relieve.

Worse: Air open. Bed in, turning over in. Eating after. *Exertion mental. Heated becoming.* Grasping cold object. Menses; before, during, after. Morning. During; motion, pains, *sleep,* stool. Morning; rising from bed. Stool before. Summer, sun in. Uncovering, undressing. Urination, vomiting after, warmth of room or stove. Warm weather.

Better: Air open. Lying.

Concomitants: Blue lips, nails. Nervousness. Pain in limbs, bones. Perspiration with and after. *Thirst.* Thirstlessness. Vomiting, bilious. Yawning, accelerated breathing.

- **FEVER: In general.** Alternate day. Burning heat. Chill; with, without; alternating with. *Cold from taking.* **Intense heat** (High fever); **delirium with;** *sleep during;* **stupefaction and unconsciousness.** Internal heat, in blood vessels. Long lasting. *Paroxysms increasing in severity.* Perspiration with or absent. Shuddering with.

Types: *Autumnal. Bilious. Cerebro-spinal.* Chicken-pox. Continued; typhoid. **Intermittent;** chronic inveterate; enlarged liver and spleen; quartan; **quotidian;** spoiled; stage partial, irregular; **tertian.** Irritative. Scarlet. Small-pox.

Stages: **Chill followed by heat;** *then sweat;* with sweat Chill; then heat without thirst; then sweat without intervening heat. Heat, followed by chill.

Worse: Anger from. Coughing. Covers, warmth. Drinking wine. Forenoon, 11 a.m. Manual labour. Menses, before, during. Morning. *Sleep during.* Summer, hot season. Warm room. Better, air open. Mental exertion. Rubbing *Uncovering.*

**PERSPIRATION. In general.** Complaints, from suppressed. Cold, debility from. **Easy.** Excoriating. **Exhausting. Greasy, oily.** Odour; sour; urine like. **Profuse;** rage during. Salty deposit. Stiffens, hose, linen. Worse: Anxiety during. Cough during. Coughing. *Day time only,* and morning. *Eating while,* after. Emission after. *Exertion;* during slight; mental. Motion on. Fever after. Headache, start of. **Night. Smoking.** Stool during. *Urination after.* Waking after. Walking while. Better: Rest when at. *Uncovering.*

**SKIN:** Anaesthesia of. Biting sensation, spots in. *Burning;* as from sparks. Chafed, infants in. Chapping. Cicatrices; break *open; painful;* become red. Coldness; icy. Contraction. *Corns; burning;* painful; **shooting; stinging.** *Cracks. Discolouration; yellow,* rings, intermittent fever in. Dry; burning; inability **to perspire,** *when exercising.* Erysipelas; recurrent, chronic. *Excoriation,* excrescences; hematodes. Formication; begins at feet, extends upward. Goose flesh. *Hairs fall out.* Inactivity. Inflammation. *Intertrigo.* **Itching;** bed in, on becoming warm; biting; burning; crawling; jerking; spots moisture. *Nevus.* Pain. Prickling. *Rough. Seborrhoea. Sensitive. Sore, feeling.* Sticking. *Stings of insects. Swellings, dropsical.* Tension. *Ulcerative pain.* Warts; painful, sensitive. Wrinkled.

Eruptions: Areola red. Biting. Blisters. Blotches. *Boils; blood;* small. Burning. **Crusty.** Desquamating. Discharges; corrosive; *destroy hair; glutinous; pus; thin; yellow. Dry.* Eczema. Elevated. *Excoriated. Granular. Gritty.* Groups in. *Hairy parts on.* **Herpetic;** burning; chapping; **circinate;** crusty; dry; **fevers in;** itching; moist; patches; scaling; suppurating; zoster; Impetigo. Itching. *Joints on.* Leprosy. Menses before. Miliary. Moist. **Overheated, from being.** *Pemphigus.* Petechiae. Phagedenic. Psoriasis. **Pimples;** itching. *Pustules;* malignant; ulcerated. *Rash.* Red scabs. Scabies; **dry;** moist; suppressed. Scaly; bran like. *Smarting. Stinging.* **Suppurating. Swelling with.** *Tubercles;* miliary; red. **Urticaria;** exercise violent after; warmth, exercise from. **Vesicular;** *bloody; red;* scurfy; small; **sudamina.**

*Ulcers:* Bleeding. Burning. Crawling with. Deep. Discharges; bloody; corrosive. Fistulous. Itching. Painful. Pulsating. Phagedenic. Sensitive. *Smarting.* Stinging. Sticky. *Superficial.* Suppurating. Suppurative pain with. *Swollen. Vesicles;* surrounded by.

# NATRUM PHOS

**GENERALITIES:** Anemia. Chlorosis. Bathing, dread of. Convulsions; emissions of semen during. *Emaciation.* Faintness; fainting; coition after. Fine, sensation as of a hair or thread. Formication, internally. Heat; flushes of; menses during. *Lack of vital heat.* Irritability. Lassitude, warm weather. *Leukemia.* Lie down, inclination to. *Loss of vital fluids.* Morphinism. Numbness; single parts of. Orgasm of blood; emotions after. Pain; stitching; tearing; twinging. *Pulsation, throbbing;* internally. Tendency to take cold. Tension, tightness. Twitching. **Weak,** emissions after; **nervous;** paralytic. Warm weather from. Yellow golden.

**WORSE:** Air open, cool, (aversion to); draft. Ascending. Coition. Cold in general; air; becoming. Conversation. Eating, before. **Emissions.** *Emotions. Exertion, of vision;* reading. Food; bitter; butter; cold drinks; cold food; *fat;* **milk;** sour; vinegar; sweets, sugar. Fright. Jarring. Light. Lying in bed. Menses; after, before. during. Motion. Music. Narcotic. **Noise. Onanism. Sexual excess.** Sitting while. Sleep; during; falling asleep on. Stooping. Storm; approach of, during. *Swallowing. Walking.* Warm room.

**BETTER:** *Eating* Pressure. Scratching.

**MIND:** Absent minded. Absorbed. Agitation. Anger, trifles at. Anxiety; fear with; future about; midnight. Bad news; ailments from; fear of. Bashful. Calmness. Careless. Cheerful. Company, aversion to. Concentration difficult. Confusion. *Delusions;* sees dead persons; hears footsteps in next room; sees phantoms, images frightful; inanimate objects are persons; that he were going to be sick or have typhoid fever. Discontented. *Dullness.* Excitement. *Fear;* of impending disease; *something will happen;* of misfortune. Forgetful; sexual excess after. Frightened easily. Hurry. Impatience; no one works fast enough to suit him. Hysteria. Ideas abundant (clearness of mind); deficiency of; evening. *Imbecility.* **Indifference.** Indolence. Irritability; before breakfast; menses during. Memory; *weakness* of. Mirth. **Prostration of mind.** Restlessness; nervousness; anxious; evening. **Sadness;** emissions after; heat during; music from. Sensitive; oversensitive, music to. Serious (earnest). Sit, inclination to. *Starting, statled;* easily; electric shocks through the body while wide awake. Stupefaction. Suspicious. Taciturn. Thoughts; diseases of; wandering. Unconsciousness. *Weeping.*

**HEAD:** Eruptions. Hair falling. Heat of head, vertex. Empty, hollow. Shocks, blows, jerks.

Headache; forehead; *occiput;* sides; *supra-orbital;* temples, to ears, to eyes; vertex and forehead. Pain; bursting; constrictive. crampy; distensive, full; drawing; heaviness; pinching; pulsating;

stitching; stunning; stupefying; tearing. Headache; paroxysmal; nausea with; with vomiting, slime, sour matter, *undigested food.* Worse, ascending; binding up the hair;' lying while; raising head suddenly; rising from lying.   Better; air open.

Vertigo; objects seem to turn in circle; gastric derangement from; mental exertion; tendency to fall; sitting while agg.

**EYES:** Pain, inner. Conjuctivitis; granular; mucus discharge; *creamy, profuse.* Dry. Inflammation; *scrofulous.* Itching. Lachrymation. Eyeballs; aching; burning; cutting; pressing; menses during; sand as from; sore; stitching, reading from. Worse; evening; while *reading; looking at fire.* Photophobia. Redness of eyes. Bathed in water as if.  Strabismus; worms due to.  Weak; light agg.

Eyelids; agglutinated; itching, margins; pain pressing, quivering; swollen; ulceration.   Pupils dilated; one contracted and one dilated.

Amaurosis (blindness). Dim. Foggy, vision. Colours before eyes; dark halo of colour around light.   Sparks, Myopia.

**EAR: Thin** deposit on external ear. Heat and redness, one sided. Crusts on concha; scaly.  Itching; burning, right; must scratch till it bleeds.

Pain; below the ear; burning; stinging, shooting; tearing; right.

Pulsation. Stopped as if. Water falling from a height into long thin narrow vessel, as if.

*Hearing acute.* Deafness. Hearing lost. *Noises in ear;* vertigo with; humming; ringing; *roaring;* rushing; waterfall like; singing; **whizzing.**

**NOSE:** Picking. Tingling. Fullness,. sense of. Tension. Itching. *Boring* into with fingers. *Epistaxis;* blowing the nose from. Coryza; *fluent* discharge. Crusts; thick; yellow. Obstruction (stoppage). Odours from or in; offensive; morning. Ozena. Pain; sore, bruised. Smell, acute.  Sneezing. Tingling. Discharge from posterior nares; tough; yellowish green.

**FACE:** Bloated; fever without. Bluish. *Circles around* eyes. Earthy. Emaciated. Pale lips. Red; alternating with pale; fever without; *alternating* sides. White about nose and mouth. Yellow. Eruptions;

chin; forehead; mouth around; pimples; *pustules.* Heat; burning; chill during. Itching; mouth around; biting; stinging. Pain. Brown spots. Sore, bruised pain in lower jaw. Swelling of submaxillary glands.

**MOUTH:** Dryness. Numbness. Prickling. Salivation. Speech difficult; throat as if closed by something, from. Taste; bad on awakening; metallic; saltish; sour. Vesicles.

Gums, bleeding; boils; ulcers. Palate, **white; *yellow;* creamy; covered with false membrane.** Teeth; caries; grinding, during sleep; looseness. Brown mucus on. Pain, boring; pressure amel., warmth external amel.

Tongue; clean and moist; bleeding; dirty white; brown at centre; yellow base; golden yellow. Hair of, sensation, and vesicles at tip. Prickling.

**THROAT:** *Yellow membrane.* Dryness. Disposition to hawk. Inflamed. *Mucus,* drawn from posterior nares; thick; yellow. Pain, burning; sore; **stitching;** on swallowing food. Swallowing difficult; can swallow only liquids. Scraping. Lump, plug as of.

Goitre; thyroid cartilage, pressed in, as if. Swelling of external throat, extending to chest.

**STOMACH:** Appetite, *increased,* wanting, diminished. Aversion to; acids; bread, and butter, fats; food; meat; milk; tobacco. Desires cravings; for alcoholic drinks, beer; *cold drinks;* eggs, fried; 'fish; pungent things.

Indigestion; fat food after. Eructations; empty (tasteless); **sour.** Waterbrash. Heartburn, Hyperacidity. Nausea; headache during.

Pain; fats from; *cramping;* gnawing; sore, bruised; 2,3 hours after eating. Sweets agg. Menses during and after agg. Fullness. Heat, flushes of. Heaviness. Thirst, extreme. Ulcers.

Vomiting; coughing; pregnancy; **acid sour;** fluid, headache during, bile; blood; curdled masses, milk; frothy; mucus. Retching.

Empty, goneness; day time; not relieved by eating; forenoon; morning; rising on; stool after.

**ABDOMEN:** Colic; child·en in; to chest; flatulent; paroxysmal; worms from burning; cramp·ng; cutting; sore, bruised; stitching. Worse; stool before; walking.

**Distension. Flatulence;** breakfast after; here and there; noisy; obstructed. Gurgling. Rumbling. Anxiety; stool after. Fullness. Marble dropped down in descending colon, as if. Cutting pain in right hypochondriac region. *Stitching pain* in liver. Sclerosis of liver, with diabetes and succession of boils.

**RECTUM AND ANUS:** Constipation; habitual, obstinate; constant desire. Constriction. Retraction. Twitching. Worm complaints.

Diarrhoea; hot weather; menses during; eating after. Flatus, afraid to pass lest feces escape. *Inactivity of rectum. Itching;* ascarides from; warm bed in. Pain. Burrowing. aching; sore; stool after agg.

Stools; bloody crumbling; difficult; hacked; hard. Ineffectual urging. **Involuntary; on passing flatus.** Light coloured. Natural first then fluid or loose. Odour, *cadaveric,* sour. Pasty. *Thin.* Shooting out. **Sour.** Urging, desire to; stools after, during. *Watery. Rice water.* yellow, fecal, brownish.

**URINARY:** Pressing pain in bladder, before urination. Paralysis. Urging to urinate (morbid desire); *coition after;* constant; frequent.

Urination; dysuria, strangury; frequent, perspiration during; unsatisfactory; *incomplete;* involuntary, night (enuresis). Retarded. Must wait for urine to start; can pass urine only when pressing at stools; must press for a long time before he can begin; must continue to press, if he stops to breathe, urine stops, until he strains again.

Stitching pain in kidneys. Prostate enlarged; emissions, stools with. *Urethra;* pain; itching in, coition after.

Urine: **albuminous,** burning; cloudy; dark; pale; red; copious, afternoon, morning; offensive; scanty; mucus; oxalate of lime.

**MALE:** Vesicular eruption. Erections; continued, frequent; painful; incomplete; sexual desire without; troublesome; violent. Wanting (impotency). Seminal discharge; *pleasure without;* smell like state urine; weakening. Seminal emissions, **nightly;** *coition after;* erections without; frequent; unconsciousness of; *every night;* spasms with; *thin,* *watery,* weakening; dreams without. Sexual passion; *increased,* erections without; diminished, wanting.

Itching (prepuce). Spermatic cord, aching, drawing; emissions after. Testes; drawing, pressing pain; swollen.

**FEMALE:** Conception difficult, due to acrid secretion from vagina. Sexual desire diminished.

*Leucorrhoea;* acrid; *copious; cream like;* honey coloured; sour odour; thin watery; yellow; menses after; rawness and itching of parts with.

Menses; amenorrhoea; dysmenorrhoea; frequent, too early, too soon; *late delayed.* Menorrhagia (copious); *protracted;* pale; watery, thin; excitement and sleeplessness with; shortening of knee cords with.

Uterus; displaced; prolapse of.

**HEART:** Atheroma. Pain in heart; alternating with other pain; with pain in great toe. *Palpitation,* audible; pulsations in different parts of body with. Bubbles start from the artery and pass through arteries, as if; lump, ball, load as of. Trembling, fluttering; agg. by ascending and eating.

**RESPIRATORY:** Pimples on chest. Pain; aching; burning; cutting; rawness; stitching; sides right and left. Pressure, deep respiration, cough during. agg. Chest; anxiety felt in; coldness; fullness; constriction; empty sensation (eating after); lump, sensation of.

Cough; irritation in larynx from; constant; dry, evening; hacking; hollow; racking; short; tickling, violent; chill during; drinking after; sitting agg.

Expectoration; bloody; **causing soreness and rawness of** lips, mouth and tongue; greenish; mucus; *offensive;* thick, viscid; yellow; taste; flat putrid, salty. Larynx; irritation; tickling; hoarseness; voice lost.

Respiration; *difficult,* asthmatic; sighing; menses during, soreness; trachea in.

**NECK & BACK:** Heaviness. Itching. Pain; *aching;* drawing; sore; stitching. Worse; breathing when; menses during; motion on; sexual excess. Perspiration. Neck; vesicles; itching. Pain; sore, bruised; sticking. Stiffness. Swelling of glands. Pain in dorsal region.

Pain; *burning,* **sore, bruised;** in lumbo-sacral region; weakness emissions after; evening.

**EXTREMITIES:** Coldness. Contraction of muscles of tendons; extensor muscles, when writing. Cracking in joints. Eruptions; joints on; vesicles. Heaviness. Itching. Numbness. Pain; tearing; joints in. **Trembling; emissions after.** Twitching. Weakness.

Pain in shoulder; drawing; pressing, rheumatic; stitching; tearing. Tension. Paralytic pain in wrists. Paralysis right hand, left ankle.

Vesicles on joints. Pimples on buttocks. Itching. Heaviness. **Numbness.** Sudden weakness. Walking unsteady. Hamstrings; tension in; contraction of, menses after. Pain in thighs, worse on ascending stairs. Bandaged sensation, in calf. Restless in legs. Ankles; weakness; in children, learning to walk. Coldness of foot; day time; during menses.

**SLEEP:** Deep Dreams; amorous; anxious; vivid. Restless sleep; during and after menses. Sleepiness; sitting while. Sleeplessness; heat during; from slightest noise; thoughts from; activity of mind from. Unrefreshing. *Waking early;* frequent; late; from slightest noise.

**CHILL & FEVER:** Chill in general; internal; one sided; shaking, Coldness, icy. Worse; cold or going into; bed in; eating after; menses during. Fever; with perspiration; bilious; worse during sleep. Perspiration; *profuse;* sour odour; anxiety during; exertion slight during; coughing agg.

**SKIN:** Biting sensation. Burning; dry. Chafed in infants. Coldness. Corns; sore; stinging. Spots; brown, liver; yellow; red.

Eruptions; blisters; burning; crusty; yellow; desquamation; eczema; herpetic; painful; pimples; flea bite like, all over body. Urticaria, nodular, rosy. *Vesicles.* Suppurating.

Erysipelas. Excoriation. Formication. Freckles. Gnawing eating.

Burning edges. Inactivity. Itching; biting; burning crawling, on becoming warm in bed. Sensitiveness. *Sore feeling.* Ulcerative pain. Ulcers; deep; crawling; yellow; *offensive discharge;* fistulous inflamed; red arcade; sensitive; stinging; stitching; suppurating; swollen; unhealthy, would not heal. Warts.

## NOTE ON PHOSPHATES

Organic phosphate is present in large amounts in all tissue cells in many forms. It is concerned with numerous metabolic changes in connection with carbohydrate, skeletal muscle and fat metabolism. It is concerned in the action of many coenzymes. High energy phosphate bonds are important in energy transfer in various tissue reactions. The reduction of adenosine tri-phosphate ATP, to adenosine di-phosphate ADP to provide energy for muscle contraction is a well known example. ADP is again restored to ATP by taking phosphate bond from creatine phosphate. Phosphates take part in regulation of H ion concentration of blood and urine.

Phosphorus is found in animal tissues in (a) nucleoproteins and nucleotides. (b) phosphatides e.g. lecithin, cephalin, (c) phosphoproteins, caseinogen, ovalbumin of egg, (d) combined with co-enzymes, (e) as inorganic phosphate in red blood cells. Skeletal muscle contains creatine phosphate, adenosine tri-phosphate, hexose and its triose derivatives.

## NATRUM SULPH

**GENERALITIES:** Abscess; fistulous. *Anemia.* Ball; globus, lump. Burns and scalds. Chorea; one sided; periodic; *right side.* Chronic disease. Convulsions, epileptic; injuries from. Dropsy; *external; internal. Emaciation.* Fainting; sitting while; stools after; walking while. Haemophilia. **Heat; flushes of; upwards. Heat; sensation of.** Infiltration. *Injuries.* Jerking, sleep during. *Leukemia.* Lie down; inclination to. Loose, torn as if.

12 F.A.

**Mercury; abuse of.** Pain; piercing; stitching internally; upward. Perspiration; complaints from suppressed. *Pulsation. throbbing; internally.* Reaction, poor. Swelling. Oedematous; smooth; **Sycosis. Trembling.** Washing; aversion to. **Weak;** *diarrhoea from,* intermittent fever from; **stools after;** walking from. *Weariness.*

**WORSE:** *Breakfast.* Cellars or vaulted places. Change of weather, cold to warm. Cloudy weather. **Wet weather. Damp dwellings.** Foggy weather; frost. Clothing. *Emotions.* Eating after.

Food; coffee; cold food; **farinaceous;** fish; **fruits;** *hot; milk; potatoes; rich;* **vegetables, green. Fright.** Grasping objects when. Lifting. *Light;* candle; gas. **Lying;** *on back; side on;* left; painless. Motion. Night air. **Noise.** Periodically. Pressure, of clothes. Reading. **Rising from a seat.** Scratching. *Seashore. Spring.* Standing. *Storm, approach of. Swallowing.* Talking by others. Touch. Twilight. Undressing after. Walking. Warmth. Warm *air; becoming, in open air, room.* Use of water in any form. *Washing with water.* **Getting drenched. Warm wet weat ier.** Weather, bright clear.

**BETTER:** Air open, desire for. Change of *position.* Cold in general (feels too hot). **Flatus passing.** Lying; *back on.* Motion. *Rubbing* abdomen. Stool, after. Stretching.

**MIND:** *Anger;* morning. Does not like to speak. Anguish; night. Cheerful (gay) followed by irritability. Confusion. *Death desire;* **must restrain to prevent injury to self.** Despair; recovery of. Discontented. *Dullness.* Estranged from her family. Fear; in a crowd; of evil, of misfortune; noise; night; *suicide of;* injury fear, he may injure himself, must restrain. Indolence, morning; breakfast after.

Industrious, desires activity. Insanity; from head injuries; paroxysmal. Irritability; when spoken to; on waking; eating amel. Sudden impulse to kill himself. Kneeling and praying. Mania; periodical. Passionate, hasty temper. Restlessness, nervousness. Sadness; from head *injuries; music from* Sensitive; music to; slightest noise to; morning. *Averse to being spoken;* morning. **Suicidal disposition;** by hanging; by shooting; **thoughts of.** Suspicious. *Taciturn.* Thinking, inability. Mental work, impossible. Wearisome. *Weeping;* delirium after, music from; open air amel.

**HEAD:** Concussion of brain. Meningitis; acute and chronic, traumatic. brain loose as if; on stooping.                    12 F.

Head drawn backward. Formication, vertex. Hair painful; when combing; when touched.

Headache; **forehead;** *occiput* to forehead; sides; temples, right. Pain; is aching; boring; digging; burning; bursting; constrictive; crushed; dull gnawing in spots; grasping; heaviness; pressing cap like, sore, bruised; stitching; tearing; wandering.

Headache; gastric causes from moving arms; wind exposure to; wandering; bilious diarrhoea with; colicky pains with; dizziness with; perspiration with; vertigo with; vomiting bile with.

Headache is worse; during eating; lying while; moving arms; reading; rest; sleep during; vomiting after. Better; cold; foot bath; perspiration; rest.

Heat of head; chill during; menses during; occiput; reading while; rising up, from abdomen. Vertex; menses during; thinking.

Injuries of the head, after. Jerking, from one side to another to right. Motions in head, on stooping. Motions of head; sideways. Perspiration; forehead; *chill during;* eating after; reading while. Sensations; creeping in scalp to vertex; falling forward or looseness on stooping; stiffness on motion. Sensitive to touch. Shocks in; sides. Twitching of muscles.

Vertigo; constipation from; head injuries after; tendency to fall to right; nausea; vomiting of bile; eating after agg.; headache during; rising from bed or sitting. Intoxicated, as if. Turning in circles, as if. Air open, amel. Vomiting, amel.

**EYES:** Pain in. Conjunctivitis; granular; pustular. Discharge; mucus; creamy profuse. Spots or specks on cornea.

Eyeballs; *burning; dryness.* Inflammation; *scrofulous. Itching, morning.* Burning tears. Painful burning, afternoon; pressing *outward;* stitching; tearing; reading from.

**Photophobia;** *chronic;* **headache during,** morning. Redness of eyes. Crawling. Watering as if. Weak.

Lids; *heavy; granular;* burning; redness; swollen; *agglutinated.* Retina; leukemic inflammation.

Amaurosis, while eating soup. Amblyopia (blurred), morning. Dim vision; eating while; fire light egg. Glittering bodies on blowing nose.

**EARS:** Heat, right side. Inflammation inside. Itching, external auditory canal. Pain behind the ear; pressing.

Pain; internal ear, right; above the ear, extending in and out; piercing; pressing out; worse, morning; warm room.

Forced outward as if. Fullness. Opening and closing like a valve; *stopped. Discharge* from ear; yellow. Hearing; acute; rumpling of paper to; lost.

Noises *in ear;* breathing when; vertigo with; chirping during intermittent fever; fluttering; *ringing; roaring;* tickling; lying amel.

**NOSE:** *Itching. Scurfy.* Epistaxis; blowing the nose from; menses before and during; sleep during; vicarious. Dryness. Crusty, scaly.

*Asthmatic breathing. Discharge fluent;* copious; crusts: *albuminous,* greenish; hard dry; purulent; like boiled starch; **thick;** *yellow,* yellowish green; watery.

Obstruction; night; sensation of. Ozena. Pain; *burning;* drawing; sore, tearing; menses during agg.

*Sneezing,* **excessive;** *hay asthma.* Thick; yellowish green discharge from posterior nares. Scraping.

**FACE:** Suffering expression. Pale, *sallow.* **Yellow;** anger after. *Herpes. Pimples;* chin on; mouth around; burning, when touched. *Vesicles,* mouth around. Erysipelas. *Itching.* Pain. *Perspiration.* Pain in jaws, extending to head. Stiffness, lower jaw. Peeling. *Swelling of submaxillary glands.*

**MOUTH:** Aphthae; from abuse of borax. Breath, *offensive. Dryness.* Heat. White slime in. Numbness. Pain as from pepper. Sour saliva. Salivation; eating after; headache during. Sensitive to touch.

**Taste bad; morning; bitter;** loss of; in morning. Vesicles; cold things amel.

Gums; blisters on; boils; detached from teeth; red; nodosities; burning pain; pustules, movable; swelling, painless; tumours painless; movable, lower gums. Vesicles.

Palate; pain, menses during; sore; touched when. Sensitive. Swelling. Vesicles.

Teeth; caries; chattering; jerks; jolts; looseness; pain, drawing. Pulsating; after eating fruits; with nose bleeding; tossing about in bed. Cold amel. Tobacco smoking amel. Elongated as if.

Tongue, **dirty**, brown; **green; greenish grey;** greenish brown, yellow; red; white. *Collection of mucus* on. Tip; **burning,** as from pepper; stitching; vesicles. Stitching pain at root. Stiff. Burnt as if, left edge.

**THROAT:** Choking. Constriction, on swallowing liquids. *Dryness;* with flow of saliva. *Hawk, disposition to.* Hawks up, cheesy lumps. Heat. *Inflamed. Mucus,* albuminous, grayish, saltish; **tenacious.** Pain; burning; sore; tearing; menses before and during. Roughness, coughing on. Lump, plug, on swallowing. Swallowing; constant disposition to; difficult. Ulcers, fauces.

Tonsils; *inflamed.* Swelling uvula. Pain; burning; drawing; pressing; to ears, sides.

Stiffness. Swelling of cervical glands. Goitre.

**STOMACH:** Appetite, *increased,* wanting. Aversion to; beer; bread; food; meat; *milk;* tobacco. *Cannot bear tight clothing. Desires, craving; beer;* **cold drinks,** food; ice or ice-cold water; boiled milk.

**Indigestion:** Debauchery in general; **farinaceous** food; wine. Distension; **eating after;** eructations amel. *Eructations;* bitter, eating after; food comes up; disagreeable; empty (tasteless); foul, incomplete; milk after; **sour;** water of. Waterbrash; afternoon; while walking. *Heartburn.* Hiccough; bread and butter after; eating after; forenoon; evening.

Nausea; constant; eye symptoms with; headache during; descending agg.; rising on; walking while; walking in open air agg.

Pain; burning; cramping; gnawing; pinching; worse, morning, night in bed, sitting while; better eating after. *Retching,* eating after. *Empty, goneness. Fullness,* distension. Heat flushes of. *Heaviness.* Pulsations. Ulcer.

*Thirst;* at start of fever only. Burning. Vehement; chill after; chill during. Extreme. Thirstless.

Vomiting; *headache during;* **pregnancy;** smoking from; vexation after. *Acid, sour.* **Bile.** Blood. *Green fluid. Mucus.* Periodic. White yeast like.

**ABDOMEN:** Colic; **flatulent;** lead; wandering; like that of diarrhoea. Extends to axilla, to back; to shoulder; to genitals. Pain; *burning; cramping;* **cutting;** digging; bearing down; pinching; sore; stitching; diarrhoea during; urging to stool, urging to urinate with.

Pain is worse; deep breathing; coughing; jarring, menses, during; pressure of clothing; standing; stool before; storm during; touch; *walking in open air;* **lying, left side.** Better by; *flatus passing; kneading abdomen;* lying on back; **pressure;** diarrhoea after.

Distension. **Flatulence;** *breakfast* **after;** noisy here and there; *obstructed;* pushing; stool during. Gurgling; gushing stools then. **Rumbling;** flatus passing before; stool before agg.

Coldness; bladder to; before stool. Constriction; bladder to; stool during; desire for stool; diarrhoea as of. Movements in, stool before. Pulsations, walking while. Tension. Typhlitis. Tremulous sensation in epigastrium.

Pain, right hypochondriac region; clawing; **sore, bruised;** shooting. Pulsation. Tension.

**Liver;** atrophy; **enlarged;** fullness, chronic. Crawling in, gall bladder; **stone colic.** Heaviness. **Inflammation, chronic.** Jaundice. Lump in. **Pain; pressing; sore;** *stitching,* throbbing. Worse; by breathing; jar; **mental labour** after; *walking while.* Better; by lying on back; on right side. **Swelling.** *Twisting.*

Mesenteric glands enlarged; hard. Tabes mesenterica. Pancreas; pain from flatulence; pressing; amel. by kneading. Pulsations.

Spleen; aching; stitching; throbbing. Umbilicus; **pain; aching; crampy.**

**RECTUM & ANUS:** *Condylomata.* Constipation, **alternating with diarrhoea;** with liver symptoms; menses before and during; **pregnancy during.**

**Diarrhoea;** aged people; women; **bilious;** *chronic;* cold drinks, cold weather or *cold food from;* in summer; **farinaceous food; fruits;**

jaundice during; **morning;** *painless;* pastry after; starchy food; vegetables; **breakfast after;** morning, driving out of bed; rising after; agg. by motion, in warm room.

Eruptions, about anus. **Flatus;** afraid to pass lest feces escape, **diarrhoea during;** difficult; **loud, spluttering offensive; stool during;** *stool urging to,* **but only flatus.** *Haemorrhage. Haemorrhoids.* Pain; stool before agg. *Prolapsus of. Ulceration.* Worm complaints. Perineum, itching.

Stools; *bilious,* bloody; *brown;* **clay coloured; copious;** difficult; **forcible, gushing; green,** turns; on passing flatus; involuntary, sleep during, urination during; knotty; light coloured. Mucus. **Odour; cadaveric,** *putrid.* Oily. Reddish. Scanty. *Sheep dung* like. Shooting out. Soft; but passed with difficulty. Thin, brown fecal; then formed lumpy, **pouring out; yellow. Watery** stools, **morning.**

Urging; desire to, but passes flatus only; constant; frequent.

**URINARY:** Paralysis (bladder). Urging to urinate (morbid desire).

Addison's disease. Nephritis; **acute parenchymatous.** Pain; cutting in ureters, piercing in both ureters with urging to urinate; sore.

**Enlarged prostate**

Painless, gleety discharge from urethra; **gonorrhoeal chronic;** *greenish yellow; with* priapism.

Urethra; pain; **burning;** anterior part and meatus; urination after, during. Stricture.

*Urine: Acrid, albuminous,* **scarlet fever after.** *Bile containing.* **Burning.** Colour; dark; pale; dark red. **Copious.** *Frothy.* Offensive odour. **Scanty.**

*Sediment; mucous; purulent;* red; *sand (gravel), white.* Specific gravity, *increased. Sugar* (diabetes mellitus), gouty symptoms with. *Viscid. Watery,* thin.

**MALE: Condylomata.** Itching. *Sexual passion, increased* (satyriasis). Swelling, odematous; penis, glans, prepuce, scrotum. Scrotum; *eruptions.* Perspiration.

**FEMALE:** Leucorrhoea; acrid; **greenish;** *purulent.* Mammae; pressing pain; retraction of nipples.

Menstruation; amenorrhoea; dysmenorrhoea. Late, delayed; protracted; short duration of; acrid; black; bloody; clotted. Ovarian cyst.

Uterus; subinvolution; pain; worse in bed, sitting or walking. Stitching in vagina.

Vulvae and labia; *condylomata;* soft, red, fleshy. Vesicles. Inflammation. Itching. Stitching pain.

**HEART:** Atheroma. Pulse; accelerated, fast. Pressing pain; eating after; pressure of hand amel. Anxiety. Oppression, morning.

**RESPIRATORY: Bronchitis;** chronic winter catarrh; asthma with.

Chest; hold must; eruptions, agg. every spring. Convulsions. Pain; pressing; **stitching;** border of lower ribs, sides; agg. during cough; **damp weather;** rising on; standing, stooping, yawning; amel. by pressure, sitting upright. Places hand to head. Spots. Blotches.

Chest; **fluttering; air open amel. Faintness after.** Fullness evening in bed. **Oppression;** amel. by lying; sitting, sunset after; walking on agg. Quaking. Trembling. Weakness; holding with both hands amel.

Trachea; mucus in; tickling.

Cough; irritation in air passages from; roughness in larynx from; tickling in larynx. Asthmatic. Dry. Night. Must hold chest with both hands. Inability to cough, from pain. Loose but violent; painful; rattling; must sit up. Deep inspiration; lying; lying on back; motion; rising on, bed from; standing agg. Air cold amel. Holding chest amel.

Expectoration; albuminous; glairy; ropy; mucoid; easy raising; **greenish.** Hard. Taste flat. Thick, viscid.

Larynx; mucus in; roughness; scraping; tickling. Hoarseness; leucorrhoea with. Husky, not clear.

Lungs; pneumonia; left lower lobe; in aged persons; delayed resolution. Phthisis; incipient; sycotic. Pleurisy.

Respiration; asthmatic; arrested. Desire, to breathe deep. **Difficult; in children.** *Loud. Rattling.* **Short, stools before. Tight.** Wheezing.

Worse; on ascending; cough with; exertion; flatulence; menses before; motion; pain during; sitting while; stormy weather; walking rapidly; wet weather. Lying; open door and windows amel.

**NECK & BACK:** Coldness; extending up. Itching, undressing while. Stiffness. Opisthotonus; spasms.

Pain; cutting; spreading upward like a fan; pressing; sore; tearing, extending down; to nape while walking.

Worse; fever during; injury, fall after; lying on side, while; motion or walking on; moving or turning head; sitting while; stretching neck; yawning. Urinate, with desire to. Urinating before.

Better; lying on right side; rubbing on; motion on; urinating after.

Neck; Pain; bruised as if, nape; drawing to clavicles, upwards, pressing; gnawing. Spasmodic drawing pain. Stiffness.

Pain between scapulae, to nape. **Cutting;** tearing; between, under; drawing below, between. Pain dorsal region.

Lumbo-sacral pain; injury after; motion amel. Cutting; sore; bruised; morning on rising, till evening.

Myelitis. Meningitis. **Injuries.** Pain; cutting; **dorsal spine;** sore, bruised tearing in cervical spine.

**EXTREMITIES:** Pimples. Urticaria. Boils in axillae. Brownish spots, inside thighs. Vesicles between thighs. Ulcers, outer side of thighs. Dry tetters, psoriasis, pimples, rawness, scabs on palms. Fingers, felon. Hang nails. Cold applications amel. Tendons affected.

Heaviness; shoulders. Inflammation of joints. Itching; undressing when; scratching amel. Lameness. Numbness.

Pain; drawing; to flexors when grasping; *joints in; rheumatic;* pressing together; sore, bruised; *tearing;* in joints; wandering, shifting.

Stiffness; chill during. Sensation of paralysis. Swelling. Tension. Tingling. Trembling; writing while. Twitching. Warts.

Stitching pain in axillae; offensive perspiration; swelling of glands. Shoulders; stiffness; heaviness; pain; boring, pressing stitching. Upper arms; compression; pain inner side; tearing pain in bend of elbows.

Pain in hands; worse on grasping anything. Trembling of hands; waking on; writing while. Weakness. Thumb sucking. Tearing pain in fingers, spinning agg.

Cracking in joints; worse on coughing; turning in bed. Pain from hips to knees; left; piercing left; pinching, only during rest. Worse; on ascending steps; motion or turning in bed; rising from a seat; in the act of sitting.

Pain in thigh bone. Weakness; in thighs; in ankles; in knees; walking while; in legs, motion during and motion amel. Sudden pressing pain in knees. Contraction; hollow of hamstring; lying on back while. Milk leg (phlegmasia alba dolens). Tendo achilles; drawing pain. Gouty pain in foot. Twitching; during sleep.

Cutting. piercing. Stitching, ulcerative pain in heels; worse, in evening, spinning while. Toes; itching, ball of; between toes.

**Sleep:** *Restless.* Yawning, frequent. Waking, headache with. Dreams; accidents; crimes (that he has committed); anxious; quarrels; sailing; unremembered; vexatious.

Sleepiness; headache during; from least mental exertion; reading while; writing when; morning. Sleeplessness; coldness from; restless-ness with; chest symptoms with; upto 1 a.m.

**CHILL & FEVER:** Chill; ascending; exposure after; getting wet from; living on water courses. Malarial; influence. Seashore, sleeping in damp rooms. **Swamps. Tropical countries.**

Chill; external; heated, overheated during. Chill; internal; *period-icity,* regular and distinct; pernicious; *quotidian; shaking;* worse; bed in; menses during; pains during; rising after. Better; bed in.

Fever; alternating with chills. Dry heat. High fever. Perspiration with. Chill followed by heat. Chill followed by heat, then sweat. Chill then sweat, without intervening heat. Uncovering agg.

Fever: Bilious **cerebro-spinal.** Chicken-pox. Continued fever abdominal; with icteric skin. Gastric. Influenza. **Intermittent, (malaria).** Remittent. Yellow.

Perspiration; *during slight exertion; fever after;* menses before and during. Complaints from suppressed perspiration.

**SKIN:** *Chafed in infants. Pale* discolouration. **Yellow (Jaundice);** anger after; new born *children.* Eruptions; moist. **yellow.** *Herpetic. Pemphigus. Pimples,* burning, moist, tensive. **Rupia.** Spring agg. Vesicular. yellow. whitish yellow. Erysipelas, smooth red and shinging. *Excrescences;* **condylomata; red.** *Formication.* Goose flesh. **Swelling dropsical.** Ulcer; *green discharges.* **Warts.** red, soft. Whitlow.

# SILICA (Silicea)

**Note:** Silicon (Si) is a widely distributed element in nature. The silicates merely give rise to a foreign body reaction, but Silica ($SiO_2$) like asbestos, causes a progressive productive reaction ending in fibrosis and associated with marked impairment of pulmonary function.

About a quarter of the earth's crust is composed of Silica. Seasand is mainly composed of it. The spicules of many sponges are made up of silica. Silicates are taken up by plants and from them Silica is often deposited on the surface or in the interior of their stems. The strength of straw is due to Silica. Silica is not found in human body, though claims are made that **it is found in ash of bones and blood.**

**Silica is a chemical rather than a mechanical irritant. In contact with body fluids, Silicic acid is produced, and it is either this or some other physical-chemical reaction which is now believed to be responsible for the tissue changes which occur.**

**GENERALITIES:** Silica has very wide spectrum of action. It acts on mesodermal, *ectodermal,* and endodermal tissues. For convenience we shall group them under different headings:

*Nutrition:* Dwarfishness. Cretinism. Tardy growth. Rickets. *Scurvy, Scrofula.* Weakness, Weariness. **Emaciation;** infants; **children;** insanity with. Atrophy of glands. Children walk late. Delicate; tender; easily enervated. Weak; feeble vital lack of heat; during exercise. Lean people. Motion averse to. Cachexia; cancer of. Obesity. Plethora.

**Blood:** Anemia; children; infants. Congestion of blood. *Cyanosis.* Hematoma. Hemophilia. **Haemorrhage;** acrid; clotted; streaked. *Heat flushes of;* during sleep. Orgasm of blood.

*Bones: Abscess.* Bare becomes. **Caries;** periosteum. **Cartilages affections of.** *Constriction.* Crumbling. **Exostoses.** Inflammation; periosteum. Necrosis. Non-union. Pain; boring; paralytic; **pressing internally; sore, bruised;** stitching. *Slow repair* of broken bone. **Swelling. Softening.**

*Fibrous tissue;* **induration;** knotty like a rope; inflammation; adhesions after operations. Muscle; indurated; relaxed; weak; awkward, *clumsy,* drops things, stumbles when walking.

**Nervous patients.** Fidgety. Grit, want of. Numbness; externally, internally; sensation, of glands; part lain on: in single or affected parts.

Pain; **beaten as if.** Biting. Boring. Broken as if. **Burning externally;** *glands;* **internally.** Constriction; *externally;* **internally;** glands in. Cutting; externally; internally; glands in. Digging. *Festering.* **Fine.** Gnawing. Goes to side lain on. Jerking. Neuralgic. Paralytic, in bones. Pinching. *Pressing,* **externally,** *internally;* inward: load as from: muscles in: together; *within outwards.* Small spots in. **Sore, bruised;** bones in; **coition after; externally;** *internally.* **Splinters, as from.** *Stitching,* in bones, glands, joints; *muscles,* tearing; **internally;** *outward. Stinging.* **Screwing. Tearing; muscles in;** cramp like or paralytic in muscles; *glands in;* downward, upward. Twinging. Twisting. **Ulcerative; glands in; internally.** Wandering, shifting.

*Paralysis:* Feeling of, externally, internally. Hemiplegia; right sided. **Organs of.** Painless. Coition after. Post-diphtheritic.

*Senses special dulled.* **Sensitiveness;** bones; glands; **internally;** *pain to;* periosteum. **Irritability** excessive; physical, irregular. Incoordinate effects.

*Sensations: Alive sensation internally.* Aura; extremities in; coldness. Ball, lump, globus. **Band, hoop,** as of a. Falling apart as if, through space; agg. lying on left side. **Fine, hair as of a.** Flowing like water, as if. Formication, internally. Ground or stairs come up to meet her. Heaviness; externally; *internally.* Full feeling. Loose, torn as if. Mould, as if forming over body. Motion, of. Pressure, simple sense of. Prickling. Short as if. Swollen sensation. Touch, illusions of. Wave like sensation.

*Sepsis.* Septicemia, *suppuration.* Pus, burrowing; foul; scanty; suppressed; thin; *unhealthy; watery; stubborn.*

**Abscess:** *Bones about.* chronic. *Fistulous.* **Glands of.** Impending, slow. Multiple, fever during. **Periosteum.**

*Ulceration; gangrenous;* **glands; phagedenic.**

**Inflammation:** Blood vessels of. **Bones.** Cellular tissue. *Glands.* Granulation exuberant. Internally. Nerves. **Periosteum. Serous membranes.** Surgical.

Injuries; glands. Cuts. To promote healthy granulation. Penetrating. Slow to heal. Splinters from. Operations, adhensions after.

Psora. *Sycosis.* **Syphilis.**

**Glands; atrophy;** *induration; inflamed; injuries;* pain in old, reopening of old; *itching;* metastasis; nodes; pain, *ulcerative.*

*Tumours;* Acuminate. Cheloid. Cryptic. Enchondroma. **Fibroid.** *Polypi.*

**Cancerous affections: Cachexia.** *Encephaloma. Epithelioma.* Noma. Fungus hematodes. Lupus. Sarcoma. **Scirrhus.** To relieve pain.

*Convulsions: Children. Clonic.* Consciousness with or without. **Epileptic;** coldness of left side before; mouse running sensation; solar plexus from; stiffness and rigidity; **unconsciousness with.** *Epileptiform;* internal; night sleep during; strong odours from; onanism after; tonic; sleeplessness and; **suppressed foot sweat** from; worms from.

Faintness, fainting; cold and taking. **Night.** Thunder storm before. While; lying on side; riding; standing; smoking.

*Pulsation, throbbing;* bones; glands **internally; night;** sitting while.

*Swelling: Affected parts of.* **Bones.** Glands; bluish; hard; hot, inflammatory; knotted like cord. *Inflammatory. Periosteum.* Receding. Dropsy; morning agg.

*Symptoms: Alternate.* Ascend. Crosswise; right upper, left lower. Changing. Erratic. Forwards. Recurring in groups. Radiating. One side; *left,* right. Wandering, shifting. Lain on parts, go to.

Mucous secretions; altered; **increased.** Secretions; *increased in general;* bland; ill effects of checked, hair destroying; lumpy; stain indelibly; thick; water. Serous membranes, synovitis. Constriction, externally internally, bones of, orifices of. *Orifices,* **affection.** Sphincter, contraction.

Bathing, dread of. Washing aversion to. **Motion aversion to.**

**Lassitude,** from conversation; from heat, of summer; sleep after. **Lie down inclination to.**

**Weak:** Feeble. Enervated. Coition after. **Emission after.** Easy. Evening. Lie down unable to. Mental exertion from. Nervous, females in. Morning, awakening after, rising when. Paralytic. Sleep after. *Stools after.* Walking from. Writing when. Weariness; evening, forenoon.

Blackness, of external parts. **Fistulae;** glands of. Glanders. Glistening.   Heaviness; **externally; internally.** Jerking, internally; bones, muscles etc. sleep during, going to. Latent disease. Lying in (puerperal state) **uncomfortable.** Magnetised, desire to be. *Mercury abuse of.* Metastasis. Morvan's disease. *Occupational disorders. Offensiveness;* body of. Perspiration; suppressed, **complaints from.** Quivering. Retraction. Spots in, complaints. Stiffness. **Stone cutters** *complaints.* **Sprains,** strains. **Tendency to take cold,** through foot. Tension; glands of; muscles; internally. Tobacco abuse of. Torpidity. **Vaccination, ill effects of.**

Trembling: **Evening, walking after.** Internally. Morning. **Night.** Senile. Upward. Writing when.

**WORSE: Morning. Forenoon. Noon. Afternoon. Evening. Night.** Midnight. *Air,* **open cool, aversion to; draft.** alone when. Ascending. Bathing cold. Bed, lying in. *Blowing* nose; sneezing; breathing when. Chill during. **Coition.** *Emission.* **Onanism. Cold in general; air; becoming, feet,** *single parts of body,* while sweating or hot; heat and; place entering on; sitting or lying on ground. Colours; bright. *Company,* society, crowds. Coryza, suppressed. Coughing. *Darkness, Dust, feathers.* Drinking; **after;** *cold;* **rapidly.** Swallowing; hasty; solids. *Eating* **after;** before (fasting); over; while. **Emotions.** Eructation. *Food; alcoholic stimulants;* beer; beans and peas; cabbage; *cold drinks, coffee,* **food,** fat; flatulent; milk, liquid; meat, **smoked; salt;** sight of; *tobacco;* warm. *Fright.* Grasping objects when. Head; shaking; uncovering. **Heat of fire;** sun; becoming overheated. **Hunger.** Idleness. **Jarring;** shaking; stepping. *Kindness, sympathy.* Lain on parts. *Light; artificial;* **day.** *Lying* **back on; bed in;**

**moist floor on; side on, left, painful.** Menses after; before; *beginning of; during;* suppressed. Moon phases **full moon;** changing; **new moon.** Mortification. Mental labour. Exertion; *physical, vision of,* reading. **Motion;** *affected parts of;* **at the beginning;** rapid, violent. Turning **over in bed.** Raising **affected part;** *arms. Rubbing.* **Running.** *Singing after.* **Rising** *after; seat from.* Riding; horse back on; **after;** wagon or cars in. **Driving in carriages.** Walking; *beginning of;* **fast;** open air in. Mouth opening. **Noise. Periodically;** at the same hour; every two or three weeks. Perspiration after. Pregnancy. Pressure; **hat of; spine on. Scolding. Scratching.** *Sitting while. Sleep;* at beginning of; *before;* **during;** *falling asleep on.* Smell. Sweat. Snuff. *Tobacco. Standing.* **Stooping.** Stools; before, during and after. **Sucking gums.** *Writing. Yawning. Talking,* by other. **Touch.** *Touching anything;* cold things. **Uncovering; single part;** *throat. Undressing* after. *Vomiting. Waking on.* Weather; humid damp; **change of; cold wet; damp;** *warm wet;* foggy; *winter; spring;* **snow air;** storm approach of, *during.* Temperature; change of. Wet, applications; **getting feet;** *weather.* Washing with water. Damp dwellings being in. Wind; cold; north.

**BETTER:** *Blowing* nose: Change of position. Cold; coffee: food. Cold in general, (feels too hot). Dancing. **Descending. Drinking.** Eating; after. Electricity. *Eructations.* Exertion. *Flatus passing.* Hanging down; **letting limbs down.** Holding or being held. **Hot application.** Light, desire for. **Lying;** back on; *bed in; side on,* painful, *painless, right. Magnetism.* **Mesmerism.** *Motion continued. Occupation.* **Pressure. Raising.** Rest. Rising. **Room in.** Rubbing. *Running.* Seminal emissions. Sitting; on first, down. Summer. *Urination.* **Walking.** continued. **Warm bed, stove.** Warm, wet weather. **Wrapping.**

**MIND:** *Absent minded.* Abstraction. Abusive. Acute, with physical weakness. *Agitation. Amorous.* Anticipation; complaints; from. *Anxiety;* conscience of; health about; climacteric about; lying while; menses, during; trifles about. *Aversion;* bright colours; reading; **spoken to when; touched being; mental work. Bashful; appearing in public, Timidity;** appearing in public. Cowardice. Bold. Calmness. Capriciousness. Careless. Censorious. Cheerful; night. Clairvoyance. **Concentration difficult.** Alone while agg. Confidence; **want of self. Confusion;** conversation agg; intoxicated as if; morning, on waking; night. Consolation agg. Contradiction; anger from; intolerant of; has to restrain himself to keep from violence. Counting continually. Critical, exacting. Death; desires; sensation of. *Delirium;* anxious; fantastic; frantic; frightful; hallucinations with.

*Delusions;* body divided. Criminals about. House full of people. People behind him. Pursued by enemies. Sees; dead persons; dogs; images; phantoms, dwells upon, **frightful,** eyes closing on, all over; needles; spectres, ghosts; thieves, in house; vermin, crawl about. Die, as if she would. Drawing her to right, something were, when walking. Fail, everything will. Fancy; illusions of. Half left does not belong to her. Injury, is about to receive. Journey, that he is on. Voices, hears. Water of. Worms creeping, as if.

*Dementia;* epileptic. *Despair,* recovery of. *Discontended.* Drunk as if. Discouraged. Duality sense of. **Dulness;** afternoon; children in; dreams after; eating amel, evening amel.; forenoon; morning.

Ecstasy. Egotism; ailments from. *Excitement. Fancies;* absorbed in; evening; *exaltation of; frightful.*

*Fear:* falling of. Lightning. Lying when. Downward motion, of. Palpitation, with. People, of. Pins, or pointed objects. Robbers. Thunderstorms. Undertaking of. Work of; *Literary. Fickle. Fidgety. Filthy. Dirty.* Foolish. Forgetful; dampness, exposure to, from. **Fright;** complaints from. *Frightened,* easily. Grasping; hand; involuntary motions of, throwing about. Guilt, sense of, crime of. *Home-sickness.* **Hysteria.** Ideas; fixed; **abundant, clearness of mind deficient.**

**Imbecility.** *Impatience.* **Indifference;** chill during. Indolence, (aversion to physical work); conversation from. Insanity. **Irritability;** children in; forenoon; spoken to, when. Jesting averse to. Jump; impulse to, in the river. Kill; desire to. Lamenting. *Laughing;* night; *sleep during;* and whining; spasmodic, hysterical. Life, weary of. Looked at; cannot bear to be. Lose her senses, gradually. *Magnetised,* desire to be. Monomania. Mania-a-potu. Puerperal mania. Memory, weakness of; mental labour or fatigue from; word for. **Mildness.** Mistakes, localities; reading in; speaking; words; misplacing; writing. Mood; changeable, variable. **Morose.** Nymphomania; menses suppressed from.

Obstinate; children, yet cry when kindly spoken to. Persevere cannot. Plans, making many. Presentiments. Premonitions. **Prostra-**

**tion** of mind, *reading from; writing after.* Quiet disposition. Religious affections *Re morse;* about trifles. **Restlessness; anxious;** driving out of bed; foreno n; headache during; **internal.**

**Sadness;** alone when; cause without; *heat during;* masturbation from; menses during or suppressed. Searching for pins. **Sensitive, oversensitive;** *mental impressions to;* noise to, slight, to; sensual impressions to; voice to; steel points, to; directed towards her. Sexual excess; mental symptoms from.

*Scolding* (abusive). Shouting. Shrieking; heat during; convulsions before; feels, as though, she must; sleep, during. Sit, inclination to. Speech; mistakes of; unintelligible. *Starting, startled; easily; sleep from;* touched *when; trifles,* at. *Stupefaction;* vertigo during. *Stupidity.* Succeedes never. *Undertakes* nothing, lest he fail. *Suicidal impulses;* by drowning; during menses, perspiration. Suspicious. Talk, sleep in, loudly. Talk; indisposed to, taciturn. **Thinking affected;** *difficult,* slow; inability of. Thoughts, sleep before going to.

*Unconsciousness; cold, after taking; conduct, automatic, during;* transient; riding while; vertigo, during.

Weeping; after noon, *night; sleep in;* spoken to when; stool during; trifles at; waking on.

**HEAD:** *In general. One sided.* Alternating sides. Any side. **Forehead. Occiput.** *Sides. Supra-orbital.* Temples. *Vertex.* Alternating with pain in arms.

Air, blowing on or flowing, night. *Alive as if something, in.* Boiling, bubbling, as if. *Crushed as if. Shattered to pieces.* Eye would be forced out, as if. Hanging as if, by a piece of string, at the nape. Lifted by hair, she had. *Nail as from.* Noise clanging, as if. Numbness, as if, forehead. Open, as if. Pulled as if, hair were. *Shaking as if; scalp of; stepping heavily; walking when.* Tingling, vibrating. Twisting, as if.

Concomitants: Appearance of lump on scalp. Chilliness. Cold feeling. Delirium. Exhaustion. Eyes, extending into. Face flushed or hot. Face pale. Hair falling. Humour, bad. Limbs heavy. Mental weakness. **Nausea.** Visual or eye symptoms. *Unconsciousness.*

From: Abdominal irritation. Animal fluids, loss of. Bathing. Head getting, cold on. *Binding up the hair. Binding head tightly.* amel. **Eye**

**strain.** Fasting. Haemorrhage from. *Hat, pressure* of. Shaking head. Spirituous liquors. Emotions, excitement.

Big. Enlarged, as if. Distensive, full. Chronic. Confusion. Eyes, extending into. *Drawing.* Hair, bristling of. *Heaviness.* **Hydro-cephalus.** *Heat;* burning; chill after; mental exertion from. Head injuries, after. Jerking. Motions in head; sitting while; step making or stumbling; walking while. Motions of head; rolling, moaning with. Nervous, exhaustion. Outward extending. Oversensitiveness. Sensitive to; air cold; draft to; scalp, hair touch to. Restlessness. Rheumatic.

**Pain:** Boring. Digging. Sore, bruised, in spots. *Bursting. Constriction.* Cutting. *Paroxysmal. Periodic;* **every day;** seventh day. Pinching. Pressing; asunder, weight as from. Shooting. *Stitching.* **Stunning.** *Tearing. Violent.* Waking up from sleep, frequently.

Worse; **ascending;** into, left. **Coition,** after. Cold taking. Combing hair. Dentition. **Draft.** Eating before. Eyes closing agg. and *amel.* Foot steps by. **Gastric disturbances. Heat during.** Lifting. Light, day light. Looking, *bright. object,* sideways, upward. **Night.** Mental exertion. *Motion, eyes* of. *Nursing infant, after.* Odour strong. Reading. Sitting. Sleep falling to. *Stepping hard. Mis-steps. Stool, pressing at,* after. Stooping. *Talking,* agg. and amel. Turning; body; eyes sideways; suddenly. Walking, air open. **Uncovering.**

Better: Darkness. Eating. Lying; dark *room in.* Nose-bleed. Rest. Vomiting. Warmth external. *Wrapping. Urination profuse.*

Paralysis of one side, coition after. **Perspiration;** on coughing; offensive; *occiput;* sleep falling to or during; **sour;** *reading while.* Stiffness; evening, in bed; occiput. Waving; occiput. Whirling.

*Head external:* Right. Occiput. Abscess. Bald; young people in. **Caries of bones.** Coldness; occiput, vertex. Drawn; backward; sideways. *Eruptions; boils; carbuncles;* crusta lactea; favus; impetigo; moist; **nodes;** *occiput;* ringworm; tubercles; *suppurative. Formication. Heat;* chill after; **night;** *mental exertion. Hold* up *unable to.* Wobbling. *Itching;* **occiput;** *spots in; warmth of bed* agg. Large. *Shocks.* Swollen; **glands of;** scalp, puffy. Twitching of muscles. Ulcers; occiput. Wens.

**Vertigo:** Back, comes up. Continuous. *Epileptic. Exertion of vision;* mental. Meniere's disease. Side, must walk, to right. Swaying towards right. With; *dulled sense; buzzing in ears;* tendency to fall, *backward, forward,* left to, *right to,* sideways; head congestion headache. **During;** *sleepiness;* unconsciousness, followed by.

**WORSE:** Afternoon. Air open in, walking. During; breakfast; dinner; eating. *Closing eyes on.* **Mental exertion.** Looking; about; *steadily;* up. Lying; on back; left side, while. Meditating. Raising, arm. *Riding in carriages.* Rising on, lying or stooping from; supine position. *Sitting, while;* up in bed. *Standing. Stooping.* Tobacco, snuff.

Better: Lying while. riding in carriages. Walking. Warmth.

Sensations: Elevated as if. *Intoxication.* Going back. Objects seem to right. Rising as if, ground were or as if raised.

**EYES:** Eruptions about eye-brows; eye-balls; lids. Hair fall out; brows. Canthi; burning, crack; eye gum; pain, pressing; pustules; red; styes, towards inner; swollen. **Cataract; foot sweat suppressed after;** right eye; office workers. Pus; in anterior chamber. *Choroid; inflammation;* suppuration, with iris involved. Neuralgia; right ciliary region.

*Conjunctiva: Discharge; bloody,* morning; *thick;* **yellow.** Inflammation; *granular; phlyctenular; purulent;* sympathetic. *Injected;* pannus.

Cornea: Abscess. Fistula. Mass of hypertrophied tissue, as if were. *Opacity;* right; *small-pox after. Painful.* Rough; spots or specks on; scars like. Staphyloma. Thickening. Ulcers; deep, indolent; scars, from; vascular.

Eyeballs: Alternating between. Burning. Cancer; **fungus; medullaris.** *Distorted. Dryness; morning,* evening. *Boils,* about. *Heat.* **Inflammation; chronic;** cold, agg; cold wet weather agg.; *foreign bodies from;* **scrofulous;** sympathetic. **Injury; after effects. Itching;** evening. Open, unable to. Movements constant. **Lachrymation;** cold air in; cough with; **open air.** Tears *burning; wind in.*

*Pain:* Aching. burning, biting etc. **Crampy.** Cutting. Drawing; backward; string with, as if, to back of head, to brain. *Sand as from. Foreign body in, from.* Occiput to. *Pressing,* outward, right. Sore, bruised. Stitching. Sudden. Tearing. Better; *urination profuse. Warmth.*

Worse: **Air cold.** Eyes, closing; Light; day; strong. Looking upward, motion of eyes. Night in bed; *turning sideways.* Vision, exertion on. Writing. 4 p.m. Hiccough, vomiting.

**Photophobia;** *chronic;* coition after; day light, morning; evening. *Pulsation;* paroxysmal. Redness; *around;* injuries after; vomiting or hiccough agg. Right. *Sensitive, cold air to.*

*Sensations:* Coldness; walking in open air. Contractive. Drawn backward, as if. Forced out of head, with brain, as if. Foreign body as of. Swimming in cold water. **Torn out, as if,** watering full of, as if.

Soreness, tendency to. Staring. Stiffness. Strabismus. Suffused. *Tension, coitin after. Weak.*

Iris; *inflammation,* adhesions with, choroid with; **hypopion** with. Jagged.

*Lachrymal canal, gland,* sac. *Discharge, sac from, pus of,* from pressure. Epiphora. **Fistula lachrymalis. Inflammation;** canal of; **glands of; sac of. Stricture of canal.** *Swollen;* canal; **gland; sac.**

*Lids:* **Agglutinated, night.** *Close, desire to; difficult to;* must; spasmodic. Eruptions; pustules. Eversion. Falling or drooping of. *Granulation.* Eyelashes, falling. *Hardness.* Heaviness. Inflammation. Inversion. Nodules, margins in. Pain, pressing. Quivering. Redness, margins. Spasm. *Styes;* induration from; recurrent. Swollen; meibomian glands; painless.

*Tumours; cystic;* nodules; tarsal. *Twitching.* Ulceration; under surface.

Orbits; caries; cellulitis; periosteitis; pressure and soreness in. Pupils; *adherent;* beclouded; contracted, chill during, perspiration during; dilated, irregular, right more than left. Retina, haziness.

Vision: **Amaurosis** (blindness); day; eating after; headache after; paroxysmal; periodic; pregnancy during; uterine affections with; vanishing of sight. Amblyopia (weak, blurred). **Dim;** *coition after; diphtheria after; headache,* after, before; menses *during,* **suppressed foot sweat;** *wiping* eye, amel. *Foggy. Hypermetropia* (long sightedness).

Illusions: Colours before. *Floating,* **muscae volitantes.** Dark, speck. Spots. Objects seem gray. Green halo around light. Rainbow. Yellow. **Dazzling.** *Flickering, during headache.* Gray cover, he was looking though. *Lightnings.* **Letters run together;** while writing. Objects run together. Sparks. Spots. Veils before. *Night, eyes closing on.*

Nyctalopia. Pale. *Paralysis of optic nerve.*

**EAR:** External: **Abscess behind.** Coldness and aching of. Boils. Moist margins. Eruptions; scaly, scurfy. Heat. Inflammation; erysipelatous; concha of; inside; margins of. *Swelling.* Twitching, left. Ulceration; *inside.*

Eustachian tubes: **Catarrh. Itching.** Inflamed. Tickling; inducing swallowing and cough.

External Auditory canal: *Boils. Boring fingers in;* amel. *Child by; sleep during.* Dryness. **Inflammation. Itching;** scratch, *swallowing* agg. Pain. Polypus. *Swelling.*

*Internal Ear:* **Caries of ossicles.** *Hypersensitive to noises. Noises,* air cold from; bubbling; blowing nose amel, chewing when; chirping; clashing; clucking; crashing, fluttering; coughing on; feet becoming cold from; lying while, night; sneezing; swallowing when; vertigo with; walking while; rhythmical, hissing, humming; *puffing;* reverberating; ringing, **bells as if,** forcing to rise and walk about at night; **roaring;** rushing, steam escaping like; rusting; **snapping,** as hearing returns; whistling, whizzing.

*Pain:* Above and below ear; to neck; to nose; sharp sounds from. Aching. Boring. *Cramp in.* Drawing. Jerking. Stinging. Throbbing, beating. *Tearing.* Worse; blowing nose; *cold application;* full moon, during; night, 1 a.m.; noise, sharp; sitting after long; *rising from a seat,* touch; vision, exertion of; weather, changing, damp. Better; motion.

*Pulsation;* lying on the ear; night.

*Sensation:* Air rushed through, eustachian tube, with tingling in middle ear. Alive, as if something in. Flowing something from. **Stopped;** *loud reports, ear* open with. *Swallowing* amel; *yawning* amel. Wind puffing out of ear.

Mastoid (behind ear): **Caries. Eruptions.** Mastoiditis. Moisture. Pain; drawing; jerking; soreness; **tearing.** Perforation; *ulceration, of* tympanic membrane.

Middle ear: Chronic catarrhal inflammation. Acute suppuration. **Chronic suppuration.** *Discharge*; **bloody;** *caries threatening;* **cheesy;** *ichorous;* **offensive; purulent; thick;** *thin;* **watery;** *yellow.* Wax; soft; increased; *thin.*

*Hearing;* **acute,** *noise to.* **Difficult,** for human voice. Lost. **Deafness;** alternate with sensibility; *catarrh of eustachian tube,* from; *change of clothing;* cold after; *cold, wet weather;* intermittent; measles after; *scarlet fever after;* **nervous;** *paralysis of auditory nerve,* from; rheumatic, gouty or scrofulus diathesis; vaccination; eating or washing, agg; *blowing nose, loud report,* yawning amel.

**NOSE:** External. bones; **caries;** *syphilitic; sore; bruised pain.*

**Abscess;** internal; sinuses. Epithelioma. Coldness. Redness; spots in. **Eruptions;** around; blood boils; crusty; eczema; *pimples; vesicles.* Heaviness. Inflammation. Formication (itching). Lupus of. *Picking till it bleeds.* Pressing. Sensitive to touch, **sore;** *blowing on; sensation.* Sunken. *Swelling. Pain, drawing;* stitching. Ulcers; *burning;* **painful.** Cracks; wings of nose; lips; corners of mouth. *Scurfy,* wings.

*Internal:* Bleeding; acrid; bright. *Epistaxis;* blowing nose from; scrofulus children, cough with; coryza with; menses absent; puberty at; *predisposition to. Blood, blowing from.* **Dryness;** *chronic, painful;* **sensation; suppressed foot-sweat after.** Small blood boils; pimples. Foreign body as if in. *Acute catarrhal inflammation,* hay fever. Inflammation; ordinary cold in head. **Coryza;** *chronic, dry;* constant discharge fluid or dry or alternating; fluent day time; **frontal sinuses to;** periodical; **easily** recurrent, *relieving obstruction;* stuffed; *suppressed;* violent attacks. Coryza; asthmatic breathing with; chest bursting with; chilliness with; cough with; urging to cough, in throat;' epistaxis with; nervous. Discharges; *bland; bloody; crusts, scabs,* high up. *painful;* **hard dry;** dripping; excoriating; flocculent; foamy; yellow; greenish, gushing; lumpy; **plugs obstructive; offensive; purulent;** slimy, **mucus of; thick;** watery. Itching. Liquids come through nose, on attempting to swallow.

**Obstruction;** alternate with discharge; *chronic, after every cold;* **foot sweat suppressed from** (Comp. dryness); *morning and fluent during* day; **pus with;** talking while. Odours, from or in; blood of; fetid; sickly. Ozema, **syphilitic. Pain; bruised;** *to brain like rays, to* forehead, **sore, bruised;** *splinter like on touch,* dryness from. *Polypus.*

Pulsation. Smell; acute; **diminished; wanting lost** (Comp. Hearing). *Sneezing;* chronic coryza with; **excessive;** combing hair from; *ineffectual* **efforts;** *urge,* paroxysmal. *Swelling.* Tickling. *Ulcers; high up; painful; right; burning.*

*Posterior nares; food sensation of, in; dryness; swallowing on.* Septum; *crusts;* pain; **ulcers,** round. *Sinuses;* **abscess.**

**FACE: Abscesses; antrum of.** Anemic, pale. Bluish, dirty looking. *Copper coloured,* Distorted. Drawn. Earthy; *haggard;* sickly. Hectic spots. Red; dark red; after eating; erysipelatous; glowing; headache during; eyes about. Swelled; hard; **toothache from.** Sickly. Waxy.

Cancer; lips; **epithelioma;** lupus; scirrhus. Chapped.

*Eruptions:* **Acne;** *comedones.* Biting. *Boils, blood.* **Eczema;** spreading; from occiput. Freckles. *Herpes.* Pimples. *Scurfy.* Syphilitic. Tubercles. Urticaria. Vesicles. *Phlegmonous,* **erysipelas. Induration.** *Heat, flashes of. Itching,* stinging.

Pain: *Prosopalgia,* attacks, *infra-orbital.* **Cold exposure** or **applications from.** *Damp weather.* To cheek bones, chest. Rheumatic. *Storm, before.* **Stormy weather.** Worse; air cold. Chewing when. *Draft,* night. Tooth-ache after. Touch. Better; **heat of stove;** *warmth;* profuse urination.

Paralysis; right side. **Perspiration;** on exertion; hot drinks after; side not lain on; sleep, on falling to. Soreness; sense of. **Spots;** pale; red; white. Cheeks; burning, glowing; pain, drawing; swelling. *Chin;* eruptions; *sticking.* Jaws; *clenched,* convulsions; necrosis of lower; pain, aching (lower), **drawing in,** crampy, maxillary articulation, pressing, sore; **stitching** (lower) *swelling* (lower); suppuration; twitching (lower), night. Maxillary sinus affection.

Parotids; *enlarged,* swelling; **abscess** *indurated;* suppurative inflammation; pain. Sub-maxillary glands; enlarged; abscess; *inflamed;* pain, *painful swelling.* Whiskers; *falling; itching; herpes.*

**MOUTH:** Lips; cancer; cracked; dryness; indurated; nodules; peeling; **ulcers.** *Cracked;* corners of mouth. **Dryness.** *Thirstless. Eruptions; corners of mouth; crusts, scabs;* around mouth. Gangrenous. Grasping at mouth. Pain; round the corners. Froth, foam from; absent during spasms; sleep during. Saliva; diminished, with thirst; frothy. Mucus slime in. Heat. Salivation. Speech difficult. *Stomacae.* Swelling; erysipelatous; after extraction of teeth.

Taste; bad, *water tastes. Bitter; food tastes; swallowing after.*
Bloody, morning. Clay like. Rotten eggs like. Fatty, greasy. *Metallic.*
Putrid. Slimy. Soapy. *Sour, eating after.* **Wanting** (loss of); *coryza, in.*

*Gums:* **Boils.** *Frequently recurrent abscesses.* Suppuration.
Bleeding. Coldness sensation. **Fistula. Inflammation.** *Pain;* **burning;**
*cold air* agg.; *pressing;* **sore;** *ulcerative;* touched when. *Swelling;*
painful; after extraction of teeth. **Tumours; painless;** movable lower
gums; **in place of two bicuspids.** *Ulcers.* **Vesicles.**

Teeth: **Abscess of roots.** *Caries.* Black film, cannot be brushed
off. Dentition; **difficult; slow;** *diarrhoea with. Dulled, blunt.* Edge feel,
as if on. *Elongated as if.* Enamel deficient. **Looseness.** *Fistula
dentalis.* Pain; burning, drawing, digging; to cheek bones, face,
forehead, temples; *neuralgia; pressing; as if held in grip; pulsating;
stitching;* tearing; ulceration at roots;   changes places rapidly; cold
drinks from; intermittent; rheumatic; *suppressed foot sweat from;*
winter. Pain, worse; masticating; cold or warm things (Comp. Merc.
sol.); *eating during. Warmth external,* or bed and **wrapping of head**
amel.

Palate; crawling; white; itching; sore; *paralysis; swelling,* suppuration with; ulcers, *perforating.*

Tongue: *Brown. White. Induration. Inflammation,* threatening
suppuration. Excoriated. Numb. Sore, spots. Swelling. **Hair of;**
sensation; **anterior part;** tip; to trachea. Trembling. Phagedenic
ulcers.

**THROAT:** Bitter, taste. **Dry,** night. *Food lodges,* in passes into
choanae. Gangrene. *Hawks;* cheesy lumps; pus etc. **Chronic
pharyngitis.** *Offensive,* **tenacious,** thick, *yellow,* mucus. **Pain;**
rawness: *splinter as from a.* Worse; **cold on becoming; empty
swallowing;** *lifting;* yawning. *Paralysis,* post-diphtheritic (Comp. Kali
phos). Sensation; **ascending into;** food of; *fullness of;* **hair** or **thread
of;** *lump, plug, ball. Swallowing difficult,* solid food gags. Swelling.

Oesophagus; gurgling, when drinking. *Sensation of* paralysis.

Tonsils: **Enlarged; inflamed,** acute, chronic: *suppuration,* predisposition. **Swelling.** *Ulcers.* Elongated uvula, swollen.

**Pain in cervical glands; swelling of, hard, suppuration.** Thyroid cartilage, swelling of. Recurrent fibroids. Ulcers. Warts.

**STOMACH:** *Appetite,* easy satiety. **Ravenous;** attack of; **chill during;** *marasmus with; pain in stomach with; relish without,* vanishing on attempting to eat. **Diminished.**

*Aversion:* Alcohol. *Food, cooked, hunger with, warm,* seen if. **Meat.** *Milk,* **mothers.** Salty food. *.Cancer. Constriction.*

Desires, cravings: Bread. Food; coarse, raw; uncooked; *cold; warm.* Ice or ice-cold water. Indistinct; knows not for what. Milk, sweets.

Indigestion; mea after. Flatulent distension. Enlarged.

*Eructations:* Bitter, burning. *Chilliness with. Empty,* tasteless. Taste like food, ingesta. Ineffectual; forenoon; stool after. *Sour. Heartburn. Waterbrash.* Hiccough; eating before and after; noon. evening, night. Induration of pyloric wall.

*Nausea:* Constant. Coition during. Drinking after. Exertion after. Faint like. Epigastrium in. Food on looking at. During; headache; *pregnancy. Stool, during, after.* Throat in. *Vaccination* after. Smoking after. Eating, while, after.

**Pain:** Chill during. Drinking cold. Coughing. Burning. Clawing. **Cramping.** *Cutting.* Gnawing. **Pressing.** Sore, Stitching, to hip joint, after lying down. Worse **being heated;** riding and rocking; stepping on; walking in open air. Better; bending double; *heat;* lying with knees drawn up. Retching, ineffectual.

*Sensation:* Anxiety, menses during. *Coldness.* Emptiness, goneness; not relieved by eating; with aversion to food. Fullness; eating so little after; eructations amel. *Heaviness.* Lump. Stone as if. **Pulsation.** Tenderness. Tension. Twitching.

**Thirst;** *burning,* **chill during;** vehement; **extreme;** with lack of appetite; heat during; small quantities for. Ulcers.

**Vomiting:** *Coughing. Drinking, cold water.* Eating while, sudden. *Expectoration on. Hawking up* mucus when. Lifting after. **Milk; mother's** after. **Nursing,** immediately after. Pregnancy. *Headache* during. Bile. Black. *Blood.* **Curdled,** masses. Food of, mucus then. Frothy. **Liquids;** cold water only; water, then food. Milk **curdled.** Salty. Stringent; sudden.

Weak, relaxed feeling.

**ABDOMEN:** *Big.* **Enlarged in children.** *Flabby. Colic, constipation* from; to small of back; to testicles; lifting agg; violent.

Pain in: Burning. **Cramping. Cutting,** *pinching. Stitching.* Tearing. Twinging, twisting. With; **leucorrhoea;** nails blue; **waterbrash.** Worse; breathing deep; **jarring;** lying, right side; menses during; *motion; walking;* stool, during, diarrhoea after, **straining at.** Better; eructation; leucorrhoeal discharge; **warmth.**

*Contraction. Cracks on surface.* Distension; children in; heat during; tympanitic. Dropsy. **Flatulence;** *obstructed;* noisy rumbling; offensive per ano; wandering. *Gurgling.* **Rumbling. Hard. Heat.** Inflammation. **Appendicitis;** *typhlitis; peritonitis; enteritis.* Retraction. Movements of fetus; **painful;** *violent. Ulcers. Volvulus.*

Sensations: Constriction, band, hoop; flatus passing amel. **Fullness.** Heaviness. Movements, in. Shattering. Quivering. **Tension.**

Epigastrium; **burning;** constant pain; crampy; stitching. pain, flatulence and pulsation in hypogastrium, and hypochondriac region.

Inguinal bubo; fistulae glands; pain, drawing, right; swelling, sensation, left; *glands.* Liver; **abscess;** enlarged; indurated; inflamed *pain, sore.* Spleen; stitching pain. Umbilicus; constriction; pain, sore, cutting; ulcers.

**RECTUM & ANUS:** Abscess (peri-rectal). Constriction; painful; stool, during.

**Constipation:** Children in. Constant desire. **Feces hard from.** Habitual. **Inactivity of rectum.** *Paralysis. Menses, before* and *during.* Must remove mechanically, with finger. Spinal affections with. Urging with. Women. Travelling while.

*Diarrhoea:* Anxiety after; **Children in;** *scrofulus.* **Cholera** *infantum.* **Chronic.** *Cold drinks or food from.* **Emaciated people in.** Hot weather. *Painless.* Vaccination, ill effects. Worse; air cold; day and night; morning; driving out of bed. Better; **wrapping; warmth of bed.**

*Fissure.* **Fistula in ano;** *alternating with chest disorders*

**Flatus:** cutting pain or pinching with; difficult; **motion from; offensive;** *rarely;* walking while agg. and amel. Haemorrhage.

*Haemorrhoids* (piles); bleeding; *external;* painful; *protruding during stool;* strangulated; *suppurating;* ulcerating; constipation with; spasms of sphincter with; worse, touch, walking. Heat, stool after. Itching; scratching agg.; *stool after, voluptuous.* Moisture; *bloody.* Pain; cramping, to testes; long lasting after stool; stitching; *sore; tenesmus;* coition agg. Stool hard after agg. Ulceration. Worms. Sensation of; lump, plug; formication; tension. Perineum; *abscess;* burning.

Stools: *Bloody,* reddish. *Copious.* Difficult; soft though; natural, recedes. *Frequent.* Dry. Hard. Knotty. *Lumpy* and liquid. Sheep dung like. Forcible. *Frothy.* Impacted. Urging; ineffectual; *abortive. Unsatisfactory.* Large. Lienteric. Mucous. Mushy. *Natural* with constipation. *Offensive. Putrid. Purulent.* Painless. *Pasty.* Thin, liquid; pouring out. Tenacious. Watery. White; *chalk like; fecal.*

URINARY: Bladder; calculi; *catarrh;* gonorrhoea suppressed from. *Paralysis.* Pain; drawing upward; *urination during.* Retention of urine; sensation of. Polypi. Plug, sensation. Urging; *day* and *night;* ineffectual.

*Urination:* Dribbling, urination after. Frequent; nervous when. Involuntary (enuresis), blow on head from; night (*incontinence*); *retarded,* must wait for urine to start; unsatisfactory. Weakness; sphincter of.

Kidney: Abscess; peri-nephric. Addison's disease. Pyelitis; calculous; chronic, *suppurative.* Pain; burrowing; griping. *Suppression of urine.*

Prostate; *enlarged; hard; inflamed, chronic,* suppuration; ball sensation, when sitting; *emissions, with or after* stools.

Urethra: gonorrhoeal, *foetid; purulent;* thick; chronic, yellow discharge. Itching. *Pain;* stitching; anterior part; agg.; *urination,* during.

Urine: *Burning.* Cloudy. *Red. Colourless.* Copious. Ammoniacal odour. Scanty. Sediment; purulent; sand; yellow. *Sugar* (diabetes mellitus).

MALE: Cowperitis. Erections; continued; delayed; frequent; *painful;* desire without; *violent;* wanting (impotency). *Moist spots* on genitals. Flaccidity. Irritability (excited). Itching; urination during.

*Seminal, discharge;* copious; voluptuous dreams with; *nightly emissions,* dribbling in sleep.

*Sexual passion* **diminished; increased, violent,** *priapism with.*

Penis & Glans: Cancer. Deadness, sense of. Denuded, glans were. Balanitis. *Itching, glans.* Pain; stitching, *red, spots. Swelling,* oedematous. Ulcers; elevated, lead coloured, sensitive edge; indolent; *mercuro-syphilitic;* painful. Prepuce; eruptions; inflammation; *itching;* burning pain; redness; swelling. Scrotum; condylomata; elephantiasis; moist eruptions; excoriation; formication; itching; moisture; perspiration; relaxed; thickened skin; red spots. Varicocele. Empyocele. **Hydrocele;** boys of; **scrofulus. Tubercles;** testes; spermatic cord. Testes; flaccidity; heat in; **induration,** right; pain, boring, cramping, pressing, squeezing; retraction; sensitive; *suppuration; swelling;* tumours; twitching.

FEMALE: **Abortion,** *tendency to;* **habitual.** Coition, nauseating. *Conception difficult* (sterility). *Desire increased; violent* (nymphomania), **spinal** irritation from. Disagreeable feeling in genitalia.

**Leucorrhoea: Excoriating;** biting; *bloody; brown;* copious; **flowing,** abdominal pains after; **gushing;** lumpy; **milky;** *offensive;* painful: purulent; thin; white; yellow; *before, after,* or *instead of menses;* causes itching; **cutting pain** (hypogastrium) with; abdominal colic, preceding and attending.

Lochial discharge; acrid; bloody, *child nurses when;* hot, ceases when lying; offensive; *red.*

*Mammae:* **Abscess;** *nipples of.* Atrophy. **Cancer;** *epithelioma; scirrhous.* Nipples; cracks on; drawn in like a funnel; *excoriation; burning; sore; stitching;* **retraction of;** *ulceration.* Distension, sensation of. **Fistulous opening in. Induration; left. Inflammation** *nipples.* Itching. *Milk,* **spoiled; child refuses** mother's; *flowing; suppressed; thin.* **Nodules.** Sensitive in; *right.* **Pain;** left; drawing from nipple all over body; sore, **bruised; stitching,** left, region of; **nurses, while the child,** agg. Perspiration, night. **Swelling; cicatrices of.** *Tumours.* Warts. **Ulceration.**

Menstruation: **Amenorrhoea.** *Delayed, first menses.* Painful. icy coldness with. *Frequent,* intermittent. *Irregular,* every two or three months. *Lactation during, nursing the child while.* **Late** and *profuse.* Lying down, ceasing on. *Protracted. Scanty flow.* Short duration of, **suppressed;** with vicarious bleeding. Menses; **acrid;** bright red, dark; *offensive;* pale; stains leaving.

Ovaries; enlarged, as if; menses before; ovaritis.

Uterus: **Cancer.** Displacement; adherent to rectum. Enlarged. *Fibroids. Menorrhagia;* **between menstrual periods;** fibroids from; nursing the child when; plethora in; standing in water from. Heaviness. Induration, cervix. Acute and chronic endometritis. Para and perimetritis. *Moles.* Pain; after-pains *bearing down in region of; labour like;* **sharp while** *nursing; sore;* menses before and during *pregnancy, during;* sitting, standing, urination, and waking on agg. *Prolapse;* lifting agg. Sub-involution. Cervical erosion and induration.

Vagina: **Fistula.** *Induration.* Acute and chronic vaginitis. Itching. Pain; cutting; pressing; sore; agg. coition during and urinating, after. Relaxation, sphincter. Sensitive. **Tumours;** cysts. *Vaginismus.*

Vulva and labiae: Enlarged, as if. Eruptions; itching; pimples; painful. *Excoriation.* Inflammation. *Irritation.* **Itching;** menses *after and during;* **pudendum** of; urination, during. Pain; burning; biting; tearing; menses during agg. erectile. **Ulcers.** Worms, in.

**HEART:** Atheroma. *Sluggish circulating.* Congestion of blood. Distension of arteries. Rupture of arteries, *apoplexy.*

Pulse: **Abnormal. Frequent, rapid.** Full. Hard. **Imperceptible. Small.** *Irregular. Quick.* Slow. Suppressed, obliterated. *Soft.* Unequal. Weak.

Pressing pain: worse, **coughing;** lying in bed, on left **side; old people in;** rising from sitting; sitting; sneezing, standing; **running;** *stone cutters in;* **suckling of infant.** *Air, warm* amel.

*Palpitation;* dinner after; motion, violent or quick agg.; exertion agg.; sitting or standing while agg.; *suppressed foot sweat from.*

Lymphangitis. Varicose; veins; ulceration.

Sensations; anxiety in the region of; heaviness; stopped as if, during sleep.

**RESPIRATORY: Asth na;** *hay asthma;* nervous; sycotic; *thun-der. Storm during worse; air, draguth of;* cold, *when heated;* wet weather.

*Bronchiectasis.* **Bronchitis.** *Chronic winter catarrh.* Sensitive to cold air.

Chest; band around; tight feeling. Suppurating cicatrices. Red spots. Dropsy. Pustular eruptions. Sternum; grasped as if, by hand; lump under. Itching. Jerks. Pain; *burning;* bursting; drawing; to left axilla, to back; *pressing; rawness;* **stitching;** intercostal, lower ribs, sides., sternum behind etc. cough, sneezing, inspiration agg.; damp weather and warm room agg. Perspiration. *Pulsation,* sternum. *Swelling.* Tight feeling around chest, as if tied with strings. Tumours, in intercostal region.

Chest internal; Alternating, rectal symptoms with. Bursting as if. *Congestion.* **Constriction** (tension); band as from; flatulence from; **suppressed foot sweat from.** Distension, sense of. Heat. *Oppres-sion;* coughing when; morning; sneezing; stool after; walking while. Orgasms of blood, heat flushes. Paralysis of diaphragm. *Pulsation. Weakness.*

*Cough; constriction.* Foreign body sensation, *irritation,* itching or rawness, tickling in larynx from. Filling up, sensation, in throat from. *Hair;* in trachea or tongue sensation from. Irritation in *throat-pit,* **trachea,** from.

Cough: *Asthmatic.* **Breathing obstructed.** *Chronic.* Deep. *Dry;* evening, loose in morning; night; loose by day. Excoriation, soreness in chest. *Hacking.* Hectic. Hernia, pain in with. *Hoarse. Hollow.* Pain in hypogastrium, inguinal region with. *Lachrymation,* with. Loose, day during; *awakening on,* in morning. *Lower* and *lower coming from.* Discharge from nose, or sneezing with. Paroxysmal. *Racking. Rattling.* Retching. Rough. *Stitches in scapulae,* with. Scraping. *Shaking. Spasmodic.* Pain in *sternum with. Suffocative.* Tickling. *Violent, wakes from sleep. Whooping.*

Cough: Worse; *air cold,* damp, cold. *Bending head backwards.* Deep breathing. Chill during. Cold; **becoming;** *drinks; food; single parts.* Crying. Dinner, after. Drinking, hurriedly after. Eating; after; hastily. Exertion. Fever, during. Heated on becoming. *Lying;* back on;

*bed in;* right side. Morning. and evening. Motion, chest of, Move, on beginning. New moon. *Retiring after.* Running. Singing. Sleep, during. Sour food. *Talking.* Change of temperature. Thunderstorm. Uncovering; **feet** or *head.* Waking on. Damp, or stormy weather. Better; abdomen warming; **warm** *drinks.*

*Expectoration: Acrid. Albuminous. Balls, in shape of. Bloody.* **Acrid** bright red; brown; pale; purulent; streaked. Brownish. Causing soreness and rawness of mouth. *Copious.* **Day time only.** Easy, raising. Eating after agg. Frothy. Gelatinous. Globular. *Granular, offensive. Greenish. Hard. Hawks up* mucus. Hot, burning. **Lumpy.** *Milky.* **Mucus;** bloody; translucent (glassy). *Offensive, foetid.* **Purulent.** Sago like. Scanty. Sediment, looks like. Starchy. Taste; greasy, oily; nauseous; putrid; salty. **Thick.** Tough. *Viscid. Transparent. Tubercles.* White. **Yellow.**

Larynx: Catarrh. *Constriction, from scratching auditory canal. Tuberculous inflammation. Irritation.* Itching. *Mucus in, ejected with difficulty.* Pain; *rawness; soreness;* tearing. Air cold, bending backwards, inspiration, lifting agg. Rattling in. *Roughness in. Scraping, clearing.* Sensitive to cold air. Swelling, fibrous, painless.

Voice: *Hoarseness;* **chronic;** *morning* agg.; paretic; weather cold, damp agg. Hollow. Husky. Rough.

*Lungs:* **Abscess.** Gangrene. Haemorrhage, frothy. *Inflammation;* **neglected, lingering;** resolution of. **Phthisis; acute; incipient;** *pituitous; stone cutters; sycotic; purulent and ulcerative.* **Ulcers.**

Pleurae; inflammation (pleurisy); **empyema.**

*Respiration: Accelerated. Arrested,* **night at. Catching. Deep,** desire to breathe. **Difficult** (dyspnea); **dust, as from.** *Impeded.* **Loud, Panting.** *Rapid. Rattling.* Shallow. Short. *Sighing,* takes deep breath. Sobbing. Suffocative, attacks. **Tight.** *Whistling.*

*Worse* (dyspnoea and other types): *Cough with. Dust. Exertion. Heat with. Lying while; back on. Manual labour.* Neck, draft of air. Night. *Pain,* during. *Rest,* during. **Running after.** Stooping. *Talking after. Thunderstorm.* Waking on. *Walking rapidly.* **Working when.** Better; motion; standing.

Trachea; crawling; hair in, sensation; **irritation;** *mucus in; soreness;* tickling in. *Irritation* and *tickling in* throat pit.

**BACK:** *Abscess.* **Coldness;** eating after; *extending down;* lying down amel. *Eruptions; carbuncles; eczema;* pimple; *pustules; painful; small-pox. Fistulae. Heat. Itching.* Numbness.

*Pain: Aching. Burning.* Cutting. Paralytic. Pressing, stone as of a. *Pulsating, rheumatic. Stitching. Tearing. Worse.* Air *draught of;* bed warm, when getting; chill during; coition; *coughing when;* driving; flatulence; **injury; jarring;** menses during; *mental exertion;* motion on; move beginning to; **nursing while; pressure;** rest during; *riding in carriage;* rising, bed from, **sitting from,** stooping from; sexual excess; sitting while; stool after; *stooping after;* **touches when;** turning when; walking on; *walking in open air; warm becoming when. Better;* bending backwards; lying, while, back on.

Perspiration; emissions after. Stiffness. *Sitting after.* Warts

Cervical region: Abscess, **old cicatrices of.** *Air, draft unbearable.* **Coldness,** creeping. Eruptions; **blood boils;** *flattened; scabs, while.* Pain; extending, **eye to, head to, occiput to, upwards, vertex;** pressing; *sore, bruised;* stitching. tearing. *Perspiration.* **Stiffness,** headache during. *Swelling of glands.* Tension. Ulcers. *Weakness of,* manual labour agg. Wry. (torticollis).

Coccyx: **Injuries.** Pain; **sore, bruised,** sitting when; **stitching;** *tearing;* touched when agg.

Dorsal region: *Coldness. Curvature of spine.* Formication. Heaviness. Kyphosis. Pain; drawing; cutting; pulsating. Pressing, as of a stone. Swelling.

*Lumbo-sacral: Psoas abscess. Caries of vertebrae. Numbness.* Pain; *aching,* waist line; burning; cramp like; crushed, as though; goes *to hip;* legs *down; lameness;* **night; pulsating;** *sore; stitching;* **tearing.** *Perspiration.* Radiating from. Tension. Stiffness. Weakness. sitting. Lying, not able to rise after.

Scapulae: *Coldness between.* Heaviness. Itching. Pain; between; *burning;* drawing, between; sore; tearing, *below, between,* walking on. Quivering. Swollen feeling. Tension. Stiffness.

*Spine and Cord:* **Spina bifida.** *Caries* (Pott's Disease). **Curvature of, pain in.** *Heat.* Myelitis. Tabes dorsalis Multiple sclerosis of cord. *Injuries.* Necrosis of vertebrae. Pain; *aching;* burning; dorsal spine in; sore. Weakness (tired feeling); manual labour, motion of arms, and sitting after agg.

**EXTREMITIES:** *Abscess; joints of;* after dissecting wounds. Alive sensation. *Alternating between upper and lower. Arthritic nodosities.* Awkwardness; drops things from hands; *stumbling when walking. Ataxia* (1). **Bursae; joints in,** *cysts.* **Carbuncles.** *Caries of bones. Coldness;* fever during (u); *menses during;* painful parts. Constriction of joints. *Contraction of muscles and tendons. Convulsion.* Cracked skin and cracking in skin (u). *Cramps, chill during curving and bowing of bones.* Emaciation of diseased limbs.     Redness in spots (1). **Distortion of joints** (1) Drawn; apart; *upwards on abdomen, in necrosis of femur* (1). **Exostosses of bones. Fistulous openings, in joints.** Heaviness. numbness with. *Eruptions; boils;* eczema; hard; *herpes; itching;* miliary; *pimples; scabs;* psoriasis (u); *vesicles,* corroding, *pustules. Inco-ordination.* **Inflammation;** *bones of; joints, synovitis. Itching.* Jerking; on falling asleep. **Lameness;** *joints of* Motion difficult (1). *Loss of power,* on waking. *Mouse running up limb;* sensation. Nodes. *Numbness;* leaning on it; lying on it; *right;* sitting.

*Pain;* Boring. Burning. *Drawing;* downwards. *Ending in jerking* (1). Festering (u). *Joints in, gouty. paralytic.* Paralysed parts in. Pinching. *Sciatica;* coldness of limbs with; hips to feet; vertebral origin. Sore. *Rheumatic;* diarrhoea chronic in (u).  Sprained as if. *Stitching;* as if asleep (u); in bones; downwards; joints in. *Tearing; jerking;* **joints in.** Up and down. Worse: Chill during. Cold. **Coition after** (u). *Over-exertion.* Lying; **bed in; customary side on** (u); affected part. Menses before (u). *Motion on, walking* (i). Move on beginning to. Taking hold of anything (u). Touch. *Uncovering.* Weather; change of; **stormy;** *wet.* Wet getting or washing (i). Writing. Rising from seat, bed from; sitting; standing; stepping; stooping; (1) Better; Hanging. Rest. (u). *Warmth.* Drawn up. Flexing limbs; motion; sitting; *warmth,* bed of (i)

*Paralysis;* painless; right; sensation of; stiffness with. **Paraplegia;** *post-diphtheritic;* sitting after. **Restlessness.** Sensitive. Shaking before epilepsy (u). Smuttiness. *Sprains;* tendency to. Pulsation, eating after. *Stiffness; joints of. Suppleness lack of* (u). **Swelling;** *bones of,* inflammatory; joints of, *white;* painful; nodular; red. Tension. *Tingling;* sitting while (i); right, side lain on (u). Trembling; epilepsy before; exertion after. *Twitching;* joints of; sleep before. **Ulcers;** black base; **bluish areola; burning; deep; itching;** joints; painless; stinging. Varices. *Weakness; joints of;* stiffness with; taking hold of something. *Walk, late learning to.*

*Axillae; right;* **perspiration, offensive.** *Shoulders;* pain, **cold and becoming;** *stitching,* downward; tearing; warm wrapping amel.; stiffness; twitching; weakness. *Upper arms;* blood rushes to; pain; swelling, *vaccination due to;* twitching. *Elbow ankylosis;* pain; weakness, paralytic. *Forearm;* eruptions; *induration;* **paralysis; red** swelling. *Wrist; ganglion back of;* injuries; lameness; *weakness,* right. *Hands; awkwardness,* drops things; *chapped; cramps, exertion on,* writing while; *inflammation; numbness, night;* pain, *tearing,* writing while. **Perspiration, copious;** offensive. Skin; **cracked;** yellow; pustules; eczema; vesicles, corroding. Tingling, night. *Trembling; holding objects on; manual; labour;* sitting while; *taking hold on; using them,* writing, *threading a needle etc.* Wens. Weakness; *paralytic;* writing when. Palms; psoriasis; felon; **perspiration;** heat; twitching.

*Fingers and thumb:* Contraction, flexor muscles. Cracked, tips. *Dryness, as if made of paper, nails about, tips.* Emaciation. *Formication.* **Helplessness.** *Numbness.* Pain. **Stiffness.** *Tingling.* Ulcers. **Nails around.**

*Nails:* brittle. **Corrugated,** *Crumbling.* **Crippled. Cracked skin between toes(i). Excoriation. Ingrowing nails (i); ulceration with.** Itching; frozen toes of. **Distorted** (u). *Blue, gray.* **white spots, yellow** (u). **Felon;** *beginning in nail; maltreatment from;* **periostitis;** splinters from; suppurating; **tendons affected;** *thumb.* Growth interrupted. *Pain; stitching; ulcerative; under.* **Roughness.** Sensation, of splinter under. **Spotted. Thick. Ulcer.**

*Buttocks;* after pains felt in; drawing pain; tension.

*Hips:* Coldness. Fistules opening. Tuberculous joint disease. *Pain;* after pains; sore; *stitching; stooping agg.; tearing,* to knees; *walking* agg. **Stiffness. Suppuration.**

*Thighs;* **caries of femur.** Bubbling sensation. **Boils.** Vesicles; during menses inside. Pain; alternating with convulsive pain in arm; bone in; *sore; tearing. Softening of femur;* **swelling; of.**

*Knees;* **bandaged as if. Gonarthracea. Coldness;** chill during; walking open air, in. Inflammation; from suppressed gonorrhoea.

**Stiffness;** standing while; walking while. **Swelling;** *dropsical; scrofulus; spongy; white* (tuberculous). Tension; *walking* while. *Weakness.*

*Legs and Calf:* Alive sensation. **Coldness;** *icy; menses during;* **warm room in.** *Contraction. Calf* in. Reddish, whitish, spots on tibia. Elephantiasis. *Milk leg,* constriction with. **Numbness** of one, pain in another. Inflammation; erysipelatous; **tibia. Swelling. Ulcers; burning;** painful. Varices; inflamed; sensitive; ulcerative. *Weakness;* descending.

*Ankles;* Sprained as if. Stepping when agg. Stitching and tearing in malleoli. **Stiffness.** Turning of. **Ulcers;** fistulus. **Weakness.**

*Foot:* Arches. **Bunions.** *Coldness; bed in;* burning with; *icy;* **menses during; mental exertion on;** *take cold through feet.* Lameness; pregnancy during. *Odour offensive,* perspiration without. **Sore, bruised;** *tearing,* back of; **walking** agg. **Perspiration;** *cold; constant;* destroys shes; **offensive,** *menses after, sour;* **profuse; suppressed. Swelling;** evening agg. and amel.; left; morning; walking while **Tickling.** Ulcers; **back of. Weakness.**

*Soles;* Callosities, tender. Corns. Itching, voluptuous, after scratching. *Pain;* **crampy;** walking while; tearing, extends above knee; *burning;* walking while. *Heels; caries; blisters; stitching; tearing;* standing while agg. **Ulcers.**

Walking; **gallinaceous, ambulatory;** *stumbles easily; tottering;* unsteady, backwards. **Weakness;** descending steps; stiffness with; *walking after.*

**SLEEP:** Disturbed by dreadful and vicious dreams. Dozing Interrupted. Position, head low with. **Restless.**

**Dreams:** *Amorous.* Anger. battles. Quarrels. **Anxious.** Assassins. *Business;* neglected of the day. Choking her, something. Confused. Cruelty. Dead of the. Death of, approaching. Disconnected. Disease; fit that he has; epilepsy. Drowning. Earthquake. **Events;** *previous day;* **long past.** Fantastic. Fights. Fire. **Frightful; sleep; falling at.** Ghosts; pursued by. Historical. *Humiliation. Journey.* Lascivious, emission with. *Love* of. Murder; *of being murdered. Nightmare.* Persistent, continued after waking. *Pleasant. Being pursued;* by cats and dogs; wild beasts. *Robbers;* fighting with. Snakes. Sleep first. Storms, at sea. Strangled, of being. Vivid.

Unimportant. Vertigo. *Visionary.* Voyages. Water, boat foundering. *Flood. Weeping.*

*Sleepiness;* but sleep cannot. *Day during. Morning.* Motion during. Thunderstorm. Walking in open air. Warm room in.

**Sleeplessness:** Pain in abdomen, from. Anxiety, from. Coition after. Coldness, of feet, from. **Eating after. late.** Midnight, before. Morning. **Orgasm of blood,** from. Overtired, when. Palpitation from. Sleepiness, with. Thoughts from; activity of mind. thunderstorm, before. Trembling in body from. Vivacity from. **Walking after.**

*Somnambulism;* get up, walks up and lies down again.

*Unrefreshing;* with abdominal pain; blood ebullitions from; chest symptoms with.

*Waking;* cough from. Dreams from, on falling asleep. 3 a.m. Erection, with desire to urinate. Frequent. Fright as from. Gastric symptoms with. Heat from. Nightmare in. Pain in limbs from. Restlessness with. Vomiting with.

*Yawning;* chill during; excessive; frequent.

Concomitants during sleep; jerks. Shrieking and screaming. Tossing about. Twitching. **Talking.** Thirst. Starting up, as in fright, trembling with.

**CHILL:** *Affected parts of.* As if cold air, blowing around waist. Emotions from. Exposure; to draught, when heated; getting wet from. External; spots in; as if hair were standing on end. Fright from. Headache, during. **Heated, overheated.** *Internal.* **One sided;** *left, before epilepsy. Shaking;* hair standing on end with. Warmth, desire for, does not relieve. Wrapping amel.; followed by severe fever and sweat. *Coldness,* **icy.**

Concomitants: Bearing down with. *Deficient animal heat with.* Pain with. Trembling with.

Worse: Afternoon, 6 p.m. Air open; cold or going into; least draught of; walking in. *Bed in; putting hand out of;* rising from; turning over in. Day, every. **Drinking.** Eating; after; while. Epileptic attacks, after. Exertion. Fright, fear. Heated, becoming. Grasping cold object. *Menses;* **before; during. Midnight after.** Pain, during. Sleep; after;

during. Stool, during. *Touch.* **Uncovering,** undressing. Waking on. Warmth of room or stove.

Better: **Drinking.** Lying. Motion. Warm room. Warmth external.

**FEVER: in general.** Seventh day. *Alternating chills with.* Burning heat; stinging. **Chill with. Cold from taking.** Dry heat. **External heat. Intense heat** (high fever). *Internal heat.* Long lasting. Multiple abscesses with. Perspiration absent. Chill followed by heat. Heat followed by chill, then sweat.

Types: *Adynamic.* Bilious. Cerebro-spinal, tubercular. Chicken-pox. *Continued fever,* typhoid etc. **Dentition during. Hectic.** Inflammatory. Influenza. *Intermittent;* long lasting heat with; tertian. Measles. **Milk** (lactation). Puerperal. Scarlet. Small-pox; black. **Thermic.** Urethral. Worms from.

Worse: Afternoon. Day every. Drinking wine. Evening, lasting all night. Forenoon; thirst and chilliness with. Menses suppressed. Mental exertion. Night. Noon. Pain in general, during. *Sleep during.* Storm, approach of. Uncovering. Washing. Better; room in.

**Perspiration: In general.** Affected parts. On the side not lain on. Single parts; axillae; hands and feet; *nape or neck.*

Cold. *Easy.* **Excoriating.** *Exhausting.* Fright from. Hot. Intermittent. Night at, phthisis of. Odour; **offensive,** of a thousand mice; *sour.* Periodical. **Profuse,** night. *Putrid.* Scanty.

Worse: *Air, in open.* Coldness after. **Coryza during.** Coughing. Day time and morning. Eating, while and after. Epileptic attacks after. *Exertion during slight;* mental. Fever, after. Menses, during. *Morning.* Motion on. Night, **midnight after.** Rest, during. **Sleep during,** on beginning to. Uncovering. Waking after. **Walking while.**

Better: **Drinking water.** Lying in bed. **Motion. Room in. Sleep.**

**Skin:** *Adherent to bones.* Barber's itch. Biting sensation. **Burning.** Chapping. Cheloid; itches when warm. Chilblains. Cicatrices; *break open;* depressed; nodular; **painful;** red become; shining; **sore, become;** *stinging and stitching. Coldness; exercise during; left side, before epilepsy;* one side, during convulsions; *menses before;* painful nerves along; suffering parts of. Contraction. **Corns;** aching; *boring;* burning; **inflamed;** painful; pressing; **sore;** *stinging;* **tearing.**

*Cracks.* Cutting. Discoloura ion; bluish, spots; brown liver spots; *pale; pale red,* spots. **Spots;** ,noist; smarting; *stinging.* **White spots** (leucoderma). *Yellow.* **Dry;** b.*rning;* **inability to perspire.** Elephantiasis.

**Eruptions:** Biting. *Blackish. Blister,* inflamed. *Boils* (furuncles); *blood;* large; maturing slowly; periodic; stinging when touched. *Burning.* **Carbuncles. Crusty;** moist; suppurating. Desquamating. Moist, white, yellow discharges. Dry. Ecthyma. **Eczema.** *Foetid. Flat.* Nodes, gummata. Hairy parts, on. Hard. **Herpetic;** burning; chapping; **corrosive;** crusty; *itching; moist;* patches; scaly, white dry mealy; *stinging;* suppurating; *tearing; zoster. Impetigo.* Itching. Jerking pain, with. *Leprosy. Mealy,* white. **Painful.** Papular. Pemphigus. Petechiae. Pocks. **Phagedenic.** *Pimples,* itching. *Psoriasis,* inveterate. Pustules, *malignant, ulcerated. Rash. Red. Rupia. Scabs. Scabies,* **dry,** suppressed mercury and sulphur with. *Scaly;* **bran like;** ichthyosis; spots. Smarting. **Stinging.** Suppressed. **Suppurating.** *Syphilitic.* **Tearing pain, with.** *Tubercles;* tuberous; syphilitic.

**Ulcerative pain with.** *Urticaria,* nodular, rosy. *Vesicular;* burning; gangrenous; hard; itching; *phagedenic;* red, areola; scurfy; smarting.

*Erysipelas;* gangrenous; swelling with. *Excrescences; fungus,* cauliflower; **haematodes;** medullary; **syphilitic.** *Flabbiness.* Freckles. *Formication. Ganglia.* Gangrene; cold; threatened with blue parts. Hard; like callosities; *parchment like; peeling off;* thickening with. Heat, fever without. Inactivity. **Induration. Inflammation; inclination to.** *Intertrigo. Itching;* air agg.; bed in; *biting;* **burning;** *crawling* scratch must; smarting; **spots.** Moisture; **spots in.** Moles. **Pain.** Purpura haemorrhagica. Sarcoma cutis. **Sensitiveness.** Soft, boggy. Sore; **becomes;** children in; feeling. *Stitching. Stinging.* Stings of insects. Stripes, streaks. Swelling; affected parts; bluish black; *burning* dropsical; hard; inflamed; pale; **spongy;** stinging. Swollen sensation. Tearing. Tension. Thick. Ulcerative pain.

**Ulcers:** Aching. Biting. *Black;* bare; margins. *Bleeding;* edges. **Bluish.** *Boring pain,* with. **Burning;** around, about; **margins;** touched when. **Cancerous.** *Cold feeling with.* **Crusty. Deep.** *Discharges; bloody; bony fragments; brownish; copious;* **corrosive;** gelatinous; *gray; green, ichorous; maggots with;* **offensive; putrid; scanty;** tenacious; *thin; watery;* whitish; *yellow.* **Elevated;** indurated margins with. **Fistulus.** *Flat.* **Foul. Fungus.** *Gangrenous.* **Glands. Indolent.**

---

**Indurated;** areola; **margins,** shiny. *Inflamed.* **Itching;** *around, about.*
*Jagged margins with jerking pain with.* Malignant. *Mercurial. Painful.*
*margins.* **Phagedenic.** Pimples, surrounded by. **Pressing.** Pulsating.
*Red areola.* Reopening of old. Salt rheum. Sensitive around; margins.
*Serpingenous.* Shining. Smarting. **Spongy, margins.    Stinging;**
*areola in;* **margins in.** *Superficial.* **Suppurating. Suppurative pain**
**with. Swollen;** areola; **margins.** Tearing with. Tension areola.
**Unhealthy.** Varicose. *White spots,* with.

    **Unhealthy.** *Warts;* fleshy; *hard;* inflamed; *large;* pain; peduncu-
lated; pulsating; soft; stinging; suppurating; withered. Waxy. Wens.
Whitlow. Worms. *Wrinkled.*

☆  ☆  ☆